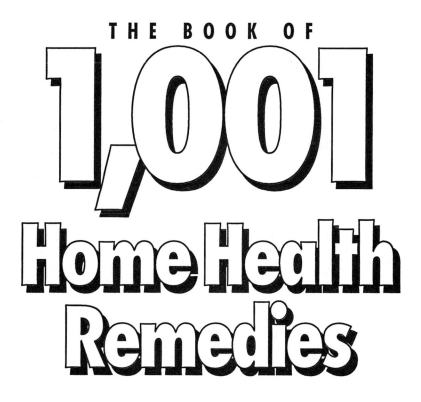

THE BOOK OF

1,001

Home Health
Remedies

THE BOOK OF

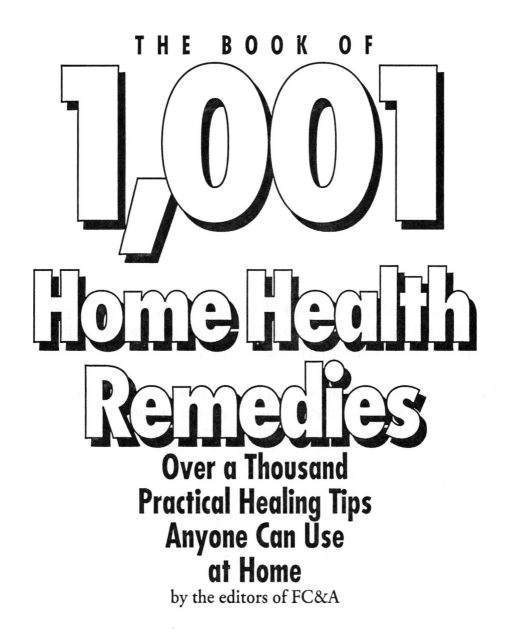

1,001

Home Health
Remedies

Over a Thousand
Practical Healing Tips
Anyone Can Use
at Home

by the editors of FC&A

FC&A Publishing
103 Clover Green
Peachtree City, GA 30269

Publisher: FC&A Publishing
Editor: Cal Beverly
Production: Carol L. Parrott
Printed and bound by Banta Company

Second printing June 1993

ISBN 0-915099-47-0

FC&A Editorial Staff ———————

Editor
Cal Beverly

Assistant Editor
Cindy B. Eckhart

Layout and Production Editor
Carol L. Parrott

Copy Editor
Linda M. Sciullo

Principal Writer
Laura N. Beverly

Contributing Writers

Madeline H. Barrow   Janet Halbert
Cal Beverly   Carol L. Parrott
Cindy B. Eckhart   Belinda Kent
Viki Brigham   Mary Jo Upton
Bruce Humphrey   Helen Holzer
Rebekah Anders   Sherry Wade

Researchers
Sherry Wade
Tricia Hammontree
Amy White

TABLE OF CONTENTS

INTRODUCTION

We've got good news for you: You are ahead of the crowd, leading the pack, winning in the game of life. Why? Because when you bought this book, you took one of the most important steps there is on the road to good health. You decided you wanted to know more about your body and how to live a healthier life.

In this world of french fries, ice cream, television and desk jobs, we've got one thing going for us—knowledge. Sure, cavemen didn't have to worry about their cholesterol count, but a pregnant cavewoman had to face a good chance of dying in childbirth.

Imagine developing diabetes in the Stone Age! And you didn't have to worry about the problems of old age back then—there was no such thing.

We've come a long way because the human race chose to learn more in order to live better. With all of today's advanced technologies and complex medicines, it seems as though doctors and medical researchers have a corner on the market of knowledge.

But it doesn't have to be that way. You've chosen to learn more, too, and our book can bring you up to date on the latest knowledge in language you can understand.

Do you know when you should never take antihistamines? Is your fluttering heart caused by your hair dye? What can you do to help prevent cancer of the breast or colon? How can you put your odds of getting heart disease way on the long side?

Can you control your arthritis by eating certain foods? Can you put a halt to your leaky bladder, body odor, dry skin, yeast infections, knee pain, hiccups?

Which old home remedies work and which ones should you never use (like putting butter on a burn)? What's the easy cure for cold sores? Is there hope for migraine sufferers? What should you do for a jellyfish sting? Should you take calcium tablets? How do you know when to trust X-rays? What's this about taking an aspirin every day? Can you get back that sense of smell you're losing?

In order to bring you the answers to these questions and more, we have spent months searching through medical journals, looking for the latest information on health issues that directly affect how we live every day. These journals are bursting with details on medical research and scientific breakthroughs, but they are written by doctors for doctors.

Wading through all the technical jargon is quite a chore. We have done the dirty work for you. In this book we've written what we learned, and we think you can read it even if you're not a genius with a medical dictionary.

This book is not one that you'll want to sit down and read from cover to cover. It is packed with cures, health tips and facts, and a quick look through it would probably give you a case of "information overload."

Read what most interests you first, especially the cures for ailments you suffer from—but don't neglect the rest of it over time. You never know when an obscure piece of information may save someone else's health, or your own.

We've included a very thorough index to help you find information on a particular topic. For instance, details about aspirin—its benefits, side effects, how it compares to other pain killers and what makes it work better—can be found in the chapters about arthritis, cancer, headaches, heart disease, pain relief, etc. The index will make it easier to find what you need quickly.

You may be surprised at some of the topics we've chosen to cover. "What is a huge section on cancer doing in a home health care book?" you might ask. "You can't treat yourself for cancer." We decided that our readers want and need to know about the big health concerns as well as the little ones. We think you'll be amazed at what medical research shows we can do to reduce our risk of all types of cancer.

It is true that you can't use some of the information in this book to "treat yourself." But just knowing it could save your life. We don't only give you the know-how to help yourself, but we give you knowledge so that you can discuss the best health options with your doctor.

For example, did you know that you should have your breast cancer surgery at a certain time in your menstrual cycle? The timing of your surgery can radically affect your chances of the cancer coming back and your chances of survival.

Many doctors either don't know or don't yet believe that changes in your hormones and in your body during the month can be so important when having breast cancer surgery, but recent medical research shows that it's undeniably true.

Obviously, you can't "help yourself" with this information in the sense that you can't perform surgery on yourself. You can't self-prescribe drugs for asthma or for the flu, either. But you can "help yourself" by talking to your doctor about your treatment.

Much of our book does emphasize self-treatment for common health problems. We know we have control over our bodies to a great extent, and we can help ourselves to better health. Of course, however, when you're sick, there's nothing quite as helpful as a doctor's care.

Use our health tips along with your doctor's advice. Always check with your doctor before you make any radical changes in your diet or lifestyle, and never change the drugs you take, prescription or over-the-counter, without your doctor's approval.

We hope you'll enjoy our book. And, most of all, we hope it will help you make better icepacks, stop a nosebleed properly, have fewer colds, eat better meals, buy the safest and best medicines, avoid some of the problems that come with aging, and simply live better lives!

God bless you!

ACNE

How to launch an attack on acne

It never fails. Whenever you have a special evening planned and you want to look your best, it happens. A pimple springs up on your face — boom, just like a spotlight for everyone to see.

And it doesn't just happen to teen-agers. It happens to some adults, even up through middle age. Ugh! What can you do?

The first thing to do is understand what acne really is — it's not just a curse of adolescence. It can happen at any age.

Acne is the clinical name given to the process that occurs when the oil glands in your skin get clogged up. You see, your skin contains oil glands (known as sebaceous glands) that produce a special oil. This oil helps keep your skin smooth and healthy and protects your skin from dirt, bacteria and dryness.

Unfortunately, the oil glands sometimes start working overtime. When this happens, the glands produce more oil than the oil ducts (the passageways that transport the oil to the surface of your skin) can handle. The excess oil begins collecting under the skin surface, and there you have the beginnings of your pimple.

The extra oil mixes with some dead cells, forming a hard plug. If this plug stays under the surface of your skin, it's known as a whitehead. If it enlarges and pushes out to the surface of your skin, it's known as a blackhead.

The dark color of blackheads is caused by a buildup of melanin, the pigment in the skin that is responsible for your skin color and for suntans.

Most girls start noticing pimples around age 11, and most boys start seeing pimples by age 13. Scientists think that the adolescent body begins producing large amounts of a hormone known as androgen. This hormone seems to cause the oil glands to overproduce the oils, thus triggering the acne.

Boys produce about 10 times as much androgen as girls, so acne is much more common in boys than girls.

Many people also inherit from their parents the tendency to develop acne. If one or both of your parents had acne, you will probably have it, too. But there is a difference in the kinds of acne that people can get.

Noninflammatory acne is the kind that most people get. This kind of acne is not severe or disfiguring. It causes a few pimples to spring up every now and then, but nothing too serious.

Other people suffer from what is known as inflammatory acne. This is a severe form of acne that has constant outbreaks that can cover the face, the neck, the back, the chest and even the groin area. The pimples formed in inflammatory acne are filled with pus, and the pimples and small cysts can cause unsightly scarring. This kind of acne is usually hereditary.

But for most people, the acne is more of an inconvenience and embarrassment than a serious medical problem. Other possible triggers of pimple outbreaks could be exposure to industrial oils and chemicals, stress and anxiety, oily makeup and shampoos, and even certain drugs.

Many people try to avoid foods like chocolate, sodas and fried foods because they say it causes acne. Scientists have not been able to prove this theory.

However, if you notice that outbreaks increase after you eat certain foods, try to avoid eating those foods.

And many women complain about more pimples the week

before or the week of their monthly period

MEDICAL SOURCES ————————————————

FDA Consumer (26,6:23)
Complete Guide to Symptoms, Illness & Surgery, 2nd Edition, The Body Press/Perigee Books, New York, 1989

How to fight pimples

To help get rid of those pesky pimples, follow these tips:

❏ Wash your face with soap and water once or twice a day. Avoid perfumed or scented soaps, and stay away from harsh deodorant soaps. These can strip your face of valuable oils that actually protect your skin, and it could lead to more pimples. Instead, use a mild antibacterial soap that will cleanse your skin without damaging it. Clean your skin gently. Scrubbing or hard rubbing might just spread the problem.

❏ Use as little makeup as possible. Using too much foundation or base often clogs the pores in your skin, leading to clogged oil glands and pimples. Try using a water-based makeup (rather than an oil-based), and apply as thin a layer as you can to allow your skin to breathe. And be sure to wash off the makeup each evening with soap and water.

❏ Don't pick at your pimples. This doesn't help them clear up any faster, and it could lead to scarring that wouldn't have occurred otherwise.

❏ Don't rest your chin, neck or face on your arms or in your hands while you watch TV, read or study.

❏ Avoid foods and drinks that seem to trigger your outbreaks (chocolate and caffeine).

❏ Drink lots of water — up to eight glasses a day. The extra liquid helps to "flush out" your system and helps prevent pimple formation. Drinking lots of water helps keep your skin (and your hair, nails and intestines) healthy.

❏ Some people think that a little bit of sunshine helps clear up their skin. However, dermatologists warn against the harmful effects of the sun and remind you that sun and heat can increase the amount of oil your skin produces.

❏ If you are taking birth control pills, ask your doctor if your brand might cause acne as a side effect. If so, ask him if you can switch brands.

❏ If your monthly period seems to trigger an acne outbreak, try to just suffer through it. There really is no smart way to adjust your hormone levels, which are triggering the outbreak. Just drink lots of water during that time and keep your skin as clean as possible to reduce your risk.

❏ If you take medications (especially medicines for epilepsy or tuberculosis), ask your doctor or pharmacist if acne is a side effect of any of your medicines. If so, ask your doctor if there is another kind of drug you can take that doesn't have that side effect.

❏ Try using one of the several over-the-counter anti-acne creams. These contain ingredients such as benzoyl peroxide, sulfur or salicylic acid that are helpful in reducing acne flare-ups.

❏ Try to avoid stressful situations that might trigger your acne outbreaks. If you can't avoid the situations, begin practicing stress-relief measures (like exercising, listening to quiet music, reading a good book or prayer). Dealing with stress and anxiety before it becomes serious can often help you avoid a stress-induced acne flare-up.

❑ If you have serious, disfiguring acne, you need to see a dermatologist. Taking medicine to improve your skin's condition can
help you avoid scarring.

MEDICAL SOURCES ————————————————————

FDA Consumer (26,6:23)
Complete Guide to Symptoms, Illness & Surgery, 2nd Edition, The
Body Press/Perigee Books, New York, 1989

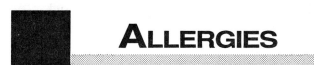

ALLERGIES

Suffering from allergies? You can run, but you can't hide

They might call it "hay fever," but it doesn't come from hay, and
it doesn't cause a fever.

The scientific name is allergic rhinitis, and it can make you feel
downright sick. The symptoms range from sneezing and a runny
or congested nose, all the way to a general feeling of fatigue and
malaise.

Most allergies come in one of two forms: seasonal or perennial.
People who suffer seasonally are allergic to the pollen of certain
plants. Trees pollinate in the spring, grass in the late spring and
early summer, and some in the late summer until the first killing
frost. House dust, molds and cats or horses are common allergens
for the perennial sufferer. They're around all the time, and if you are

allergic to them or to smoke or pollution, your hay fever might never let up.

The only way to get complete relief from allergies is to avoid what bothers you. That's easier said than done, since you can't always pinpoint the culprit, especially when it is airborne. Moving to a different locale won't help either, since you might find a host of new allergens waiting there for you.

Seasonal allergy sufferers should stay inside with the windows shut as much as possible during the allergy season. Air conditioner filters also help remove pollen from the air.

Most people are able to find relief by using antihistamines and decongestants for the symptoms of allergies. Your doctor or pharmacist can advise you about the correct dosage of antihistamines and decongestants.

It's easy to mistake allergies for a cold.

But you should suspect an allergy is your trouble if your symptoms fit one of the following categories:

- Last for more than a week.
- Go on all the time (house dust or mold).
- Start up and stop at the same time each year (pollen).
- Get worse around cats or horses.

Talk to your doctor or pharmacist to find relief for your allergy symptoms.

MEDICAL SOURCES ————————————————————

U.S. Pharmacist (14,5:46)
FDA Consumer (23,4:17)

How to figure out what you've got

Allergic rhinitis — no, it is not something suffered by a wild, horned animal from Africa.

It is what more than 60 million Americans suffer from each year. And it pretty much covers and includes most forms of allergies.

Seasonal rhinitis is the kind that causes you to suffer from allergic reactions at specific times throughout the year: usually early spring, early summer and late summer. Seasonal rhinitis is often referred to as hay fever, and the different dusts and pollens in the air during the three allergy seasons cause all the familiar symptoms of hay fever.

People can develop seasonal allergic rhinitis at ages as young as early childhood and on through adolescence and early adulthood. Symptoms usually diminish as you grow older, but they never completely go away.

Perennial allergic rhinitis causes symptoms throughout the whole year. Offending culprits include house dust, molds and dust mites. These things are not linked to changes in seasons.

People suffering from both types of allergic rhinitis complain of the same types of symptoms. Those who have just mild sensitivity complain of itching around the mucosal membranes inside their nose or eyes. These people often make their situation worse than it really is by constantly rubbing their nose or eyes and irritating the already-sensitive skin.

People with greater sensitivity suffer from the same itching, but they also suffer from sneezing, watering eyes, runny nose and other cold-like symptoms. Often they suffer from weakness, fatigue, chronic cough and itching throat, loss of appetite and sense of taste or smell, and decreased attention span.

Occasionally these symptoms can develop into the more serious cases of sinusitis, nasal polyps or ear infections.

Unfortunately, there are no real cures for allergic rhinitis — there are only different ways to control it and to keep it from getting worse.

MEDICAL SOURCE ───────────────────────

U.S. Pharmacist (17,7:38)

How to control your allergy symptoms

The following tips will help you manage your case of allergic rhinitis:

❑ Try to figure out what you are allergic to: pollen, grass, hay, dust, house mites, etc. Then try to stay away from the things that trigger your symptoms. You'll probably never be able to completely get away from them, but you can try and minimize your exposure.

❑ If your allergens (the things you are allergic to) are located outside (pollen, grass, etc.), then stay inside as much as you can during the seasons that disturb you the most (early spring, etc.). Keep your doors and windows closed and run the air conditioner. If possible, put an air filter system on your air conditioner so that it filters dust and pollen from the air as it cools it. Also try using a dehumidifying machine if your climate is very humid. A cool, low-humidity environment also helps prevent dust mites (a common allergen) from growing. The cool air also helps prevent household molds from growing (many people are allergic to molds).

❑ Always use your air conditioner in your car, and avoid riding with the windows down or in a convertible.

❑ Keep your pets outdoors as much as possible. If you allow them inside, keep them from getting on the furniture and going into your bedroom.

❑ If your allergens are mostly indoors (dust, mold and dust mites), try enclosing your mattress in zippered plastic covers. This keeps dust mites from living in your mattress stuffing and causing your allergic symptoms. Also consider buying and using synthetic pillows instead of feather pillows. Dust mites will inhabit the stuffing in synthetic pillows just as quickly as feather pillows, but you can wash the synthetic pillows in hot water and kill the dust mites.

❑ Wash your bed sheets and mattress pads often in hot water to kill any dust mites living there.

❑ Move books and toys to closets instead of leaving them out to collect dust. And when you do dust, dust with a wet cloth that picks up the dust instead of a dry cloth that just stirs up the dust.

❑ Carpet and venetian blinds are huge dust collectors. If possible, remove them from your house. Hardwood floors do not promote the growth of dust mites. And although dust collects on the wood floors, they are easy to clean. Try using throw rugs that you can wash in hot water from time to time. The throw rugs will cut down on dust and moisture in the room, and an occasional washing will get rid of any wayward dust mites.

❑ Find and repair any leaking faucets or pipes around the house to prevent the growth of molds.

❑ Do not smoke, and do not allow others to smoke in your home or in your car.

❑ Do not use kerosene heaters, fireplaces or wood-burning stoves, and try to avoid homes where they are used.

❏ If you have wreaths decorated with dried flowers, put them outside. Dried flowers can aggravate your allergies, and they collect a lot of dust.

❏ Try using over-the-counter medications to treat your symptoms.

MEDICAL SOURCE ──────────────────────────

U.S. Pharmacist (17,7:38)

Antihistamines and decongestants: which ones to use

❏ **Antihistamines** help soothe itching eyes and runny noses. They start soothing your symptoms right away, and they stay in your system for three to six hours. The most troublesome part of using antihistamines is the sleepiness they cause. Many people choose not to use them for that reason. Always avoid driving and operating machinery while taking antihistamines. If you find that one kind of antihistamine doesn't help your symptoms, try a different brand before you give up on them altogether. To get the best effects, some doctors recommend that you take antihistamines throughout the entire pollen season. Always follow the package instructions. Taking too many or too few will prevent the best results. People with the following disorders should not use antihistamines unless instructed by their doctors: asthma, peptic ulcer, narrow-angle glaucoma, and symptomatic prostatic hypertrophy.

❏ **Decongestants** also help soothe symptoms from allergic rhinitis. Often, decongestants will reverse the sleepiness caused by antihistamines if you take them together (or take a drug that contains both). You can get decongestant tablets, liquids and nasal sprays. You can use the pills and liquids for long periods of time. But never use the nasal spray for longer than three days at a time. After three days, the decongestant can start to cause congestion. Use the pill or liquid forms instead. People suffering from diabetes, hyperthyroidism, heart disease and high blood pressure should use decongestants cautiously. Always follow the package instructions carefully to get the best results.

MEDICAL SOURCES ───────────────────────────

U.S. Pharmacist (14,5:46 and 17,7:38)
FDA Consumer (23,4:17)

Safety tips for antihistamine and decongestant usage

Antihistamines help control the itching and sneezing caused by allergies. If antihistamines upset your stomach, try taking them with milk or a light snack.

Antihistamines might cause drowsiness, especially if taken with alcohol, tranquilizers or sedatives.

Do not take antihistamines if you have:

- glaucoma
- asthma
- chronic pulmonary disease
- shortness of breath
- difficulty breathing
- difficulty urinating because of enlarged prostate

Decongestants help clear nasal congestion. They come in pill or capsule form like antihistamines, or in nose drops or sprays.

Use the decongestant spray for three days only. Longer use

might make your congestion worse.

Only one person should use a decongestant spray (don't share the bottle — it can spread infection). You should discard it when you're finished.

Do not use a decongestant if you:

> • take medication for high blood pressure or depression
> • have heart disease, thyroid disease, diabetes or difficulty urinating because of an enlarged prostate

MEDICAL SOURCES ———————————————————————

U.S. Pharmacist (14,5:46)
FDA Consumer (23,4:17)

Athletes and allergies — could your performance be suffering?

Hay fever, seasonal allergies, and minor cases of the common cold — they affect millions of Americans every year. And every year, many of those Americans treat their symptoms with over-the-counter antihistamines and decongestants.

Most of those people are familiar with the warnings on the packages (drowsiness, fatigue, etc.) and don't drive or operate heavy machinery while taking the medications. However, one segment of the American population unwittingly continues to put itself in danger — the athletes.

Many athletes — both serious, highly trained athletes and the amateur weekend warriors — take allergy medications regularly to get rid of their allergy or cold symptoms and be able to continue in their sporting activities. Most of these people wouldn't think of driving a car while taking medication that causes drowsiness, for example; but they don't realize that many sporting activities can be just as dangerous.

Most over-the-counter antihistamines cause drowsiness, fatigue, delayed reaction times, poor motor coordination and loss of concentration. For this reason, most antihistamine packages warn against driving and using heavy equipment. But none of the packages warn against taking a long bicycle ride on a busy road—but the cyclist who is drowsy and uncoordinated because he took an antihistamine is in just as much danger.

In addition, many over-the-counter decongestant medications cause restlessness, insomnia, irritability, headaches and tremors. What the packages don't warn you about, however, is that the decongestants can use up your body's water stores. That means an athlete can easily suffer from dehydration while out training, especially during hot, dry weather.

Over-the-counter allergy medications (antihistamines and decongestants) have many published side effects that all allergy-sufferers, including athletes, should not ignore. These side effects can negatively, and even dangerously, affect an athlete's performance.

Athletes should avoid any athletic activities that require hand-eye coordination, concentrated attention span, quick reaction times, and coordinated motor skills while taking those medications. If the athlete cannot take a break from his training schedule to let the medication wear off, then he should avoid taking the medications to begin with. Check with your doctor about medications that can help relieve your allergy symptoms without affecting your athletic performance.

MEDICAL SOURCE ————————————————

The Physician and Sportsmedicine (20,6:112)

Is your hair dye causing your heart to flutter?

Trying to "wash that gray out of her hair" was almost a deadly mistake for one 59-year-old woman from California.

She had been dyeing her hair for a number of years with no problem until one day after applying the solution to her hair, her eyes began to swell, she became itchy and hoarse and began having heart palpitations.

She decided to switch to another brand of hair dye and buy an antihistamine just in case she had a reaction.

As it turned out, she did have another allergic reaction, but the antihistamine did the trick and she recovered quickly.

She decided to try her old hair color one more time, and this time it really did her in. Her vision became blurred, her face and hands swelled, and she got dizzy and shaky. She couldn't breathe and fainted.

Paramedics arrived and, with an injection of adrenaline, saved her life. She had a rare, yet severe, allergic reaction to a chemical in the hair dye.

An allergic reaction usually occurs after the first or second exposure to an allergen (the agent or substance causing the allergic reaction). However, allergic reactions may not occur until after years of exposure.

So, don't dismiss any unusual symptoms you might experience just because you have used a product for several months or years.

And don't be fooled into thinking you're safe just because you have used a product before.

The most common allergic ingredient in hair dyes is a synthetic organic compound called p-phenylenediamine.

It is found in most permanent hair colorings.

If you are worried about having an allergic reaction, but would still like to color your hair, use these precautions: do a patch test every time you use permanent coloring, wear gloves to protect your hands, avoid rubbing the dye into your scalp, and wash off any dye that touches your skin.

You can also try to avoid p-phenylenediamine. Most semi-permanent hair colors, including "cellophanes," do not contain this substance.

Be sure to check the label for contents.

MEDICAL SOURCE —————————————————

In Health (5,2:28)

Say goodbye to runny nose and hay fever?

Medicines to swallow and allergy shots aimed at irritants have been the common way to ease the symptoms of allergies — until now.

Research is currently under way to develop a vaccine that blocks allergic reactions before they have a chance to get started.

The University of Birmingham, England, conducted experiments with 10 rats severely allergic to egg whites. Six rats received the vaccine, then all 10 were fed egg protein.

Five of the vaccinated rats had no allergic reaction, while all four of the unvaccinated rats suffered serious symptoms, resulting in death for two of the rats.

The vaccine was successful in five of the six test rats.

Although the vaccine sounds promising, it is still in the testing stage.

MEDICAL SOURCE —————————————————

Science News (138,22:341)

Shy about your runny nose?

Do you have a runny nose, red eyes, and a strong fear of meeting new people? Recent evidence indicates that there might be a link between hay fever and shyness.

A group of University of Arizona investigators studied a group of college students and found that those who considered themselves extremely shy also suffered from more hay fever, depression, fearfulness and fatigue.

In another study at Harvard University, researchers suggested that hay fever and shyness are both controlled by the same transmitters and chemicals in our brain that regulate mood, smell and immunity.

So, if you suffer from shyness, get your handkerchief ready — you may have an increased vulnerability to hay fever.

MEDICAL SOURCE ─────────────────────────

Science News (138,17:262)

Can allergies hurt your heart?

Researchers at the University of California-San Diego believe that men with allergies run a higher risk of heart attack.

Many people who have allergies produce high levels of an immune system protein called Immunoglobulin E (IgE).

Researchers believe that the IgE might somehow disrupt the blood circulation and contribute to heart disease or heart attack. If you have allergies, ask your doctor if monitoring your heart would be beneficial.

MEDICAL SOURCE ─────────────────────────

American Heart Association news release (March 14, 1991)

ANGINA PAIN

Put the squeeze on angina pain

It's the most common symptom of coronary artery disease, and you know it's there when the squeezing, pressing pain begins, usually in the center of the chest, and then moves to the shoulders and arms.

Doctors say the pain is normally triggered when you make your heart work harder. Physical exercise is one example of putting extra demands on your heart.

To avoid the pain of severe angina attacks, doctors say, do these things:

- Stay calm. Avoid emotional upsets.
- Keep comfortably warm. Avoid extreme cold.
- Use moderation. Don't try overly vigorous exercise.
- Keep it light at the table. Don't eat heavy meals.

Angina attacks are usually lessened with a program of mild to moderate exercise; a low-fat, high-fiber diet; and stress-reduction techniques.

If, however, you have angina pain when your heart is not working harder, it may be a warning sign of a more serious form of coronary artery disease.

Naturally, you should ask your doctor about any heart or chest pain and how to manage any angina attacks.

MEDICAL SOURCE ─────────────────────────

Complete Guide to Symptoms, Illness & Surgery, 2nd Edition, The Body Press/Perigee Books, New York, 1989

Arthritis

Use these remedies for arthritis flare-ups

Here's how you can take the initiative in battling that relentless enemy, osteoarthritis.

❑ **Rest:** The first and best weapon against arthritis is a good balance between rest and exercise. Getting a good night's sleep, plus morning and afternoon rest periods, helps take pressure off weight-bearing joints and rests tired muscles.

❑ **Balance your rest** with gentle exercise, experts suggest. Exercise builds muscle strength and helps prevent stiffness and loss of motion. One of the best forms of exercise for people with arthritis is swimming in a mildly heated pool. Even if you can't swim, you can still enjoy gentle exercise in the shallow part of a pool, researchers suggest.

❑ **Heat** also helps. Use heat to relieve the pain that comes with osteoarthritis. Try soaking in a warm tub and using a heating pad or hot pack to help ease pain in sensitive joints. Elderly patients should avoid hot tubs and whirlpools, however, because the water is often too hot and can cause unnecessary strain on the heart.

❑ **Massage:** Gentle massages can also help to relieve your stiff, aching muscles. Using heat and massage regularly provides great relief from arthritis pain without the extra cost of professional therapy.

❑ **Ease up** when it hurts. One of the best methods of relieving arthritis pain is simply reducing the stress on the sensitive joints.

❑ **Get the right** appliance. Walkers and properly fitted canes can help improve your balance, relieve over-tired muscles and provide stability. But the cane or walker must "fit" you and your needs. A cane or walker that's too tall or too short can magnify arthritic pain and discomfort.

❑ **Ease stress,** improve safety. Simple devices in the home can also help ease stress on arthritic joints and improve safety. To get around better, consider using raised chairs and toilet seats, shower chairs, grab bars in bathrooms and nonslippery rugs and bathmats. Take away the need to stretch by installing lowered closet shelves and bars. And replace buttons and zippers with Velcro closures to help ease the stress on arthritic hands and arms.

All of these commonsense tips are easy and inexpensive. They're good ways to help relieve osteoarthritis pain and promote more independence in everyday activities.

For more information, contact the Arthritis Foundation, P.O. Box 19000, Atlanta, Ga. 30326. Ask for their free booklets, "Arthritis: Basic Facts," "Taking Care: Protecting Your Joints," and "Coping With Pain."

MEDICAL SOURCE —————————————————————————
Senior Patient (2,1:55)

How to change your eating habits to combat arthritis pain

A special kind of fasting (eating sparingly or not eating certain foods) is an effective way to treat rheumatoid arthritis, but most people tend to have relapses when they start eating normally again.

Now, you might be able to sustain the benefits of fasting with a special diet. Here's what worked for some other people during a scientific study.

Researchers studied 27 people on a special diet and 26 people who ate normally.

Those on the special diet fasted for over a week, then were put on a vegetarian diet for a year.

The diet included herbal teas, garlic, vegetable broth, watered-down potatoes and parsley, and juice extracts from carrots, beets and celery.

During the next phase, they were put on a gluten-free vegan diet for three to five months.

A vegan diet is a vegetarian diet that omits all animal sources of protein.

Gluten-free means that they didn't eat any food containing wheat, rye, oats or barley.

During this diet, they were asked not to eat food that contained gluten, meat, fish, eggs, dairy products, refined sugar or citrus fruits, salt, strong spices, alcoholic beverages, tea and coffee.

Gluten is vegetable albumin — prepared from wheat and other grains.

The diet was then changed to a diet consisting of dairy products and vegetables (lactovegetarian diet) for the remainder of the study.

After only four weeks at the health farm, the diet group showed a significant improvement: fewer tender and swollen joints, less stiffness, and more grip strength. These benefits were still present a year later.

The special-diet group also lost more weight than the regular-diet group.

But the reduction in weight explains only a small portion of the improvement, the report says.

Some people's arthritis might be triggered or aggravated by food allergies, the report says.

Talk to your doctor about what kind of diet is best for you.

MEDICAL SOURCE ─────────────────────

The Lancet (338,8772:899)

Double doses of this vitamin can help bring arthritis relief

Taking daily doses of vitamin D might provide a "D"-ouble solution for people suffering from psoriatic arthritis.

Symptoms include dry, scaly, inflamed skin in addition to aching arthritic joints. It's a "double disorder" with double the pain and irritation.

But now there might be double relief in the form of a vitamin.

Scientists evaluated 10 people who suffered from active psoriatic arthritis.

Each person "rated" the amount of pain, stiffness or discomfort from the arthritis, and the researchers took pictures of the psoriatic sores on each person.

Each participant in the study began taking a half-microgram of vitamin D3 each day.

Researchers increased the dosage by a quarter-microgram per day every two weeks until the participants reached a maximum dose of two micrograms of vitamin D3 each day.

Researchers evaluated the 10 people once a month for six months. During each evaluation, the study participants were asked to rate their arthritis pain, and researchers took more pictures of their painful skin patches.

After six months of vitamin D3 therapy, seven of the 10 people reported improvement in joint pain. Of the 10, four people had substantial (greater than 50 percent) improvement and three had moderate (about 25 percent) improvement. Two of the participants were unable to complete the study.

Some of the study participants also said that their skin sores got better. However, the improvements varied and didn't reflect changes in the arthritis symptoms.

Although the study involved only a small number of people who suffer from psoriatic arthritis, researchers suggest the positive benefits of vitamin D3 therapy are impressive.

All other therapies used for psoriatic arthritis (anti-inflammatory drugs, steroids and gold salts) have potential harmful side effects.

We produce vitamin D3 in our skin naturally, as do many animals. Oils from fish livers are rich in D3. Some multivitamins and fortified foods contain vitamin D3.

Scientists are hopeful that vitamin D3 will provide a safe, natural way to combat the pain and irritation from psoriatic arthritis.

MEDICAL SOURCE ———————————————————

Arthritis and Rheumatism (33,11:1723)

What's the right amount of vitamin D?

The Recommended Dietary Allowance for vitamin D is five micrograms per day for people over age 25. People under 25, expectant mothers and nursing mothers need about twice that amount.

The supplements used in the study above represent at maximum only about 20 percent of the RDA. For comparison, a quart of enriched cow's milk contains about 10 micrograms of vitamin D.

Be careful about overdosing on this vitamin. Intakes of only about five times the RDA (a little over 50 micrograms a day) has produced toxic reactions in young children.

MEDICAL SOURCE —————————————————————

Recommended Dietary Allowances, 10th Edition, National Academy Press, Washington, D.C., 1989

Walking can help relieve the pain and stiffness of arthritic knees

If you have been suffering from the stiffness of osteoarthritis, now you can relieve your pain and stiffness with a few steps — literally. The simple act of walking seems to help improve the stiffness and relieve the pain that comes with osteoarthritis of the knees.

Osteoarthritis is a disease that affects over 16 million people in the United States today. The progressive disease affects the joints, causing stiffness, achiness and occasional loss of motion.

The knee joint is frequently affected, and many people complain that they can't get around like they used to because their knees are so stiff.

But researchers think they have found a way to relieve some of that stiffness. Recent research suggests that the simple exercise of walking will help loosen up the knee joints in people who suffer from osteoarthritis.

To test the effects of walking on osteoarthritic joints, the investigators recruited 102 volunteers who were over age 40 and who suffered from osteoarthritis of the knees. The volunteers were divided into two groups: one group began an eight-week program that involved walking three times a week (30 minutes at a time), classes on osteoarthritis, and support groups.

The other group received classes on osteoarthritis and support, but no exercise program.

After the full eight weeks, the volunteers in the exercise group reported improvement in the amount of pain they had and improvement in how well they could get around. No one reported that the walking increased the pain or stiffness — the results were overwhelmingly positive. The volunteers were also healthier than when they started, and most could walk a good bit farther than they could when the study began.

On the other hand, the volunteers in the no-exercise group experienced little or no improvement in their symptoms.

The results from the study should encourage people who have stiff knees from osteoarthritis to start on a simple walking program.

Taking those first, simple steps might be your key to getting rid of your stiffness and getting back into life the way you used to know it.

MEDICAL SOURCE ———————————————————

Annals of Internal Medicine (116,7:29)

How and when to use heat and cold for your pains

Whether you have arthritis or you're a weekend gardener who has overdone a good thing, the correct use of heat or cold therapy can be your ticket to temporary relief from minor aches and pains.

Cold therapy temporarily deadens nerves that carry pain and also reduces swelling and inflammation. Heat therapy helps relieve stiffness and pain by increasing circulation in the affected area.

Another popular technique used for pain relief is a contrast bath

— alternating use of heat and cold.

To get the best results from heat or cold therapy, it's important to use them correctly.

Here are a few tips to help you use heat and cold safely and effectively.

Before using heat or cold:

❑ Check with your doctor or therapist, especially if you are sensitive to cold or heat.

❑ Avoid using heat or cold on areas where you have poor circulation or vasculitis (inflammation of a blood or lymph vessel).

❑ Make sure your skin is healthy and dry.

❑ Use extra padding between your heat or cold source and areas where the bone is close to the surface (wrap the heating pad or cold pack in a towel or cloth).

❑ Allow your skin to return to normal temperature between treatments.

While you are using heat or cold:

❑ Avoid using creams, lotions or heat rubs on your skin with heat or cold packs.

❑ Time yourself. Using heat or cold too long can hurt you. (Ask your doctor about the best length of time for cold or heat therapy.)

❑ Stay awake, and don't lie on top of the heat or cold pack.

❑ Remember that a bath or shower that is too hot may make you tired or dizzy.

What to look for after use:

❑ Normal skin will be a uniform pink color. Watch out for warning signs of blisters or dark red or red and white areas.

❑ Check for any new discoloration or swelling.

Talk to your doctor or therapist about how heat and cold therapy might fit into your overall plan to relieve arthritis aches and pains.

MEDICAL SOURCES ———————————————————————

Arthritis Today (3,3:22)
Arthritis Writings, Winter 1989

Ibuprofen vs. aspirin: It's a tie!

In recent years, thousands of arthritis sufferers have relied on prescription forms of ibuprofen for relief from joint pain and inflammation.

But new information suggests that ibuprofen is actually no more effective than that good, old standby ... aspirin.

Researchers at the Indiana University School of Medicine tested arthritis sufferers to see whether aspirin, a low dose of ibuprofen, or a high dose of ibuprofen was most effective at relieving arthritis pain.

They found that aspirin was equally effective as either amount of ibuprofen in a four-week study.

Since arthritis strikes up to 80 percent of people age 65 and older, this is good news, indeed.

If you currently use ibuprofen for relief of arthritis symptoms, check with your doctor about the possibility of substituting aspirin.

MEDICAL SOURCE ———————————————————————

The New England Journal of Medicine (325,2:87)

Acetaminophen to the rescue

The old phrase, "You can't win for losing," has a lot of meaning for some people taking medications.

Many times, taking medicine for one problem only seems to create new problems. If you suffer from osteoarthritis of the knee, this could very well be true for you.

Many doctors treat the pain that comes from osteoarthritis of the knee with large doses of anti-inflammatory drugs. However, that pain is not always caused by inflammation of the joint.

Sometimes the joint pain can come from other causes, such as stretching the joint ligaments, muscle spasms near the joint, microscopic fractures of the bones in the joint, or simple bone irritation due to the formation of scar tissue.

If the pain is not caused by inflammation, then treatment with high doses of anti-inflammatory drugs is obviously not necessary.

The problem with using large doses of anti-inflammatory drugs is that those drugs frequently cause negative side effects, such as nausea, stomach irritation and ulcers.

Using simple pain relief drugs often can help remove the discomfort of osteoarthritis of the knee without causing the negative side effects.

Researchers recently tested the effectiveness of simple pain relievers that did not contain anti-inflammatory agents and compared the results with pain relief from anti-inflammatory drugs.

About 200 people who suffered from knee-joint pain associated with osteoarthritis participated in the study.

Half of the people took daily doses of 4,000 milligrams of acetaminophen (a very weak anti-inflammatory agent), and the other half took less than 2,500 milligrams of ibuprofen (an anti-inflammatory drug) daily.

After four weeks of therapy, each group reported a 10 to 12 percent reduction in joint pain — both types of pain medicine helped relieve the pain and discomfort.

However, the group taking the ibuprofen (the anti-inflammatory drug) reported more nausea, stomach upset and bloody bowel movements.

The results of the test indicated that simple pain medications without anti-inflammatory agents were effective in relieving some of the joint pain associated with osteoarthritis of the knee without causing the negative side effects.

Since some of the pain that comes with osteoarthritis of the knee is caused by inflammation, the researchers suggest starting with a pain reliever like acetaminophen, and if no improvements result, then try a pain reliever with an anti-inflammatory agent.

Ask your doctor which pain relievers are best for you.

MEDICAL SOURCE ———————————————
Emergency Medicine (24,1:104)

The 'angel' herb soothes arthritis

According to legend, this herb was given to humans by angels as a cure for the plague, and so it got its name, Angelica. It is a tall member of the parsley family, and many people use it as an attractive border around their herb gardens.

But it can do more than border the garden. Angelica has been used in folk medicine as an expectorant cough medicine, a diuretic, an antiflatulent, and even a remedy for rheumatism.

Today, the herb is available commercially in the form of candied or crystallized stems.

You can use the dry leaves to make herbal teas or as scent in your potpourri basket. The leaves and stalks make marvelous cake decorations, and when cooked with rhubarb, Angelica helps reduce the tartness from the rhubarb.

MEDICAL SOURCE ————————————————————————

The Lawrence Review of Natural Products (February 1988)

Sodium fluoride therapy linked to arthritis?

If you are receiving treatment for osteoporosis, you might have an increased risk of arthritis.

A new treatment for osteoporosis, called sodium fluoride therapy, has been linked to an increase in rheumatoid arthritis.

The case of a 68-year-old woman who began sodium fluoride treatment for her osteoporosis has recently been reported.

In addition to her osteoporosis, she also suffered from rheumatoid arthritis, but had not experienced any recent flare-ups and her condition was stable.

But, within a few days of starting the treatment, she experienced extreme inflammation and stiffness of the joints and tiredness.

When she stopped the sodium fluoride therapy, she was back to normal within a week. She tried two more times to take the sodium fluoride.

Both times her arthritis worsened dramatically after just a few days and returned to normal when she stopped the therapy.

If you suffer from osteoporosis and need treatment for your condition, but you also suffer from rheumatoid arthritis, check with your doctor to see if another solution might be better for you.

MEDICAL SOURCE ————————————————————————

Archives of Internal Medicine (151,4:783)

Popular arthritis drug causes liver damage

You're suffering from arthritic pain and discomfort, and you're desperate for relief. So when your doctor suggests drug therapy, you are willing to try it.

If, however, he suggests the arthritis drug Voltaren, you might want to think twice.

Apparently, this popular arthritis drug has been linked to seven cases of hepatitis in patients within four to six weeks of taking the drug.

In fact, one of the seven patients, a 65-year-old housewife, actually died as a result of complications caused by the liver problems linked to the drug.

The other six people, all middle-age or elderly people, obtained relief from their liver disorders after they stopped using the drug.

Voltaren is a member of the nonsteroidal anti-inflammatory drug class and is one of the top-selling arthritis drugs in the nation today.

Scientists are not sure why the drug causes liver problems, leading to hepatitis and even death, and they strongly urge careful monitoring of all people using the drug and immediate discontinuation of the drug if signs of liver problems develop.

MEDICAL SOURCE ————————————————————

Journal of the American Medical Association (264,20:2660)

Stiff, achy joints? It might not be arthritis at all

Afraid your stiff, achy joints could mean rheumatoid arthritis? It could just be a simple, curable virus.

This virus has sometimes been mistakenly diagnosed as rheumatoid arthritis because its symptoms include chronic joint disease.

In a two-year study conducted by Dr. Stanley J. Naides of the University of Iowa in Iowa City, the tiny human virus parvovirus B19 was found to be so common that 40 to 60 percent of adults worldwide already have its antibodies. It's called chronic arthropathy to distinguish it from true arthritis.

Adults with chronic arthropathy seem to suffer an influenza-like illness along with stiff joints, while in children the virus can appear as a facial rash that resembles slapped cheeks.

The condition affects more women than men and is especially widespread for those in the nursing, teaching and day-care professions.

The B19 infection can cause a critical shortage of red blood cell production, according to Dr. Naides.

Persistent nonproduction of red blood cells can result in bone marrow suppression (the body's failure to produce bone marrow).

Those particularly vulnerable to chronic arthropathy are fetuses, people with chronic anemia, sickle cell anemia or AIDS.

The good news is the B19 virus can be fought with blood transfusions or by administering gamma globulin (a protein formed in the blood that helps in the body's ability to resist infection).

If you suspect your aching joints might be caused by parvovirus B19, check with your doctor.

MEDICAL SOURCE ————————————————————
Research Resources Reporter (15,8:1)

Asthma

Getting your breath

Maybe you dream that you are underwater and cannot breathe. The dream is so real that you wake up.

But it feels as if you never woke up. You force your lungs to pull in precious air. Not nearly enough.

The squeaking and whistling sounds come from your throat and chest like a dying gasp.

The problem is getting your breath. The disease is asthma. The cause is complex and uncertain. There is no miracle cure. But, there is help.

Some things that can trigger asthma attacks

❏ Cold or flu

❏ Stress or emotional problems

❏ Cold or dry air

❏ Exercise

❏ Pollutants in the air

❏ Perfumes

❏ Allergens, feathers, animal danders (tiny scales from hair, feathers or skin), pollens and molds

❏ Metal salts (platinum, chrome, nickel)

❏ Wood dusts (oak, western red cedar)

❏ Alcoholic beverages

❑ Flour, coffee, tea

❑ Foods containing sulfiting agents (fruit juices, salads, shellfish, fresh and dried fruits)

❑ Monosodium glutamate

❑ Tartrazine (food additive)

❑ Enzymes (those in laundry detergents)

❑ Certain chemicals used in solvents, paints and plastics

MEDICAL SOURCES ————————————————————

Complete Guide to Symptoms, Illness & Surgery, 2nd Edition, The Body Press/Perigee Books, New York, 1989
Your Good Health, Harvard University Press, Cambridge, Mass., 1987
Harvard Health Letter (16,7:5)

How to manage an asthma attack

Not being able to breathe can be very frightening, especially for those who have asthma.

Sometimes anxiety can cause even more rapid and shallower breathing that can aggravate asthma and interfere with your inhaler.

Here are some tips to control the anxiety that sometimes accompanies an asthma attack.

❑ Sit down and drink a glass of water or other flavored drink. It can distract you and slow down your breathing.

❑ Breathing exercises can help you control your breathing. Sit down and take a long, slow, deep breath. At the same time, push on your upper abdomen with your hands folded. Let the air out slowly with your lips "puckered." Keep your lips almost completely closed to cause resistance. Do this exercise approximately three times. Once your breathing is slowed down, your inhaler is likely to be more effective.

MEDICAL SOURCE ─────────────────────

Ambulatory Care Alert (1,3:4)

Using inhalers

Many asthma sufferers get relief with inhalers. There are two major types, steroidal and bronchial dilators.

❏ The steroidal inhalers reduce the sensitivity of the airways so they will be less likely to react to allergens such as mold and dust mites.

❏ The bronchial dilators reduce swelling almost immediately so air can be drawn into the lungs. Some doctors prescribe one or both of these. Follow your doctor's directions, and read the label on your medicine. Eighty-two percent of people admitted to the hospital due to severe asthma did not use their medicine correctly.

MEDICAL SOURCES ─────────────────────

Drug Therapy (22,3:19)
Postgraduate Medicine (92,3:95)

Cleaning tips to asthma-proof your home

❏ Wash your walls and woodwork with a diluted chlorine bleach solution. This should remove microscopic molds. Wear a breathing mask while you do this.

❏ Filter your inside air. Air cleaners can remove some asthma-triggering microscopic particles from the air.

❑ Use a built-in vacuum cleaning system. It releases less dust into the air.

MEDICAL SOURCE —————————————

Postgraduate Medicine (91,1:225 and 91,4:215)

Exercise without fear of an asthma attack

Your legs are dimply and untoned, and you're starting to get a spare tire around the middle. You'd love to exercise to tone up your muscles, but the thought of exercise scares you—the last time you tried (back when you were in elementary school), you had such a scary asthma attack that you swore off exercise forever.

The attack you experienced back in grammar school is known as "exercise-induced asthma" (EIA). People who experience EIA complain of chest tightness, wheezing, shortness of breath, and the inability to get in enough air during or immediately after they've exercised. They feel like they are choking to death.

Around 80 percent of all asthmatic people have experienced an episode of EIA, and they all agree that it is a frightening and unpleasant experience to go through. That's why many people who have asthma refuse to exercise.

There are even some people who have no symptoms of asthma at all except when exercising, and that gives them even more reason to avoid exercise — stay away from what causes the problem.

But, researchers are now suggesting that you can exercise, even if you have asthma, and not have to suffer from EIA. You just have to change the way you've been exercising.

Recent scientific studies indicate that the right kind of physical exercise in asthmatic people greatly increases their heart and lung health. It also increases their self-esteem and decreases the amount of energy it takes to do certain tasks. Thus, it makes exercising easier.

The more you exercise, the more your lungs expand to allow you to breathe, and the harder it is to induce an EIA episode. In other words, people in bad shape suffer from exercise-induced asthma quickly and upon almost no exertion. People in good shape from exercising have to be working extremely hard to trigger an episode of EIA.

Scientists maintain that people suffering from mild to moderate asthma can perform and tolerate most forms of physical exercise or physical activities — if they develop their exercise program carefully.

Follow these simple steps to design your own exercise program:

❑ Take the medicines your doctor prescribed regularly. This will help you get good control over your asthma symptoms, including those caused by exercise, pollen, dust, etc. If you do not take your medicines properly, you are setting yourself up for problems when you try to exercise.

❑ Take a puff or two from your inhaler about 15 minutes before you begin exercising, just to open up your lung passageways a bit.

❑ Begin warming up before you start any strenuous exercises. Do some light stretching for about five minutes, then do some more moderate to vigorous stretching for another five minutes. This brings your total warm-up time to about 10 minutes.

❑ Start your exercises or your physical activity. This could be walking, cycling, aerobics, swimming, or any other type of aerobic exercise. Go slowly for about 15 minutes, trying to keep your heart rate and pulse rate low. If you start having symptoms of EIA, try to continue exercising at the same rate (or a little slower) and work through them. Inhale a puff from your inhaler if necessary to help the symptoms pass.

❏ After the symptoms pass, start pushing a little harder on your exercises. Push as much as your body will let you—you can tell when you need to slow down.

❏ After the hard portion of your workout, start a slow cool-down process. Slow your rate and intensity of exercising gradually over a 10– to 30–minute time period. If you slow down too quickly, your lung airways will react suddenly and trigger an episode of EIA. This is a crucial time during the exercise process. Many people tolerate the exercise well but then stop exercising too quickly and trigger an asthma attack. Take your time, and you'll be able to avoid an attack.

❏ If you exercise outside, try to avoid air pollutants (smog, etc.) and pollen as much as possible. For example, do not run on busy streets, because the exhaust from the cars will aggravate your lungs. Remember that pollen counts are usually the highest in the mornings. Try exercising inside during high-pollen or high-smog days.

❏ Wear a scarf or mask over your mouth and nose if you exercise outside during cool or cold weather. This helps to warm and moisturize the cold, dry air you breathe and will help prevent your lungs from reacting.
Also, try breathing through your nose as much as possible. Breathing through the nose warms, moisturizes and cleans the air more than mouth breathing, and this can help prevent an asthma attack.

❏ Try to exercise in warm, humid environments. A gymnasium

that is a little hot and moist is much easier on your lungs than a cool, dry, air-conditioned gym. Also, swimming is a marvelous exercise because of the warm, humid environment. People suffering from asthma (even serious cases) should consider swimming as a regular exercise, because the warm, moist air helps avoid asthma attacks. Try to breathe through your nose, even though the air around the pool is warm and moist. Breathing through the nose is just another safety precaution to take to help avoid an asthma attack.

❏ Always carry your medications with you to the gym, to the pool, or in your pocket if you cycle, jog, etc. Having your medication at your fingertips can help prevent serious asthma attacks if necessary. You can use some medications at the start of the attack, and keep it from getting out of hand.

❏ People with asthma should check with their doctor about an exercise program that is safe for them.

❏ If your children have asthma, show them how to properly warm up and cool down before and after exercising. Make your children's physical education teachers aware of your children's special needs and encourage the teachers to allow and motivate your children to participate in sporting events, if they take the proper precautions.

A little time spent teaching your asthmatic children how to exercise properly and avoid episodes of EIA will help to keep your children physically fit and allow them to enjoy the simple pleasures of childhood games without the fear of an asthma attack.

MEDICAL SOURCES ─────────────────────────

The Physician and Sportsmedicine (20,3:159 and 20,6:42)
FDA Consumer (26,6:3)

Breathless from your workout in cold weather?

Do exercise and cold weather leave you short of breath?

Well, you're not alone. Almost 80 percent of people with asthma have what is called exercise-induced bronchospasm.

Some of the symptoms of this asthma complication include a coughing attack and tightness in the chest during or shortly after exercise.

Exercise-induced bronchospasm appears to be most common during running or jogging. It's believed to be a hyperreactive airway response to increased and rapid inhalation of cold, dry air. It is probably caused by the loss of heat and water.

Researchers conducted a study to find out whether using a mask that retains heat and moisture prevents exercise-induced bronchospasm.

They studied six people who had asthma and exercise-induced bronchospasm. Researchers gave them no asthma medication for at least six hours before exercise.

They were randomly given masks during exercise. Almost everyone showed an improvement in exercise-induced bronchospasm with the mask.

The mask seems to be promising during exercise but probably not practical in all cases.

If you cannot use a mask during exercise and have to rely on your inhaler for relief, some doctors have recommended that you use a beta-adrenergic inhalant approximately 15 to 20 minutes before you exercise to reduce the symptoms of exercise-induced bronchospasm.

And if this doesn't help, try warming up for about 15 minutes, then use a second dose of your inhaler. Researchers say this usually works long enough for you to finish your workout.

If you use a beta-agonist for relief, see the new cautions in this chapter.

MEDICAL SOURCES ────────────────────────

    Postgraduate Medicine (91,3:155)
    British Medical Journal (6825,304:479)

A preventable cause of asthma?

Researchers are pointing fingers at a bacterium known as Chlamydia pneumoniae. Some scientists believe this bacterium might be an important, preventable cause of asthma.

Studies indicate a positive relationship between exposure to this bacterium and your chance of suffering from asthma, bronchitis and wheezing.

Apparently, 30 to 50 percent of adults throughout the world have been exposed to Chlamydia pneumoniae. Your risk of exposure is highest if you are over the age of 30.

Nearly 30 percent of people in the study who were exposed to Chlamydia pneumoniae developed breathing problems, compared to only 7 percent of people not exposed.

Other threats to breathing are microscopic insects (dust mites) which live in every home. They live in carpets and anywhere there is dust.

A severe threat to some asthmatics is the common mold Alternaria alternata. This is one of the most common mold spores in the air found in the United States, especially in the midwestern grain-growing areas.

If you are allergic to this mold, you might be at a much higher risk of respiratory failure, according to recent studies.

In one study, 10 out of 11 people (91 percent) with asthma who had a past history of respiratory arrest showed that they were allergic to Alternaria alternata.

Among those who had no past history of respiratory arrest, only 31 percent showed an allergic reaction to this type of mold.

People with asthma who have been tested and are allergic to Alternaria alternata may be at a much higher risk of respiratory failure, according to the report.

Other risk factors that should be added to the list are the time of year and pollen.

When pollen and mold-spore counts are at their highest, death rates due to respiratory failure are also at their highest.

If you suffer from asthma, check with your doctor to see if you are allergic to this mold.

Other causes of respiratory problems might be exposure to allergens or chemicals in the workplace, medication or animal dander to which you might be overly sensitive.

MEDICAL SOURCES ——————————————————————

Journal of the American Medical Association (266,2:225)
The New England Journal of Medicine (324,6:359)

Asthma drugs harm patients?

Some asthma drugs may be doing more harm than good, and they might even increase the risk of death from asthma.

Based on a recent study, researchers are finding evidence that could link the asthma drug fenoterol with increased complications among asthma patients.

Fenoterol is a member of the class of drugs known as beta-agonists. These drugs work by relaxing constricted muscles around tightened airways. This allows the airways to open up a bit and enables easier breathing. However, scientists are concerned about the long-term effects of the drug on asthma sufferers.

Many asthmatic people use such beta-agonist drugs as salbutamol or terbutaline frequently throughout the day to help keep their airways clear and open. The beta-agonist drugs provide short-term relief, but they do not treat or help the underlying problem.

In fact, researchers fear that the routine use of the beta-agonists could increase inflammation of the airways and cause eventual scarring. The scar tissue would further damage the airways and possibly increase the risk of death from future asthma attacks.

In other words, the short-term effects of the drug are helpful, but the long-term, cumulative effects could be deadly.

The drug fenoterol is not available in the U.S. at this time. However, many asthmatic patients use similar inhaled drugs such as salbutamol or terbutaline from the same beta-agonist class.

Scientists are not currently suggesting that all beta-agonist drugs should be discontinued.

However, to help avoid the possibility of long-term damage to the lungs, some researchers are advising doctors to discourage their patients from using beta-agonists so heavily and frequently.

Instead, researchers recommend the use of inhaled steroids. Inhaled steroids offer more long-term benefits by fighting inflammation rather than providing short-term dilation of constricted airways.

Here are examples of beta-2 agonists.

- Proventil
- Brethaire
- Ventolin
- Alupent
- Bronkometer
- Isoproterenol HCL
- Ephedrine Sulfate
- Bronkaid Mist (over the counter)
- Primatene Mist (over the counter)
- Medihaler-Iso

MEDICAL SOURCE ————————————————————————

Science News (138,24:373)

The problem with beta-agonists

Over the past ten years deaths due to asthma have risen 30 percent.

The medical community has not been able to determine the cause of this sharp increase in asthma-related deaths.

Dr. A. Sonia Buist, who represents the American Asthma Education Program, suggests the treatment that helps relieve asthma symptoms for the short-term "may make things worse."

Recent reports indicate that regular use of some of the most widely used asthma drugs can increase your risk of fatal asthma attacks.

Regular use of these medications might hamper the body's natural defenses against inflammation by lessening the mast cells' histamine-producing activity, researchers suggest.

Dr. Stephen Hoffman believes that an asthma attack is composed of two reactions in the body.

The first is bronchospasm, which is a tightening of the muscles of the airways (bronchi).

This tightening can be caused by inhaling irritants that provoke mast cells to release histamine and cause muscle contraction. The contraction of the airway muscles cuts down the amount of air that can be breathed in or out of the lungs.

Bronchospasm (called the early response) is usually accompanied by coughing and wheezing and can last up to two hours.

The other, and possibly more important reaction, is linked to chemical reactions during the body's immune response.

This reaction is known as the late response and might occur hours after the early response (bronchospasm). It can last up to 12 hours.

In the lining of the bronchi the mast cells are joined by other cells called eosinophils, which release prostaglandins, leukotrienes and other chemicals. These chemicals cause the lining of the bronchi to become inflamed and swell even more.

Normally, this inflammation helps fight foreign bodies in bronchial tissue. In the case of an asthma attack, it is like a false alarm. The reaction is worse than the danger from the foreign substance.

So, once an asthma attack has begun, the body creates conditions that can make the next attack even worse.

The most widely prescribed medication for asthma is the beta-2 agonist, which stimulates the beta receptors to dilate the bronchi and blood vessels. It also lessens the histamine production of the mast cells. This medication interrupts the early stage of an asthma attack.

The bronchodilator medication could actually make your asthma worse, scientists say.

Some doctors recommend the use of inhalers that contain corticosteroids, which interrupt the late response. Other doctors prescribe cromolyn, which interrupts both the early and late response.

A Harvard Medical School researcher believes that anyone using a bronchodilator on a daily basis should also use anti-inflammatory medication.

Other side effects of bronchodilators include bronchial irritation, increased heart rate, nervousness and increased blood pressure.

Do not discontinue any medication without talking with your doctor.

MEDICAL SOURCES ————————————————

Medical World News (33,1:34)
Harvard Health Letter (16,7:5)

Asthma sufferers: Take a big, deep breath — but don't forget to remove your inhaler cap!

Watch out asthma sufferers, you could be getting more than your breath back from your inhaler!

It's the middle of the night and suddenly you can't breathe.

Half asleep, you reach for your inhaler and take a deep breath. ... But wait, you forgot to take the cap off!

Sounds hard to believe?

It was true for one 25-year-old asthma sufferer who woke during the night with shortness of breath. In his groggy state he forgot to remove the cap from his inhaler and then swallowed it.

Although this man was able to remove the cap, he caused considerable damage to his vocal cords.

Most breathing problems for asthma sufferers seem to occur at night.

Therefore, doctors advise you to take extra care when using your inhaler at night or when you are sleepy.

Doctors estimate that 20 to 75 percent of patients using metered-dose inhalers use them improperly.

Be careful to use your inhaler correctly.

MEDICAL SOURCE ———————————————————————
The New England Journal of Medicine (325,6:431)

Toothpaste can 'take your breath away'

Brushing your teeth will freshen your breath, but it might also take your breath away.

Take the case of the 21-year-old asthmatic woman.

She had been treated, without success, for six weeks for coughing, wheezing and breathing difficulties.

Nothing helped until she switched from a paste-based toothpaste to a gel-based toothpaste.

Then, her symptoms disappeared overnight.

When tested with a paste-based toothpaste again, she began wheezing within 10 minutes.

The only difference between the contents of the gel-based and paste-based toothpastes is the type of artificial flavoring used, according to Proctor and Gamble, which manufactures both varieties.

The gel-based toothpaste contains a mild spice-blend flavoring, while the paste-based contains wintergreen or spice-mint.

When this was discovered, the woman admitted that chewing

gum containing wintergreen or peppermint also leaves her "breathless."

If you experience some unexplained breathing difficulties after brushing your teeth or chewing gum, check with your doctor about possible allergies.

MEDICAL SOURCE ————————————————————

The New England Journal of Medicine (323,26:1845)

ATHLETE'S FOOT

How to fight the fungus

Athlete's foot is a nasty little fungus from the ringworm family that lives between the toes, producing scales and cracked, bleeding skin.

Sometimes it spreads to the soles of the feet, which become thick and scaly.

The symptoms of athlete's foot include itchy, peeling skin on the feet, particularly between the toes, and foot odor.

The fungus earns its name because those who spend any amount of time in sweaty socks and shoes — athletes — are most susceptible to the problem.

To prevent athlete's foot:

❑ Wash your feet daily with soap and warm water, cleaning all dirt from under the nails and between the toes.

- ❏ Dry each toe separately, paying particular attention to the gaps between the toes.

- ❏ Powder your feet with an antifungal powder.

- ❏ Powder your shoes and socks with an antifungal powder.

- ❏ Wear clean cotton or wool socks. Don't wear sweaty, soiled socks. Soiled socks can provide an inviting environment for fungus to thrive.

- ❏ Avoid nylon socks, pantyhose and plastic shoes.

- ❏ Wear open shoes or sandals if your feet feel sweaty.

Doctors say antifungal footbaths don't help much. They also say to avoid ointments.

MEDICAL SOURCE —————————————————————

The Columbia University Complete Home Medical Guide, Crown Publishers, Inc., New York, 1985

BACK PROBLEMS

Helpful tips to avoid low-back pain

- ❏ Try to maintain your spine's normal curves.
- ❏ Get a good desk chair and sit straight up; don't slump.
- ❏ If you work at a computer, be sure the screen is at eye-level.
- ❏ Your chair should support you as you lean forward.
- ❏ Don't stay in the same position for very long periods of time.
- ❏ Get up and stretch, and walk around every hour or so.
- ❏ To lift something from the floor, get close to the object, bend your knees, and bend at your hips. Don't arch your back and stretch.
- ❏ When unloading your dishwasher, pivot on your feet so that you keep your hips and shoulders in a line, and bend at the knees and hips.
- ❏ To reach a high shelf, put your feet in a staggered stance (one foot in front of the other), then push off your back foot onto your forward foot as you reach up, keeping your hips and shoulders in line.
- ❏ To get out of a chair or couch, slide forward to the edge of the seat, and use your legs and arms to lift your body up.
- ❏ If you read in bed, place pillows under the small of your back and behind your neck so you can recline, not slump.

MEDICAL SOURCE ————————————————————

In Health (4,2:46)

Bed rest adds insult to injury

The last time you hurt your back, did your doctor tell you to take some painkillers and go to bed for several days?

The painkillers might be appropriate, but new studies suggest that longer bed rest can actually make things worse. For years, many doctors have treated sharp, low-back pain with long periods of bed rest.

Extended inactivity from bed rest can cause a loss of flexibility and weakness of back muscles, the report says. That, in turn, might cause you to re-injure your back when you resume your normal daily activities.

When doctors prescribe lengthy bed rest, back-pain sufferers seem to have more days of disability and miss more days from work, the report says. Adding insult to injury, your back usually doesn't feel much better, either.

For people who have acute low-back pain with no neurological (nervous system) problems, bed rest of about two days should be enough, the new report suggests.

Then you should try to resume your normal activities gradually.

If you do have nerve problems, you should see a specialist.

Nerve problems, for example, might show up as tingling, numbness or loss of reflex responses in a leg or foot. These are serious and require medical attention without delay.

Talk to your doctor about what kind of back treatment is best for you.

MEDICAL SOURCE ——————————————————————
Southern Medical Journal (84,5:603)

BAD BREATH

Beating back bad breath

The first step to banishing bad breath is to keep your mouth squeaky clean, since bad breath is often caused by the decomposition of food left between the teeth.

Dentists recommend the following:

- Brush your teeth at least twice daily with a soft toothbrush.
- Massage carefully your gums around the teeth with the soft bristles. Use a rotating motion that doesn't pull your gums away from the teeth.
- Brush your tongue (the top part).
- Floss your teeth as thoroughly and as regularly as you brush them. Dentists usually have no preferences between waxed and unwaxed flosses. Either kind is good. If you have a dental bridge or other permanent dental appliances that make it difficult to use regular floss, try any of several brands of "super" floss. One end is stiff for easy threading between tooth and gum. Another part is fluffy, like a miniature bottle brush, to clean out hard-to-reach crevices. The third part is regular floss.

You should also have your teeth professionally cleaned at least twice yearly. During those cleanings ask the hygienist to show you how to brush and floss most effectively.

Diet helps in the battle against halitosis (bad breath). Parsley and peppermint, for instance, are natural breath sweeteners, while onions and garlic often foul the breath.

Though mouthwashes won't get at the causes of bad breath, they can momentarily freshen the breath.

If your bad breath persists, it could be due to a gum or sinus infection or a stomach upset. Also, infected tonsils often cause bad breath.

MEDICAL SOURCE ───────────────────────

The Marshall Cavendish Illustrated Encyclopaedia of Family Health, Marshall Cavendish House, London, 1986

BED-WETTING

How to 'dry out' your bed-wetting child

Bed-wetting is defined as the involuntary discharge of urine during sleep by children older than 3. The problem tends to run in families and is more likely to occur among boys. The good news is that most outgrow it before adolescence.

Bed-wetting is a mysterious problem because it is not clearly understood exactly what causes it.

It's fairly obvious why a child begins or continues to wet the bed during the night if the family moves or there's a new baby or a divorce or some other frightening — to the child — event.

But in many instances, the causes or problems are far more subtle.

First, you will want to have your child thoroughly examined to rule out any potential diseases. At all times, you should strive for a low-key approach that encourages the child. After all, the child doesn't wet the bed on purpose; it's an unconscious act.

Next, try the "dry-bedtime" approach. Restricting the child's fluids in the evenings can be helpful if you don't make an issue of it. That is, if you try to reason with a very young child about the wisdom of restricting fluids, you'll probably make him want a glassful of liquid.

Instead, provide a juicy orange instead of a glass of milk for an evening snack. Of course, if the child is old enough to participate in solving the problem, then include him in discussing the overall program.

Waking a child up and taking him to the bathroom may work with some children.

Some parents report success with an alarm clock set to go off every two hours. The time between the alarm settings is increased gradually as the child begins to associate the alarm with urination and subsconsciously begins to control himself.

Others are successful with an alarm system in the bedding that goes off whenever liquid touches it.

Often, older school-age children break the habit when they want to go to a sleep-over party or away to camp. It sometimes eases the child's fears if he can first spend the night at a sympathetic relative's home before launching into camp or sleep-overs.

The child who continues to have the problem should be referred to a child counselor, regardless of whether he appears to have other psychological or emotional difficulties.

MEDICAL SOURCES ————————————————

Dr. Spock's Baby and Child Care, 6th Edition, Pocket Books, New York, 1992

The Oxford Companion to Medicine, Vol. 1, Oxford University Press, New York, 1986

BLACK EYE

Ease the black-eye blues

A so-called black eye is actually a bruise of the cheek, eyelids and eyebrow.

To lessen its effect, immediately apply cold compresses and an icebag.

Once the discoloration is fully developed, however, the cold compresses and ice bag will have little or no effect on lightening the bruised areas, though they may help the swelling and the pain.

A blow hard enough to produce a black eye could also injure the eyeball or the optic nerves. There is more cause for concern if your vision is blurred or you begin to see double.

Therefore, you should have your black eye examined by an ophthalmologist (a medical doctor), who may prescribe an eye patch, antibiotics or painkillers.

In any event, do not attempt to force open an eye that has been swollen shut after an injury. In fact, don't press on it in any way.

Try taking some vitamin C to reduce the time it takes for the color to fade away.

MEDICAL SOURCE ————————————————

The Columbia University Complete Medical Guide, Crown Publishers, Inc., New York, 1985

BLADDER CONTROL

Help control leaky bladder with low-impact exercises

Ladies, you don't have to give up your exercise program because of a leaky bladder.

You might be able to reduce incontinence by strengthening your vaginal muscles and by switching from high-impact to low-impact sports programs.

You can strengthen vaginal muscles by contracting and relaxing the pelvic-floor muscles for 10 seconds at a time several times a day.

Or, you could try a new device called vaginal weights. Vaginal weights are inserted like tampons. Gravity then pulls on the weights forcing the vaginal muscles to push the device back into place.

The weights are worn 20 to 30 minutes daily. Ask your doctor about this new health product.

A University of Michigan Medical Center study on exercise-related bladder control among women revealed that one-third of those women studied experienced some degree of bladder leakage. Also, 89 percent of the women exercised at least once a week.

Incontinence is usually a female problem because women's muscles are weakened during childbirth and because men have a longer urethra, which helps prevent leakage.

The women in the study ranged in age from 17 to 68.

The study indicated that the more vaginal births a woman has had, the higher the likelihood for incontinence during exercise.

But, leakage incidents were reduced during participation in

low-impact sports.

Those who leak during a coughing bout or when they are lifting are more apt to leak during exercise.

Exercise leakage occurs most frequently when you are running or doing high-impact aerobics because your bladder is harder to control during a bouncing activity.

"It's the repetitive impact that's a problem," says Dr. John O.L. DeLancey, an author of the study as well as assistant professor of obstetrics at the University of Michigan.

"We would not necessarily tell people to stop exercising. Instead, we tell people to change their form of exercise," he says.

Low-impact exercises with less bouncing activity include swimming or bicycling.

Consult your doctor before starting any exercise program.

And remember: Bladder control is a common problem for many women, so you shouldn't feel uncomfortable discussing it with your doctor.

MEDICAL SOURCE ─────────────────────────

The Physician and Sportsmedicine (19,1:15)

BLISTERS

Say bye-bye to blisters

Almost everyone has a story to tell about walking in a pair of shoes that rubbed huge, painful blisters.

In fact, the most common blisters are those caused by friction, though blisters can also be caused by insect bites, burns, viruses, bacterial infections or chemical irritations. You should seek medical treatment for blisters other than those caused by friction or minor burns.

The friction blister, commonly found on the hands or feet, is rarely dangerous, though it can be painful.

Do not attempt to burst the blister unless it is particularly large or painful.

In those instances, sterilize a needle with a match and gently pierce the blister. After it drains, cover it with a bandage and keep it covered until it heals — about three or four days.

To prevent blisters on the feet:

- Wear well-fitting, comfortable and substantial shoes for long walks.
- Avoid walking shoes with internal ridges or ankle supports that rub.
- Choose woolly socks that are soft and have no ridges.
- Break in new walking shoes gradually.
- Keep your feet clean and dry.
- Don't wear old, hard or rough socks.
- For everyday wear, choose sandals.

To prevent blisters on the hands during physical labor:

- Wear soft, thick gloves.
- Change grip often.
- Harden up your skin with denatured alcohol three times a day for several weeks before doing manual labor.
- Don't work with rough, abrasive materials, such as concrete blocks, without gloves.
- Grip implements loosely.

MEDICAL SOURCE —————————————————————

The Marshall Cavendish Illustrated Encyclopaedia of Family Health, Marshall Cavendish House, London, 1986

BLOOD PRESSURE

The bad news is: Heart disease is the leading cause of death in America. The good news is: It's one of the most preventable causes of death in America.

Heart disease kills one person every 34 seconds in the United States, says the American Heart Association. If you can feel those seconds ticking by, destroy your time bomb yourself before it explodes.

Along with high cholesterol, lack of exercise and smoking, high blood pressure is at the top of the list for making that heart disease time bomb tick.

You can lower your high blood pressure naturally, even without prescription blood pressure drugs.

Are you sure that you don't have high blood pressure?

Your doctor has told you that your blood pressure level is fine, so you aren't worried. But you may need to check it again.

In the past, most doctors said you had high blood pressure if your diastolic blood pressure was high. ("Diastolic" is the bottom, lower number in the blood pressure figure.)

Now, researchers are saying that systolic blood pressure (the top, higher number) is much more important, even when the diastolic blood pressure is normal—around 90 millimeters of mercury (mm Hg).

That means that a lot more people may have high blood pressure than was previously thought. And, the older you get, the less important the bottom blood pressure number is. As you get older, your arteries stiffen, causing your systolic pressure to go up. This stiffening doesn't raise your diastolic pressure; in fact, it can even go down.

The Systolic Hypertension in the Elderly Program studied 2,365 people with a systolic pressure of 160 to 240 mm Hg and a diastolic pressure of 90 mm Hg or less. The researchers treated these people with blood pressure lowering drugs, and gave a placebo to a control group.

Compared to the control group, the group receiving the drugs had 36 percent fewer strokes and 35 percent fewer deaths due to coronary heart disease. These are people who would have had almost normal blood pressure levels according to the old way of figuring.

To get an accurate systolic blood pressure level, you may want to check it more than once. Systolic blood pressure levels can be high at one time and low at another, especially if you are over age 60.

MEDICAL SOURCES

Archives of Internal Medicine (152,110:1977)
Journal of the American Medical Association (268,10:1287)

Lower your blood pressure the natural way

Do you have high blood pressure or think you're at risk for high blood pressure? Help yourself with these four steps:

> - Exercise at least 30 minutes three times a week.
> - Lose at least 10 pounds.
> - Eat a diet low in salt (under 6 grams per day).
> - Consume no more than two alcoholic drinks a day.

Numerous studies show that exercise alone reduces systolic pressure (the upper number in a blood pressure reading) by an average of 11 mm Hg and reduces diastolic pressure by an average of 8 mm Hg. Regular aerobic exercise can be much more effective in decreasing hypertension than blood pressure drugs.

MEDICAL SOURCES

Medical World News (33,11:9)
Postgraduate Medicine (92,6:139)

Lowering your blood pressure when you're slim and trim

If you are overweight, a smoker or a heavy drinker, you're probably not surprised when you get a high blood pressure reading. You know what you need to do to lower your blood pressure and your risk of heart disease.

But what if you're a thin nonsmoker who drinks very little alcohol and you still have high blood pressure? Don't be frustrated: You can benefit from certain changes in your diet even more than an overweight person can.

Increasing your intake of dietary fiber, potassium, magnesium, vitamin C and calcium will help prevent high blood pressure, studies suggest. And only thin men seemed to get any benefit from the calcium.

A California study showed that people who were lean, under age 40 and moderate drinkers were able to reduce their risk of high blood pressure by 40 percent simply by eating foods that contained at least 1 gram of calcium per day.

The best way to lower your blood pressure through your diet is to eat more fruit, researchers suggest. The fiber from the fruit works better than cereal and vegetable fiber when lowering systolic blood pressure.

The more strawberries, blueberries and peaches the men ate, the lower their systolic blood pressure. Strawberries also helped lower diastolic blood pressure.

The researchers don't know why fruit fiber worked better than other fibers, but they suspect that fruit might contain some unknown ingredients that help lower blood pressure.

MEDICAL SOURCES————————————————————————

Circulation (86,5:1475)
Science News (142,21:340)

High blood pressure? Have a banana!

Eating foods high in potassium can actually lower your blood pressure, researchers say. That's one reason potassium-rich fruit is the food of choice for people with high blood pressure.

In one study, a test group increased the amount of potassium-rich foods they ate by more than 60 percent a year. As a result, these people were able to cut by more than half the amount of medicine they took for high blood pressure. To get this much potassium, the test group simply ate three to six servings of fruits, vegetables, peas and beans a day. Skim milk is also a good source of potassium.

Dr. Louis Tobian suggests that potassium lowers blood pressure by preventing thickening of artery walls. The thickening slows down blood flow and can trigger strokes or heart attacks.

To protect yourself against high blood pressure, eat your potassium-rich string beans and apples every day.

MEDICAL SOURCES ─────────────────────

British Medical Journal (301,6751:521)
Annals of Internal Medicine (115,10:753)
Hypertension (19,6:749)

Hypertension medication only temporary?

If you're taking medication to help lower your blood pressure, you might not need to feel chained to these drugs for life.

Many doctors thought that once you started drug treatment for high blood pressure, you were on them for life.

However, a study suggests that some people might be able to stop taking their medications and still maintain normal blood pressure measurements.

Based on the British study, eight out of nine people with high blood pressure who stopped taking their medication under strict medical supervision had normal blood pressure measurements even up to two years later. However, doctors stress that maintaining a normal blood pressure usually includes maintaining a more healthy diet and a practical exercise plan, as well as losing weight or quitting smoking if those were risk factors involved.

Doctors also stress the extreme importance of regular follow-up visits among the people who are weaned off hypertension medication.

These people need to stop in to the doctor's office every two to three months for blood pressure checks just to make sure everything is going well.

If you are taking medicine for high blood pressure, never stop taking it without your doctor's advice.

Your doctor will know how to slowly wean you off the medication and help you establish a regular follow-up plan to ensure your best health.

MEDICAL SOURCE ───────────────────────────
Medical Tribune (32,18:10)

Some substances that can cause your blood pressure to increase include:

• oral contraceptives
• corticosteroids
• sodium-containing antacids
• some over-the-counter appetite suppressants
• decongestants
• some nonsteroidal anti-inflammatory drugs
• cocaine

MEDICAL SOURCE ───────────────────────────
FDA Consumer (25,10:28)

Crunchy way to help lower your blood pressure

Crunching celery might do more for you than satisfy your appetite.

Celery, an old Oriental remedy for mild hypertension, apparently is still effective.

Scientists discovered that celery contains a chemical that opens the blood vessels, which in turn lowers your blood pressure. Researchers caution against using the celery cure alone. Celery contains sodium and other chemicals, which at high doses can be harmful to your body. Check with your doctor about including more celery in your diet.

MEDICAL SOURCE ───────────────────────────────

Science News (141,19:319)

Is hypertension cure worse than disease?

Some who use prescription drugs to control high blood pressure might answer yes to that question.

Many people complain that their blood pressure medicine causes them to feel "down" and tired. They say they don't sleep well, they have a hard time concentrating, or they feel less "sharp."

Nearly four out of every 10 people quit taking their high blood pressure medicines because of the side effects, according to some studies.

However, Dr. Joel E. Dimsdale reports that often these complaints might actually be confused with the effects of high blood pressure itself.

In fact, researchers have proved that even when a placebo (substitute pill that contains no medication) is given for high blood pressure, it causes these same side effects in almost one out of every four people tested.

People believe they feel worse after taking their medicine just because they are paying closer attention to their symptoms, believes Dr. Dimsdale.

Dr. Dimsdale makes a couple of suggestions that might improve your results from high blood pressure medicine.

❑ Have your spouse or someone who lives with you discuss your hypertension with you and your doctor. Your spouse has probably noticed your symptoms and can help you give a more accurate picture of your high blood pressure symptoms and your reaction to medicine.

❑ Adopt a positive attitude toward your treatment. Many people do feel better after taking high blood pressure medicine and suffer no bad side effects.

Be sure to talk with your doctor if you are concerned about hypertension or side effects from your high blood pressure medicine.

MEDICAL SOURCE ───────────────────────

Archives of Internal Medicine (152,1:35)

Feeling down? Check your blood pressure

Because of the dangers associated with high blood pressure, it seems that everyone is trying to lower their blood pressure. But scientists now think that blood pressure that is too low might not be good for you, either.

Scientific evidence suggests that low blood pressure can cause medical symptoms such as fatigue, dizziness and headaches, as well as anxiety and depression.

A recent study linked low blood pressure to both tiredness and feelings of faintness or lightheadedness.

Most people experience lower blood pressure in the mornings after they have been lying down for hours. To avoid the dizzy headrush, lightheadedness and faintness when getting out of bed, many doctors recommend rising slowly to a sitting position in bed. Rising too quickly results in a quick drop in blood pressure.

While you are sitting, yawn, stretch and take deep breaths to help increase the heart rate. This helps raise your blood pressure. Then, slowly rise and stand, continuing to take deep breaths for a moment.

If you feel dizzy upon standing up after you have been sitting for a while, remember to stretch, breathe deeply and rise slowly out of the chair to avoid a sudden drop in blood pressure.

Older people might need to drink a lot of water each day to avoid getting a low blood volume from dehydration. This can also contribute to low blood pressure.

Regular exercise also helps prevent blood pressure that is too low. Exercise keeps the heart muscle strong and beating regularly. People experience drops in blood pressure when the heart is not beating quickly enough. Exercise helps avoid a heartbeat that is too slow.

If you are taking medication or on a diet to help lower your blood pressure, do not stop your routine without talking to your doctor. If you think you suffer from low blood pressure, call your doctor. She can help determine whether your blood pressure is healthy for you.

MEDICAL SOURCE ─────────────────────

British Medical Journal (304,6819:75)

BODY ODOR

Common sense about unpleasant body scents

First, it's important to remember that you — just like everyone else — naturally and automatically have an individual odor, caused by your own sweat.

Second, sweat is the way your body regulates its temperature. While sweating varies from person to person depending on the individual's activity and nervous tension levels, no one escapes sweating.

Occasionally, a very strong body odor can be a warning sign of a serious medical condition or skin infection. If you worry about your body scent, check with your doctor.

Otherwise, to prevent body odor:

❑ Bathe or shower daily, especially after exercising, to prevent sweat buildup.

❑ Ladies, you might want to shave your underarms so the sweat doesn't become trapped in the hair.

❑ After bathing or showering, dry the skin thoroughly, using a clean towel that isn't too soft, since a towel that is a little rough does a better job.

❑ Avoid using a lot of perfume or scented powder, which frequently combine with the sweat to produce a stale odor.

❑ Apply deodorant or antiperspirant regularly.

❑ Wash your clothes regularly.

❑ Wear comfortable, loose clothing.

❑ Wear cotton underwear that lets the skin breathe.

❑ Don't bathe too frequently — more than once or twice a day — or else you will kill off healthy skin bacteria and make the problem worse.

❑ Certain vegetables, such as parsley, contain chlorophyll, a natural deodorant that helps to prevent body odor.

❑ Conversely, other foods such as onions, garlic and some types of cheeses seem to make body odor worse.

MEDICAL SOURCE ————————————————————————

> *The Marshall Cavendish Illustrated Encyclopaedia of Family Health*, Marshall Cavendish House, London, 1986

BOILS

Boo to boils: how to avoid and treat this problem

Boils are infections of the tiny pores called follicles from which hairs grow. The infections are caused when the follicles become infected with bacteria, and an abscess or swelling filled with pus forms.

A carbuncle is a boil with two or more heads. Most often boils and carbuncles arise on the neck, face, armpits, groin or buttocks where clothing rubs.

You are most susceptible to boils when you're overworked, anemic or undernourished. Alcoholics and those who eat a lot of fat also tend to have boils.

The infection thrives in oily, blocked-up pores. The skin becomes hot, red and swollen. The center of the swollen area contains pus. Once the pus is released and the central core of tissue is gone, the boil heals within a week. Occasionally, a boil will heal without bursting.

To prevent boils or carbuncles, improve your diet by cutting some of the fat. Also, if you tend to be anemic, eat more iron-rich foods. You should also improve your overall diet and eliminate alcoholic beverages.

Other prevention techniques include:

- Bathing daily and drying the skin thoroughly.
- Using an unscented powder after bathing and drying to prevent greasy buildup in your pores.
- If you're susceptible to boils, avoid nylon underwear and tight collars.
- Wash your clothes regularly.

To treat boils:

- Apply a dressing to a draining boil frequently.
- Don't pick at a boil or squeeze one before a head forms.
- Don't squeeze a carbuncle or large boil.
- Don't attempt to disinfect the skin with a household disinfectant.

If the boil or carbuncle is particularly large or painful, seek medical attention.

MEDICAL SOURCE

The Marshall Cavendish Illustrated Encyclopaedia of Family Health, Marshall Cavendish House, London, 1986

BONE PROBLEMS

Calcium — should you or shouldn't you?

A decade ago, few people even knew how to pronounce osteoporosis.

Now, many women and a lot of men have realized the dangers of this potentially crippling bone-loss disease and are seeking ways to fight back.

One warrior is the nutrient calcium. But, there are questions: Does the type of calcium you take matter? What can it do for you? What won't it do for you?

Calcium seems to be as popular as vitamin C once was. Over-the-counter sales of calcium supplements are nearly $200 million each year. Most of the people who are taking these supplements are women trying to prevent the onset of osteoporosis.

Increasing or supplementing dietary calcium can help prevent osteoporosis, but it is important to know that calcium cannot reverse bone loss.

Calcium is safe when taken as directed, according to researchers. It is the most abundant mineral in the body. More than 99 percent of calcium is stored in your bones to strengthen and support your skeleton.

Calcium is responsible for helping the body transmit nerve signals, maintaining strong bones, helping blood to clot, keeping the heart healthy, and other important biochemical processes in the body.

One of the factors that hinder the absorption of calcium in the body is a diet high in fat. The additional fat in the digestive system combines with the calcium to form a "soapy scum" that causes less calcium to be absorbed into the body.

Eating a diet that is too high in grains, cocoa, spinach and soybeans can reduce calcium absorption. Foods high in protein can cause more calcium to be passed out of the body by the intestines.

Aluminum-containing antacids, anticonvulsants, magnesium and phosphates can also reduce calcium absorption.

Dietary calcium is usually preferred over calcium in pill or powder form.

The reason? Foods with calcium also contain additional minerals and elements which can help your body use the calcium. Getting your nutrients by eating and drinking the right foods is the preferred way, and certainly the most "natural."

Some foods that contain calcium are dairy products; sardines (they have edible bones); and green, leafy vegetables (except spinach).

Calcium is best absorbed when your body has an ample supply of vitamin D. If you cannot eat dairy products, supplements might be an alternative for you.

Calcium supplements from bone meal or dolomite might contain dangerous amounts of lead.

These amounts of lead can be unhealthy for children, the elderly and women of childbearing age.

Natural calcium carbonate from ground oyster shells or factory-made is a good alternative. Calcium citrate is usually better absorbed by the elderly because of reduced stomach acid.

Check to see how quickly and completely your tablet dissolves. Place your calcium tablet in approximately six ounces of vinegar. A tablet that dissolves within 30 minutes or less should be easily absorbed by your body.

When buying your calcium supplements, remember that calcium carbonate is only 40 percent calcium.

This means if you take a 500 milligram calcium carbonate pill you are getting only 200 milligrams of calcium. And, calcium citrate contains only about 20 percent calcium. Be sure you are getting the proper amount.

The recommended daily allowance for both men and women over age 25 is 800 milligrams. Talk to your doctor before taking any dietary supplements.

MEDICAL SOURCE ─────────────────────────

U.S. Pharmacist (16,4:26)

Enriched OJ provides diet with lots of easily absorbed calcium

When you have breakfast, make sure you don't leave out a glass of orange juice. You could be depriving your body of its most easily absorbed source of calcium.

When you don't get enough calcium from your diet to meet your body's day-to-day calcium requirements, your body resorts to pulling calcium from your bones.

This results in bone loss, and it leaves your bones weak and brittle.

One easy way to avoid this is to add calcium-enriched orange juice to your diet.

Calcium-enriched orange juice contains a form of calcium known as calcium citrate malate. This form of calcium is readily absorbed and used by the body. Calcium citrate malate is especially helpful in preventing bone loss from the spine.

Talk with your doctor about adding calcium-fortified orange

juice to your diet.

MEDICAL SOURCE ————————————————————

The New England Journal of Medicine (323,13:878)

Possible side effects of calcium supplements

Although side effects are uncommon, there are some things you should know.

❑ Some side effects could be bloating, stomach gas, nausea and constipation.

❑ Too much calcium taken with an antacid could cause the milk-alkali syndrome, which is excess stomach gas and possible kidney trouble.

❑ Another possible painful problem is increased chance of kidney stones, especially if you have already had them.

MEDICAL SOURCE ————————————————————

U.S. Pharmacist (16,4:26)

Some calcium tablets hold possible health hazards

In an effort to prevent or retard the development of osteoporosis (the brittle-bone disease), many men and women have begun taking calcium supplements and antacids that contain high amounts of calcium.

However, they may be getting more than they bargained for.

Apparently, some antacids and calcium-supplement pills contain potentially dangerous levels of manganese.

Manganese is a trace metal that is important in the human body in microscopic or "trace" amounts. Too much of this metal can be hazardous to your health.

Dangerous levels of manganese can cause problems in the nervous system, such as impaired coordination, tremors and even psychiatric problems.

Some researchers claim that some antacids and calcium supplements contain levels of manganese high enough to cause these problems.

The safest way to obtain enough dietary calcium is to eat a diet full of calcium-rich foods and avoid dietary supplements.

MEDICAL SOURCE ─────────────────────────

Pharmacy Times (57,1:21)

Keep your 'D' high

Women who have reached menopause and don't get adequate amounts of calcium and vitamin D are in danger of losing bone mass during the winter months.

The reduced exposure to the sun in winter months causes a drop in vitamin-D production. This change can stimulate a rise in the parathyroid hormone, which regulates calcium and phosphorus metabolism. This change can harm bone density.

Researchers conducted a study of 249 healthy, postmenopausal women to find out if vitamin-D supplementation during the winter can prevent bone loss.

All of the women were given calcium supplements to bring their intake to 800 milligrams a day (the current recommended dietary allowance for men and women age 25 or older). Half were given supplemental vitamin D and half were given a placebo (fake pill) for a year. Researchers measured each person's bone density for the months of July to December and for January to June.

Both groups had increased spinal bone density between summer and winter months and decreases between winter and summer months.

But, the vitamin-D group showed significantly less bone loss from winter to summer.

In other words, adequate vitamin-D supplementation during the winter, in addition to calcium, helps improve overall spine density for postmenopausal women, suggests the report.

Talk to your doctor before starting any dietary supplements.

MEDICAL SOURCE ————————————————————

Modern Medicine (60,1:69)

Salt away this wisdom: just say no

Researchers suggest that restricting the amount of salt in the diet seems to help reduce bone loss in women past the age of menopause.

To test this theory, 59 women who were past the age of menopause agreed to lower their dietary salt intake for one week to determine whether their salt intake affected their bone loss.

Bone loss usually occurs when the body does not get enough dietary calcium to maintain the proper level of calcium in the bones.

When this happens, it pulls calcium out of the bones, leaving the bones brittle and breakable.

Calcium can also be pulled out of the bones when there is too much salt in the body. The body flushes this "pulled out" calcium through the urine. Scientists can measure the amount of bone loss by measuring the amount of calcium in the urine of women at risk for osteoporosis.

Since urinary calcium is related to the amount of sodium in the urine, researchers attempted to lower calcium loss by lowering the sodium loss. To do that, the researchers cut back on salt. The women gave urine samples before and after one week of reduced salt intake.

Scientists found that the amount of calcium in the urine was greatly reduced after a week of restricted salt intake only in the women who started out with a high level of sodium in their urine.

Those women who maintained low-sodium diets before the study did not produce significantly lower levels of urinary calcium after the study.

However, scientists speculate that one out of every four women past the age of menopause maintain a sodium intake high enough to put them at risk for increased bone loss.

That means that one out of every four women past the age of menopause would benefit from a low-salt diet.

Although there is no known cure for the crippling bone loss of osteoporosis, a low-salt diet might turn out to be one of the best ways to prevent it.

MEDICAL SOURCE ────────────────────────

Archives of Internal Medicine (151,4:757)

Are fluoride side effects worth the health benefits?

Some studies have shown that taking fluoride supplements along with calcium supplements can help reduce the number of hip fractures in women and men who suffer from osteoporosis.

But are the side effects of the fluoride supplements worth the benefits? Fluoride treatments aren't worth it if the dosages are too high.

People who take between 50 and 74 milligrams of fluoride daily usually suffer from side effects such as discomfort and pain in the digestive tract, pain in the hips and legs, and bone fractures. Those who take under 50 milligrams daily have few side effects.

So if your fluoride tablets are a problem, ask your doctor to check the dosage.

A lower dosage could eliminate the side effects and still give you the protection from bone fractures that you need.

MEDICAL SOURCE ——————————————————————

The New England Journal of Medicine (323,6:416)

Diuretic slows down bone loss

Suffering from high blood pressure and worried about osteoporosis?

A group of drugs called thiazides might help in both areas.

Thiazides are a class of drugs that act as diuretics and are commonly prescribed to help lower blood pressure.

Although thiazides have been associated with several negative side effects, recent medical studies show that thiazides also help reduce bone loss in men and women.

This "positive side effect" helps lessen the chance of a serious bone fracture. Bone loss is caused when the body takes calcium from the bones.

This reduces the weight and strength of the bones and increases the risk of serious fractures. Thiazide diuretics have actually reduced the speed of this dangerous bone loss.

Many brand name blood pressure medications contain thiazide. The drugs that contain at least 50 milligrams of thiazide seem to be the most effective at maintaining good, strong bones.

If you are currently taking a diuretic drug that contains thiazide, talk with your doctor about the side effects — both negative and positive.

Ten drugs that contain thiazide

Capozide

Dyazide

Minizide

Esidrix

Prinzide

Vaseretic

Enduron

Diucardin

Diuril

Oretic

MEDICAL SOURCE ————————————————

British Medical Journal (301,6764:1303)

Faster healing for broken bones

Broken bones are more than just painful — they are horribly inconvenient. Wearing a cast around and possibly even using crutches for six to eight weeks isn't anyone's idea of a good time.

So, if you knew of a way to speed the healing of the broken bone, would you try it? If you said "yes," then you need to leave your carton of cigarettes at home. In other words, stop smoking.

Recent studies indicate that smoking delays the healing of broken bones. Healing times are fastest for nonsmokers, intermediate for ex-smokers and longest for current smokers.

Why put yourself through the misery? Researchers suggest that if you stop smoking while you are in the cast, your bones will heal faster and you will have a better chance of a complete recovery.

MEDICAL SOURCE ───────────────────

The Physician and Sportsmedicine (20,5:33)

Broken bones misdiagnosed in the elderly

Do X-rays really show the whole picture?
Not for this 79-year-old woman.
She had been having pain in her left leg near her ankle for about two weeks. The swollen area was red and warm. The doctor couldn't see any broken bones from the first X-ray. She had what the doctor thought was an infection in her leg. So the doctor decided to treat her with an antibiotic to clear up the infection.

After three weeks her leg didn't show any signs of improvement, and she was unable to walk because of severe pain. A repeat X-ray showed a nondisplaced fracture (fracture in which the bone has not moved out of place) of the lower part of the shin bone or tibia.

For four weeks she wore a cast on her leg, then she gradually started walking again.

This case is typical of many undiagnosed cases of broken bones. Elderly people with osteoporosis can experience a fracture of a weakened bone without having any typical symptoms.

Common places for fractures to occur are in the ribs, hip, thigh, knee, ankle, wrist or spine.

Arthritis sufferers might shrug off pain in their bones as being symptoms of their arthritis, when sometimes it can be fractured bones. This can result in unnecessary suffering when diagnosis and treatment are delayed.

Sometimes doctors can miss the diagnosis of a broken bone

because the fracture might not show up on the X-ray until changes known as callus formation take place several weeks later.

A new procedure called scintigraphy appears to be eliminating these misdiagnoses. Scintigraphy shows fractures that an X-ray can miss. The recovery rate is much faster when fractures are found early. If you are experiencing a sudden onset of pain in a bone or joint, see your doctor right away.

MEDICAL SOURCE ———————————————————

Arthritis and Rheumatism (34,7:912)

Parents, be specific with your kids after injuries

Ask a teen-ager his definition of rough play, and it's guaranteed to be different from his parent's idea of rough play. And sometimes that can cause some serious health problems.

For example, one teen-age boy recently had a cast removed from his arm. The bone was healing properly, and the doctor and parents advised the boy to avoid football, wrestling and other rough activities.

The boy followed the instructions according to his teen-age mentality and promptly refractured his arm doing military-style push-ups the very same evening. You can certainly imagine his defense: "But, I wasn't playing football. ..."

The moral of the story: Your kids need things spelled out in fine detail when it comes to matters of their health. Taking the extra time to carefully explain things will help you avoid future injuries due to the differences in the adult mind and the child's mind.

MEDICAL SOURCE ———————————————————

The Physician and Sportsmedicine (20,5:64)

BOWEL PROBLEMS

Tips to help relieve irritable bowel syndrome

To say the least, it's an embarrassing situation.

Your body keeps alternating between diarrhea and constipation. To make matters worse, you've noticed more bloating and excessive flatus (passing gas).

You haven't changed your diet lately, so what could it be?

You might be suffering from an illness known as irritable bowel syndrome (IBS). In fact, about 15 percent of the population suffers from symptoms of IBS.

Irritable bowel syndrome masquerades under many different names — nervous indigestion, nervous diarrhea, dyspepsia, spastic colon, functional colitis and others.

Each of these terms has been lumped under the name — irritable bowel syndrome (IBS). And each of the names suggests the same thing — it's an extremely unpleasant sickness that demands immediate care.

Irritable bowel syndrome affects twice as many women as men, usually beginning in early adulthood, although it can last for many years.

Irritable bowel syndrome is just what it sounds like — your bowel is "irritated." In other words, your large intestines are acting up. But doctors don't really know why the intestines do that. And until they find out why, all they can do is figure out who has IBS and try to make them more comfortable.

The first step, then, is to recognize the symptoms of irritable bowel syndrome:

❏ IBS usually causes abdominal pain that is linked to alternating episodes of constipation and diarrhea.

❏ Bouts of diarrhea are usually marked by a sense of urgency—badly needing to go to the bathroom—and an increase in the number of times you need to go to the bathroom. The amount of stool that you actually pass is small, and occasionally IBS sufferers notice that they only pass gas or mucus without passing stools.

❏ Many people suffer from early-morning diarrhea, and they complain of having to make several trips to the bathroom after breakfast.

❏ Those who are not suffering from diarrhea pass stools that are hard, dry and pellet-like. You might occasionally notice a feeling of an "incomplete bowel movement," or you could experience three or four days of constipation followed by several loose, "break-through" stools.

❏ The abdominal pain and cramping usually is located on the left side of the abdomen. And sometimes pain can radiate up through your shoulders, chest and back.

❏ Many people become bloated and experience excess gas.

❏ About half of the people with irritable bowel syndrome also complain of nausea, vomiting, heartburn and belching.

❏ IBS can start at any age, but it usually bothers people who are between the ages of 20 and 50, and it seems to afflict women twice as often as it does men.

❏ If you are experiencing fever, anemia, dehydration or weight loss along with some of the other symptoms, you probably do not have irritable bowel syndrome. Fever, anemia, dehydration and weight loss are usually not symptoms of IBS.

What can you do about it?

The first thing you need to do is realize that IBS is an inconvenient and occasionally embarrassing condition, but it really is not a serious illness.

The next thing to do is to keep a close watch on the things you eat and drink. Keep an accurate journal of your diet for a few weeks — what you ate and drank for every meal, and every in-between-meal snack. Also, keep a private journal of your bowel movements during that same few weeks. Try to figure out whether there are any foods or drinks that seem to be triggering your episodes of irritable bowel syndrome. Drinks like fruit juices, coffee and wine seem to bother some people. And many people try to avoid fatty foods, fried foods and spices. Figure out what you need to cut out of your diet to help settle your intestines.

Now, add some more fiber to your diet. Most Americans eat only 15 to 20 grams of fiber each day. We need about twice that much every day. Eating more fiber will improve your bowel habits (especially constipation) and help relieve some of the symptoms of IBS. You can add bran cereals, oat bran and high-fiber vegetables to your diet to increase the amount of fiber you eat each day.

Or you can use the over-the-counter fiber supplements to help boost your fiber intake.

Psyllium powder is an excellent fiber supplement, and some of the commercial brands of psyllium powder include the following: Correctol, Fiberall, Metamucil, Perdiem, Serutan and Syllact. Your doctor or pharmacist can recommend a fiber supplement for your diet.

If you are having an embarrassing problem with flatulence, the key is to avoid the foods that cause the flatulence. Listed below are some examples of foods that are big offenders, moderate offenders, or relatively safe:

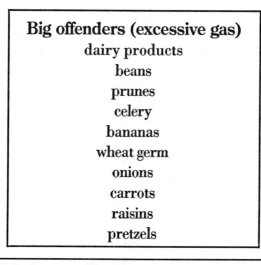

Big offenders (excessive gas)
dairy products
beans
prunes
celery
bananas
wheat germ
onions
carrots
raisins
pretzels

Moderate offenders (moderate gas)
breads
apples
citrus fruits (oranges, lemons, grapefruit)
potatoes
pastries

Relatively safe (low gas)
meat (beef, chicken, turkey and fish)
eggs
rice
lettuce
broccoli
nuts
cauliflower
cucumbers
potato chips
Graham crackers

A final way to help reduce your episodes of irritable bowel

syndrome is to lower your stress with daily exercise. Occasionally, stress can affect your bowel habits. Regular daily exercise helps reduce stress and keeps your body healthy.

MEDICAL SOURCE ─────────────────────────

Modern Medicine (57,5:100)

Simple home remedies to help relieve painful bowel problems

IBS usually causes symptoms such as abdominal pain, diarrhea or constipation, abdominal distention (bloating), flatulence (excess gas) and nausea.

Scientists haven't been able to find a "germ" or virus that causes IBS. Many researchers think that it is usually caused by emotional factors, such as depression or stress.

Since there really is no definite medical cause, what can you do about it? Here are some easy tips to help manage IBS:

❑ Avoid chewing gum, carbonated drinks and other foods that cause you to swallow air.

❑ Avoid drinks containing caffeine or alcohol.

❑ Avoid tobacco products.

❑ Avoid all foods that seem to cause you discomfort (gas, heartburn, etc.).

❑ Breath mints and other candies that contain sorbitol or mannitol may increase flatulence or diarrhea.

❑ Laxatives may worsen the situation. Ask your doctor's advice on how to use them, if at all.

❑ Heating pads or a hot-water bottle can help relieve abdominal pain and cramping.

❏ Be sure to tell your doctor about all other medications you use. Some may aggravate your condition.

Be sure to tell your doctor if your symptoms don't improve after a few days. More serious conditions may need more professional treatment.

MEDICAL SOURCE ─────────────────────────────

U.S. Pharmacist (15,8:43)

New kind of 'natural' treatment for people with bowel problems

People with colon and bowel problems now might find some relief with "nutritious" enemas. Doctors are experimenting with enemas that contain amino acids, which are chief components of proteins.

Dr. Richard Breuer, associate professor of medicine at Chicago's Northwestern University, and his co-workers tested whether enemas with a solution of short-chain fatty acids (amino acids) could benefit people with bowel diseases.

Researchers gave the enemas to a group of 41 people with ulcerative colitis. Twenty-one people treated themselves for six weeks with an enema of acetate, propionate and butyrate (short-chain fatty acids) along with saltwater solution twice a day. The other 20 people used only enemas of saltwater.

Results clearly showed improvement in 10 of 17 people who were treated with short-chain fatty acids, compared with only six out of the 20 who were given saltwater.

Short-chain fatty acids are essential to the makeup of colon cells, according to the report. People with ulcerative colitis have abnormally low levels of short-chain fatty acids in their bowel movements, the report states.

These enemas appear to help the colon repair itself and heal the damage caused by the inflammatory process. Such an approach hasn't been tried before.

Ulcerative colitis is an inflammatory disease where ulcers occur on the mucous membrane of the colon. It is most often characterized by bloody diarrhea. It's called chronic because it flares up, then subsides, then flares up again.

Crohn's disease is also a chronic inflammatory disease, but it occurs in the lower small intestines and colon. It also can occur anywhere in the digestive tract. Symptoms of Crohn's disease include chronic diarrhea, abdominal pain and fever.

MEDICAL SOURCE —————————————————————————
Medical World News (32,12:19)

BREAST PROBLEMS

Breast disorders range from nuisances to dangers

There are several varieties of breast discomfort, most of which are annoying but harmless.

Mastodynia is the monthly swelling and painful tenderness that may precede a woman's menstrual period. The effects of mastodynia can frequently be relieved by wearing a bra — if you don't — or by wearing a bra made of a stretchier material.

Also, many women find relief from the overall feelings of premenstrual tightness and puffiness by avoiding excessive salt, sugar, coffee, tea and alcohol.

As you age, breast swelling can become chronic, even remaining after menstrual periods have ceased.

Nevertheless, some lumpiness is normal, which is why it's so important for women of every age to examine their breasts regularly.

Fibrocystic disease occurs when the normal changes that take place every month as a mature woman's breasts prepare for milk production become exaggerated.

As women age, it becomes more difficult for the lymph system to absorb the fluid in the breast tissue after every monthly cycle. The fluids become trapped and form cysts, which may persist or disappear after a couple of periods or disappear and re-appear a year or so later.

Fibrocystic disease can be intensely painful. Also, women who suffer from fibrocystic disease are much more likely to develop breast cancer.

The treatment for fibrocystic disease includes caffeine restriction and added vitamin E. Your doctor or health care provider may also prescribe hormone therapy.

In addition to self-exams, women who are older than 40 or women who have a history of breast cancer in their families should have regular mammograms.

MEDICAL SOURCE ────────────────────────

The Columbia University Complete Home Medical Guide, Crown Publishers, Inc., New York, 1985

BREAST-FEEDING

Avoiding problems with breast-feeding

Breast milk provides the best possible nutritional and emotional beginning for your child. That's because your milk contains all the nutrients your newborn needs and is more easily digestible and absorbed than any other infant food.

Breast-feeding compared to bottle feeding means saving time, effort and money.

Furthermore, there's never a problem with storage or spoilage. Many pediatricians say that breast-feeding protects the baby against infections, as well as allergies.

The breast-feeding mother is more apt to regain her prepregnant figure quicker because breast-feeding causes the uterus to contract more readily.

Emotionally, breast-feeding is the most natural and effective way of understanding and satisfying the needs of your child. It also strengthens the bonds of love between the newborn and his mother.

The best start for breast-feeding is to make sure the baby is not bottle-fed in the hospital. Tell your doctor that you plan to breast-feed and ask her assistance.

Make certain everyone in the hospital nursery knows not to give your baby a bottle. You might find that a hospital with a rooming-in feature is your best choice if you plan to breast-feed.

Next, your breasts need to be stimulated by the baby's sucking to produce and keep up a good supply of milk. It takes several days after birth to establish the milk, so don't give up; just keep putting the baby to the breast.

To help your body produce a good supply of milk, drink plenty of fluids and eat a healthy, well-balanced diet. Some doctors say that a few extra calories might be in order since the body will use more calories than usual in milk production.

Much of what you eat or drink will pass into the baby's milk, so it's important not to drink alcoholic beverages or to take any kind of drugs unless the doctor takes your nursing status into account.

Most mothers who are breast-feeding for the first time worry that they won't have enough milk. Normally, the more the baby nurses, the more milk the breasts produce.

If your baby appears healthy, if his crying is within normal limits, if he is steadily gaining weight, and if your pediatrician seems satisfied that your baby is progressing, relax. Remember that perfectly healthy babies' weights and appetites fluctuate from day to day.

MEDICAL SOURCES ——————————————————

> *The Womanly Art of Breast-feeding*, La Leche League International, Franklin Park, Ill., 1987
> *Dr. Spock's Baby and Child Care, 6th Edition*, New York, 1992

Microwave dangers for nursing mothers

Using the microwave to heat up the bottle might be quick and easy, but it could be harmful for your newborn. Microwaving human milk can destroy many of the milk's components that are so beneficial for your baby.

More and more women who are working outside of the home use breast pumps to express and then store their breast milk for the baby to drink while they are at work. You can safely refrigerate breast milk for a few days and even freeze it for up to a month.

It's the warming-up process that you need to be careful

about. If you heat the milk to temperatures well above the normal body temperature (37 degrees Celsius or 98 degrees Fahrenheit), you could be destroying many of the beneficial properties of the milk.

Breast milk contains many different things that in some ways make it more desirable than infant formula. One of the most important components is what we call antibodies.

Antibodies are part of your body's natural defenses and immune system, and they attack any viruses or bacteria that get into the bloodstream to help protect you from illnesses and diseases. Antibodies are one of the first lines of defense against illnesses.

Antibodies take time to be produced, however, and a newborn will not develop a full "army" of antibodies for several months. Fortunately, some of the mother's antibodies can be given to the baby through the breast milk.

The problem is that microwaving might destroy those important, disease-fighting antibodies.

Breast milk also contains enzymes known as lysozymes. These enzymes are also important members of the natural "army" your body has to fight against disease. Babies who are nursed get the benefit of the mother's lysozymes through the breast milk. Unfortunately — you guessed it — microwaving seems to damage these valuable enzymes, too.

In recent studies, researchers found that heating breast milk to high temperatures that are common in the microwave (72 to 98 degrees Celsius or 162 to 208 degrees Fahrenheit) can result in a 96-percent loss of lysozyme activity and a 98-percent loss of the function of some types of antibodies.

Microwaving the milk seems to decrease the amount of disease-fighting forces and increase the risk of infection from poisonous bacteria.

The scientist also noticed some (but not as much) damage to disease-fighters in the milk even when the microwave was set on low temperatures. They suspect that the temperature and the effects of the microwaves that the microwave oven produces work together to harm the milk.

Many researchers advise nursing mothers to avoid using the microwave to heat any refrigerated or frozen breast milk. Instead, slowly warm the bottle of milk in a pot of water, being careful to warm the bottle slowly and evenly, avoiding high temperatures.

MEDICAL SOURCE ———————————————————

Science News (141,17:261)

BRONCHITIS

Blow away breathlessness when you blow up a balloon

Blowing up balloons probably is something you haven't done since your youngest child started high school and you said good-bye to childhood birthday parties.

But, if you suffer from bronchitis, you might need to take the art of balloon blowing back up. It could help relieve some of your symptoms.

People with bronchitis, emphysema and other chronic lung diseases often complain of breathlessness because their lung tissues aren't working as well as they used to. The tissue in the lungs is damaged and scarred, and people suffering from lung diseases just can't get as deep a breath as they need. That makes them feel tired and weary and like they can't ever quite catch their breath.

People with lung disease often realize that they can't do the types of activities they used to do because they get too short of breath. Simply walking out to the mailbox becomes a major chore for some.

Many doctors will tell you that there are different forms of physical therapy available that can help you restore some of that lost lung capacity. But that therapy is expensive, complicated and time-consuming. So, unfortunately, most people don't get any therapy, and they are left with their breathlessness and diminished activities.

But researchers might have found a way to improve your condition, using the simple blow-up balloon.

Researchers tested their ideas using 28 volunteers (average age of 65) who each suffered from chronic bronchitis. The researchers measured each volunteer's lung capacity, and they found that all of the volunteers suffered from some degree of breathlessness.

Half of the volunteers received balloons. They were instructed to blow up the balloons to a diameter of 20 centimeters (almost eight inches) 40 times a day for eight weeks. The other half of the volunteers did not receive balloons. They just went about their normal activities.

At the end of the eight weeks, the researchers measured the lung capacities of all the volunteers again. They found that the volunteers who had inflated the balloons for eight weeks had a huge decrease in their symptoms of breathlessness — they were able to breathe much more easily. The volunteers who did not use the balloon still suffered from the same amount of breathlessness.

The volunteers who blew up the balloons also reported an improved sense of well-being and a greater ability to walk around without losing their breath.

The researchers are not sure whether the improvement comes from a strengthening of the lung muscles or from a decreased sensitivity to breathlessness. However, they suggest that balloon inflation is an easy and inexpensive way for people with bronchitis and other lung diseases to decrease their breathlessness at home.

Other tips to help reduce your symptoms of bronchitis include:

- Stop smoking, and try to stay away from others when they are smoking. Inhaling smoke from your own cigarette or from someone else's cigarette will harm your lungs and make it harder for your body to recover from bronchitis.
- Drink lots of fluids. This helps loosen up any mucus in your lungs and helps you to breathe easier.
- Take a hot shower. The steam also helps loosen up mucus in your lungs.

MEDICAL SOURCE ─────────────────────────

British Medical Journal (304,6843:1642)

BURNS

Hot tips to cool off your burns

Everything was going fine ... until your loose shirttail got hung on the handle of the pot, and you accidentally pulled the pot of boiling water off the stove.

Your whole left leg feels like it's on fire as soon as the hot water hits you. The question is, what should you do? What do you do after you burn yourself?

Here are some hot tips for you to follow when you or one of your family members gets burned.

❑ Look at the burn and decide how serious it is. You can have first-, second- or third-degree burns, and your treatment will depend on how serious it is.

First-degree burns are the least severe, and you can usually treat these at home without even calling the doctor. These burns are red and painful, but the skin is not broken and there are no blisters. Examples of first-degree burns are mild sunburns, brushing up against a hot iron, or touching a hot casserole dish without a potholder.

Second-degree burns are a little more serious than first degrees. These burns are also red and painful, but, unlike first-degree burns, here you have blisters and weeping or oozing of the burn. Examples of second-degree burns are more serious cases of sunburn, touching your hand against the hot eye on the stovetop, or getting burned with a drop of hot glue from a glue gun.

Third-degree burns are serious matters. These burns can be charred or white-colored. And sometimes they don't seem to hurt because the nerves in the skin have been damaged. These kinds of burns can be caused by actually coming into contact with fire, electricity, strong chemicals or acids spilled on your skin.

If you have a third-degree burn, see your doctor as soon as possible. Any delay can set up the perfect situation for infection, and that could be very dangerous.

❑ If you have a first-degree burn, dry the burn tenderly after you've soaked it in cool water for up to 15 minutes. Then cover it loosely with some gauze for about 24 hours and let it start healing on its own. After the 24 hours is up, try something like aloe vera cream or lotion to help relieve some of the stinging or itching

Try to keep the burn protected, and do not take extremely hot showers. If the burn starts to itch as it heals, take an antihistamine, such as Benadryl, or use some anti-itch cream to relieve the itch. Try not to scratch. If the burn doesn't get better in about 10 days, or if it gets worse at any point, call your doctor.

❑ If you have a second-degree burn, soak it in cool water and carefully and gently dry the burn with a clean towel. Then cover the burned area with a layer of antibiotic cream.

Do not touch the burn with your fingers — use rubber gloves or a sterile tongue depressor blade (the kind the doctor uses) or even a cotton swab to apply the cream. Cover the antibiotic cream with a nonstick dressing, and keep the dressing in place with some gauze.

Wash off and then reapply the antibiotic cream two or three times a day, covering the wound with gauze each time. If you have blisters, do not try to "pop" the blisters. Leave the blisters intact — they will go away on their own. If a blister pops, clean it off with soap and water, then put some more antibiotic cream on it.

When the burn begins to heal and the blisters go away, you can treat the burn like a first-degree burn and use aloe vera or sunburn-relief spray to ease any stinging or burning. Remember not to scratch if it begins to itch.

❑ If you have a third-degree burn, see your doctor as soon as possible.

❑ When treating your burn, forget about any old wives' tales—do not put butter, shortening, yogurt or other things on a burn. These things could cause infection and make the situation worse than it was in the first place.

❑ Do not use sprays that cause numbing or anesthesia of the skin in an effort to relieve the pain — the sprays can actually make the burns hurt worse.

❑ Make sure your tetanus immunizations are up-to-date. If they are not, get whatever booster shots your doctor says you need.

❑ Know when to see your doctor. In some cases, home remedies for burns are not enough to assure proper healing.

Call your doctor if:

- You have a third-degree burn.
- You have burns on the face, eyes, hands, feet or pelvic area.
- Your burn begins to look infected. Your burn is probably infected if it starts to get warm, red and swollen again, or if you see any brown, yellow or green fluid or pus.
- Your burn does not begin to heal in about 10 days.
- Call your pediatrician if your children get burned.

Treating minor burns is usually a simple procedure. But the best treatment is to avoid them altogether.

Call your local fire department (on the nonemergency line!) and ask them to pay a visit to your home or workplace for a safety inspection. They can help you cut down on your risks of burns and household fire accidents.

With the help of your fire department, plan an escape route for your family in the event of a fire and teach it to your children.

MEDICAL SOURCE ─────────────────────────
American Family Physician (45,3:1321)

BURSITIS

How to bury bursitis pain

The bursa is a tiny sac located where the tendons pass over areas of bone around your joints. When the bursa becomes inflamed, bursitis results. This can happen in the course of such diseases as gout or rheumatoid arthritis, which involve the synovial membranes, after a trauma to the area or during an infection.

In severe cases, doctors place the area in splints and prescribe rest and cortisone therapy.

To avoid bursitis:

❏ Avoid kneeling for long periods of time.

❏ Never shuffle on your knees when you are in a kneeling position.

❏ Apply elastic athletic bandages to your knees after kneeling if the knees seem sore.

❏ Use rubber kneepads when gardening or scrubbing floors or elbow pads when leaning on the elbows for extended periods of time.

❏ Pad any area that will be subjected to pressure. For instance, pad the shoulders if you will be hiking with a backpack, and wear thick clothing if you're planning to carry heavy objects.

❏ Avoid tight, badly fitting shoes, especially if you have bunions.

❏ Sit on a cushioned surface instead of a hard surface to prevent buttock bursae.

To treat bursitis, use ice packs in combination with an elastic bandage. If there's no improvement in a couple of days, check with your doctor.

MEDICAL SOURCES

The Oxford Companion to Medicine, Vol. 1, Oxford University Press, New York, 1986
The Marshall Cavendish Illustrated Encyclopaedia of Family Health, Marshall Cavendish House, London, 1986

CANCER

Healthy habits lead to cancer prevention

Cancer.

Just hearing the word sends chills up your spine.

But you don't have to just sit helplessly, not knowing what to do to avoid it.

The best way to avoid cancer is to prevent it.

And you have the ideal means of protection right at your fingertips: Your own healthy habits can be the natural key to cancer prevention.

Smoking is responsible for almost a third of all cancers. Poor diet causes another third of all the cancers in the United States.

So here are simple ways you can protect yourself:

- **Stop smoking now, and your chances of avoiding cancer will begin to improve right away.**
- **When you're planning your meals, choose a wide variety of foods that have more fiber and less fat.**
- **For early detection of cancer, talk to your doctor about the tests that are right for you.**

To find out more about cancer prevention, detection, treatment or rehabilitation, call the Cancer Information Service toll free at 1-800-4-CANCER from 9 a.m. to 10 p.m. Eastern Standard Time. The National Cancer Institute provides this service.

It's beyond the scope and intent of this book to try to tell you how to "treat yourself" for cancer or even cancer symptoms. You simply can't and shouldn't treat yourself for such a serious condition. Expert medical care is required, from diagnosis to treatment to rehabilitation.

However, there are a number of things that you can do to help prevent cancerous conditions from arising, and we tell you about several of them in this section. This information is based on recent medical research, but it can't take the place of your own personal doctor, nor should it.

Foremost, you should immediately seek medical advice if you have any of cancer's warning signs or if you suspect you have the disease. There is no substitute for competent medical help on a timely basis.

MEDICAL SOURCE ————————————————————

FDA Consumer (24,10:14)

Eat these five times a day to prevent cancer

Broccoli or some other kind of fruit or vegetable, that is. And you need it five times each day, says the National Cancer Institute.

The new "5-a-Day for Better Health" program supported by the National Cancer Institute is designed to encourage Americans to boost their daily consumption of fruits and vegetables from less than three to at least five times each day.

Why? you might ask.

Because the scientific evidence for the cancer-fighting effects of fruits and vegetables is growing.

Although fruits and vegetables are helpful in fighting many types of cancer, a recent review suggested that a fruity and leafy diet seems to be most effective against lung, mouth, stomach, colon, rectal, bladder and cervical cancers.

Researchers state that for adults who don't drink heavily and don't smoke, the one choice that seems to influence their long-term health prospects more than any other is their diet.

The director of the "5-a-Day" program, Jerianne Heimendinger, estimates that if all Americans started eating four or more daily servings of fruits or vegetables, about 25 percent of all diet-related cancers could be prevented.

MEDICAL SOURCE ─────────────────────────────

Journal of the National Cancer Institute (83,21:1538)

Microwaved vs. raw — broccoli in the fight against cancer

The protective chemical found in broccoli is called sulforaphane. Studies suggest it causes the body to beef up production of enzymes that neutralize cancer-causing substances. And the good news is that it withstands microwaving.

Some other sulforaphane-rich foods include: cabbage, kale, cauliflower, brussels sprouts, ginger, onions and bok choy.

Develop a taste for raw or microwaved broccoli as well as other sulforaphane-rich foods as a part of your normal diet.

It might be the healthiest thing you do all year!

MEDICAL SOURCES ─────────────────────────────

Medical Tribune (33,7:14)
Science News (141,12:183)

Vitamin C boosts immune response to cancer risks

Drink your orange juice or eat a tangerine for powerful protection against cervical, stomach, colorectal, breast and other kinds of cancer.

Based on recent studies, Dr. Gladys Block of the U.S. National

Cancer Institute's Division of Cancer Prevention and Control suggests that vitamin C offers significant protective effects from these cancers.

She also notes that there seems to be a link between low levels of vitamin C and a higher risk of some cancers.

Vitamin C seems to offer its protective effects by blocking the production of cancer-causing substances in the body. Apparently, vitamin C can act as a kind of "scavenger" and hunt down and destroy cancer-causing agents in our blood and tissues.

Vitamin C also seems to stimulate immune cells in the body, which helps strengthen the body's fighting response to dangerous substances.

The Recommended Daily Allowance for vitamin C, for people over the age of 50, is 60 milligrams. Vitamin C is readily available in fruits (especially citrus fruits), vegetables and potatoes. However, eating the foods raw is the best way to get the vitamin C, because cooking in water or heating causes the food to lose a good portion of its vitamin C.

MEDICAL SOURCES ─────────────────────────

Journal of the National Cancer Institute (83,6:396)
U. S. Pharmacist (15,8:49)

Spice to the rescue

Count the cancer-fighting potential in these spices, and it all adds up to good health!

Two new warriors have emerged in the fight against cancer: Saffron and Nigella sativa or "black cumin" (an unrelated cumin look-alike).

Studies reveal that these spices inhibited cancer-forming tumors in mice.

Saffron contains carotenoids, the orange-yellow pigment found in carrots that is associated with lowering your risk of cancer.

So, if using these spices adds up to better health, you might want to add saffron and black cumin to your diet.

MEDICAL SOURCES ————————————————————

Nutrition and Cancer (16,1:67)
Prevention (44,4:25)

Blisters on the eyes could be early warning signs of trouble

When waxy, yellow blisters develop on the eyelids, there may be trouble somewhere else in your body.

These blisters are called amyloid deposits, and your doctor can surgically remove them from your eyelids. But the blisters might signal the appearance of amyloid deposits in other organs of the body.

They may also indicate the presence of a form of bone cancer called multiple myeloma.

See your doctor right away if you notice such changes in your skin.

MEDICAL SOURCE ————————————————————

Journal of the American Medical Association (266,19:2693)

Don't put your bladder on hold

"Holding it" could mean trouble for your bladder. When it comes to using the bathroom, that is.

Frequent urination might be a key to preventing bladder cancer.

This news is especially important for smokers, because a cancer-causing chemical called 4-aminobiphenyl (ABP), found in cigarette smoke, might be a prime cause of bladder cancer, researchers say.

Researchers studied animals whose bladder cancer resembles that in humans.

Those that urinated every four hours had one-third the cancer-causing substances in their bladder compared with those that urinated every eight hours.

According to Fred F. Kadlubar of the National Center for Toxicological Research, the liver breaks down ABP into a carcinogen.

The carcinogen is filtered from the blood by the kidneys and accumulates in urine stored in the bladder.

The longer this chemical remains in the bladder, the stronger your exposure is to this cancer agent.

To lower your risk of bladder cancer, take frequent urination breaks and stop smoking, researchers suggest.

MEDICAL SOURCE ———————————————————
Science News (140,8:125)

High-fiber diet reduces breast cancer risk

Based on recent laboratory studies, researchers are suggesting that adding high-fiber foods to a high-fat diet will have a significant reducing effect on the development of breast tumors.

International studies show a strong link between a typical high-fat diet and breast cancer development in women in all countries except Finland.

Finland is an exception because, while Finnish women eat a

high-fat diet just like the typical American diet, they also eat a large amount of fiber.

The high-fiber intake of the Finnish women seems to modify the otherwise bad effect of their high-fat diet.

Based on this observation, scientists conducted a study on laboratory rats to determine the effects of dietary fiber on breast cancer. In the study, the scientists took four groups of rats and fed them the following: Group one received a high-fat diet; Group two received a high-fat diet with an extra-fiber diet; Group three, a low-fat diet; and Group four, a low-fat diet with an extra-fiber diet. The rats remained on these diets for about 15 weeks.

The laboratory rats fed high-fiber diets experienced the development of fewer breast cancer tumors than the rats fed low- or no-fiber diets.

Scientists have known that a high-fat diet can increase a woman's risk of developing breast cancer. However, this study shows clearly that the addition of high-fiber foods significantly reduces the tumor-promoting effects of a high-fat diet.

Although this study was conducted on rats, scientists suggest that additional dietary fiber may function as an anti-tumor agent for humans as well.

MEDICAL SOURCE —————————————————————

Journal of the National Cancer Institute (83,7:496)

Lower risk of breast cancer with wheat diet

Ladies, wheat-bran muffins are good for more than your mid-morning snack. They could lower your risk of developing breast cancer.

A diet high in wheat bran may help reduce estrogen hormonal levels in women who have not experienced menopause yet. And a lower level of estrogen could mean a lower risk of breast cancer.

Scientists performed a study on about 60 premenopausal women to test the effects of wheat bran on estrogen levels. They discovered that the women who ate three to four wheat-bran muffins a day for two months lowered their blood levels of estrogen.

Wheat bran helps lower estrogen levels by reducing the number of bacteria in the intestines that cause the hormone to re-enter the bloodstream, researchers think.

High levels of estrogen in the blood have been linked to an increased risk of breast cancer, so the reduced levels associated with a high intake of wheat bran help reduce that risk of developing breast cancer.

Corn-bran and oat-bran muffins did not have the same effect on lowering estrogen levels.

Women past the age of menopause might also benefit from wheat bran. The report suggests that a high intake of wheat bran helps prevent the development of a second tumor in postmenopausal women who have already been treated for breast cancer.

So, enjoy that mid-morning wheat-bran muffin snack.

MEDICAL SOURCE ———————————————————

Medical Tribune (32,19:2)

Simple vitamin treatment helps breast cancer

A new treatment for some forms of breast tumors might be around the corner.

Vitamin-D ointment applied to the nodules of women with

advanced or cutaneous metastatic breast cancer (cancer that has spread to the skin) shows promising results.

A study reported that approximately one-third of the women who completed a six-week, vitamin-D treatment program experienced a 50-percent reduction in the size of the cancerous area.

Doctors monitored the test group closely for hypercalcemia, a side effect of the treatment. That's when too much calcium gets into the bloodstream.

Two of 19 women tested developed this condition and discontinued therapy. However, the other women experienced positive results.

MEDICAL SOURCE ───────────────────────────────

The Lancet (337,8743:701)

Lumpectomy vs. mastectomy—Does procedure affect survival?

Radical mastectomy — women dread ever having to face this procedure, but thanks to modern research, you might not ever have to. What was once considered to be standard procedure is no longer recognized as the best treatment for all types of breast cancer.

Removal of the entire breast along with some of the tissue in the adjacent armpit can leave women with depression, anxiety and sexual dysfunction.

For 25 years, Dr. Bernard Fisher of the U.S. National Surgical Adjuvant Breast and Bowel Project (NSABP) has been questioning the benefits of total mastectomy.

He has been trying to determine whether a woman with a cancerous lump in the breast increases her chance of living longer by undergoing mastectomy.

Would removing only the lump (lumpectomy) give the woman as good a chance to survive?

Dr. Fisher has gathered evidence that he feels justifies use of conservative surgery rather than procedures that can leave the chest bony and scarred.

His most recent conclusions add further support to his earlier convictions.

Nine-year follow-up studies strongly indicate that mastectomies fail to alter the ultimate outcome once a breast cancer sets its course.

Dr. Fisher's concept is that breast cancer is a systemic disease (it involves more of the body than just the breast). He believes that the type of local treatment of a cancerous lump, whether by mastectomy or lumpectomy, is unlikely to affect survival time significantly.

Dr. Fisher studied women for nine years and found that, following lumpectomy, 43 percent of the women had a recurrence of the tumor in the operated-on breast. Those women who had lumpectomy plus breast irradiation (radiation therapy) had only a 12 percent rate of local recurrence.

But no matter which treatment group the women were in — whether mastectomy, lumpectomy or lumpectomy plus irradiation — there was no significant difference in the rate of spread of the cancer to another site or in survival time.

Dr. Fisher concluded that there was no cause-and-effect relation between recurrence of cancer in the affected breast and spread of the cancer to some other site.

Recurrence in the breast did, however, indicate a more aggressive type of cancer that would be more than three times as likely to appear at some other site than cancers that did not recur in the breast.

Mastectomy and breast irradiation lower the rate of recurrence close to the original site, but do not lower the risk of spread to another site, according to researchers.

Radical mastectomy appears to be no more effective than breast-conserving surgery for improving your survival time.

Breast-saving surgery is good news.

But the persistent high death rate from breast cancer is still alarming. One in every 10 women will develop breast cancer. Just last year, more than 150,000 cases were diagnosed.

Early diagnosis of breast cancer is extremely important. Mammography, which is a low-dose X-ray of the breast, can detect cancer up to two years before you or your doctor could discover a lump.

Cancer removal at an early stage can be a relatively minor surgical procedure. Chances of a complete cure are good, researchers say.

Mammograms are proving to be so valuable in diagnosing unsuspected cancers that doctors are urging all women over 35 to have one.

Many doctors suggest that after the age of 50, women need to have a mammogram at least once a year. Mammography will detect about 90 percent of breast cancers. Widespread screening programs can prevent up to 30 percent of breast cancer deaths, these doctors say.

Mammography is the best method available for detecting breast cancers in their early stages.

MEDICAL SOURCES —————————————————

The Lancet (338,8763:327)
FDA Consumer (25,6:10)

Facts concerning breast cancer

- Ninety percent of breast cancer occurs in women over age 39. Risk of developing breast cancer increases as you get older.
- Women who have never had children have a greater chance of developing breast cancer.
- Women who've had both ovaries removed before age 35 seem to have a reduced risk of developing breast cancer.

MEDICAL SOURCE ——————————————————

Better Homes and Gardens, Woman's Health & Medical Guide, Meredith Corp., Des Moines, Iowa, 1981

Cancer surgery: Timing can save your life

Timing is everything when it comes to surgery for breast cancer, new research indicates.

Scientists suggest that a woman should time her breast cancer surgery to coincide with the mid-point of her menstrual cycle. Such timing might extend her life.

British researchers compared 19 women operated on during mid-cycle (days 7 to 20) and 22 women who had surgery around the time of menstruation (days 0 to 6 and 21 to 36). Those women who had surgery at or around the start of their menstrual cycles had four times the rate of both relapse and death.

Mid-cycle operations in women whose cancer had spread beyond the breast produced almost the same rate of survival as surgery done at the time of menstruation on those without metastatic (spreading of) disease.

Scientists speculate that monthly changes in hormone levels in a woman's bloodstream affect the number of natural killer cells in the bloodstream.

Fewer killer cells on patrol equals a greater chance of a cancer spreading, researchers think.

They also believe that a woman's immune system is at a low ebb, with fewer killer cells, near and during the menstrual period, possibly to help the egg become implanted in the womb.

A woman's immune system seems to kick into high gear in mid-cycle (between days 7 to 21), peaking in the middle with the maximum number of killer cells in the bloodstream. These armies of killer cells might be more efficient in mid-cycle at hunting down and killing any cancer cells that escape during surgery.

Thus, the study suggests, the best time for surgery is during mid-cycle.

In this study, day zero of the cycle is the first day of menstrual flow. Menstruation occurs on an average of every 27 to 28 days, although time may vary from 18 to 40 days.

Although rescheduling of operations could lead to some short-term delays, the disadvantage will probably be outweighed by the potential long-term benefits, these researchers speculate. An earlier American study produced the same findings.

If you are concerned about breast cancer surgery, talk with your doctor about the timing of the surgery and your own menstrual cycle. Many doctors still don't believe such timing has any significance.

MEDICAL SOURCE ——————————————

The Lancet (337,8752:1261)

Weight loss increases cancer survival?

If you have a family history of breast cancer and you are overweight, cut your long-term cancer risk by shedding several pounds.

That's the potential good news.

Women who were obese at the time their breast cancers were diagnosed had a four-out-of-10 chance of developing breast cancers again within 10 years, according to the researchers at the Centers for Disease Control in Atlanta. Normal-weight women had a 10-percent smaller risk of recurring breast cancer, the report says.

The risk was even greater for women with so-called node-negative cancers. Obese women with cancers that were confined to the breasts and had not spread to nearby lymph nodes had a six-in-10 chance of a recurrence. The researchers defined obesity as being 25 percent or more over ideal weight for height.

Doctors followed 923 women for 10 years after their initial diagnoses of breast cancer. All the women had undergone breast removal.

More than half had gone through menopause before discovering their cancers. Ages ranged from 24 to 95, with nearly four out of 10 being 60 or older.

Almost without exception, the overweight women had larger tumors at first diagnosis than the normal-weight women. Of the entire group, nearly seven out of 10 were first diagnosed as having a common type of cancer called infiltrating-duct carcinoma. Four out of 10 had lymph-node involvement.

In the study group, generally speaking, the older the woman was, the more likely she was to be overweight.

The disadvantage of being fat might even outweigh the advantages of earlier detection of cancerous tumors, CDC researchers indicate.

Usually, earlier detection means longer cancer-free survival times. But carrying too many pounds apparently cancels out that benefit, the report suggests.

"Weight control may have a substantial effect on breast cancer mortality and on mortality associated with other chronic conditions," the report says.

MEDICAL SOURCE ──────────────────

Annals of Internal Medicine (116,1:26)

Vitamins could be your 'ACE' against colon cancer

Pass the spinach, oranges and whole grains! The vitamins A, C and E contained in these foods can help protect you from colon cancer, according to Italian researchers.

Dr. Gian Maria Pagnelli reports the results of vitamin tests with a group of people who had surgery to remove pre-cancerous growths called adenomas from their colons.

For a period of six months after surgery, half the group took large doses of vitamins A, C and E, and the other half did not. Then researchers checked all participants again for changes in the colon that might signal a new growth of cancer. Dr. Pagnelli and the research team found that these vitamins did reduce colon cell changes that can develop into cancer.

The nutrients A, C and E must be taken together for the vitamin therapy to work, researchers believe, although they're not sure why. More studies are needed to determine the long-range effects of large amounts of these vitamins.

The official adult Recommended Dietary Allowances for these vitamins are as follows: vitamin A, 1000 micrograms (one milligram) for men and 800 micrograms for women; vitamin C, 60 milligrams for men and women; and vitamin E, 10 milligrams for men and 8 milligrams for women.

Until we know more about using vitamins to prevent cancer,

you can help prevent colon cancer by including some natural, healthful vitamin sources in your daily diet.

The chart below has some suggestions.

MEDICAL SOURCE ─────────────────────

Journal of the National Cancer Institute (84,1:47)

Examples of healthy vitamin sources to protect your colon

Vitamin A	Vitamin C	Vitamin E
spinach	raw, leafy vegetables	whole grains
liver	tomatoes	nuts
milk	citrus fruits	vegetable oils
egg yolks	green peppers	margarine
carrots	red peppers	wheat germ
squash	potatoes	soybeans
sweet potatoes	strawberries	dark green, leafy
peaches	apricots	vegetables

Talk to your doctor before beginning vitamin therapy or making changes in your diet.

MEDICAL SOURCE ─────────────────────

Diet and Health, National Academy Press, Washington, D.C., 1989

Ingredient in your jellies could 'preserve' your life

The stuff that helps turn fruit into jelly might help you lower your risk of colon cancer. This natural, safe and inexpensive product comes from the peel of citrus fruits and apple pulp. It's called pectin, and it's the fiber that puts the gel in your jellies. And it seems to offer double-barreled protection against both colon cancer and high cholesterol.

Researchers have known for some time that certain parts of fruits and vegetables offer health benefits. In fact, the type of fiber found in fruits and vegetables that is known as "cellulose-derived fiber" helps cut the risk of colon cancer by about 50 percent in laboratory tests.

However, pectin now seems to offer even more health benefits than cellulose-derived fiber. Research shows that rats fed a 10-percent pectin diet experienced the same 50-percent decrease in colon cancer incidence as those fed a diet with cellulose-derived fiber.

However, those on the pectin diet also experienced the additional benefit of a 25- to 30-percent decrease in cholesterol levels. And, lower cholesterol levels help protect you from problems such as high blood pressure and heart disease.

In other words, the cellulose-derived fiber is good for protection against colon cancer alone. In addition, the pectin is good for protection against colon cancer and against high cholesterol.

Scientists think that pectin helps protect against colon cancer by interfering with cancer-causing agents in the colon. And it helps lower cholesterol by preventing the small intestines from absorbing extra fats.

Researchers suggest that in order to achieve the level of protective effects of pectin seen in the research, you would need to eat a lot of fruits and vegetables — even up to 15 apples a day. So, scientists are exploring the possibility of adding pectin to food products to create "pectin-fortified" foods.

Until then, however, even eating a small amount of fruits and vegetables each day will give you some protection. For double-barreled protection against colon cancer and high cholesterol, start with an apple a day, but don't stop there.

Adding more fruits and vegetables to your diet will help give you maximum health benefits.

The easiest way to get enough pectin in your diet might be to add it to your desserts. A single bowl of a gelatin dessert has more pectin than an apple. Other natural sources of pectin are grapefruit, oranges, sour plums, Concord grapes, gooseberries and vegetables such as carrots and cabbage.

Eating prunes, which contain pectin, also helps lower your cholesterol. In fact, studies report that eating 12 prunes each day can help lower your cholesterol in just four weeks.

MEDICAL SOURCES ————————————————

> *Journal of the National Cancer Institute* (84,6:438)
> *Science News* (141,12:180)
> *Medical Tribune* (32,7:12 and 33,7:14)

A pineapple a day might keep the doctor away

Fiber is fiber, right? Not according to a report which found that Polynesian people living in the South Pacific have a lower incidence of colorectal cancer perhaps due to the type of dietary fiber they eat.

Fiber in our diet is supposed to protect us from cancer by absorbing cancer-causing substances. However, how this happens is still a mystery.

In the study, Polynesian populations in the South Pacific were compared to European descendants living in the same area. The Polynesians' dietary fiber came from eating taro, pineapples, yams, and bananas. The European descendants ate food like potatoes and cabbage.

Will a pineapple a day keep the doctor away? This study seems to suggest so!

MEDICAL SOURCE ———————————————————

Nutrition and Cancer (17,1:85)

Regular use of aspirin slashes risk of colon cancer by half

If you are concerned about your risk of developing colon cancer, help might be as close as your medicine cabinet.

Most people now accept that an aspirin a day helps keep heart attacks away. New research indicates that it also helps in the fight against colon cancer.

Lynn Rosenberg of the Boston University School of Medicine conducted an 11-year study including 1,326 people with large bowel cancer (either colon or rectal cancer), 1,011 people with other forms of cancer, and 3,880 people with no history of cancer of any kind.

The people who used aspirin regularly cut their risk of colon cancer in half. The researchers defined regular use as at least four times a week for at least three months.

Scientists also discovered that the protection you might get from aspirin doesn't last. After a year of non-use, even if you had previously taken aspirin regularly, your risk of cancer is the same as if you had never taken aspirin.

Colon cancer is one of the leading causes of cancer deaths in the United States.

MEDICAL SOURCE ———————————————————

Journal of the National Cancer Institute (83,5:355)

Oat bran reduces acidity in the digestive system, decreases risk of colon cancer

Pour on the oats to lower your acid levels. Studies suggest that acidity in the colon may be a risk factor for colorectal cancer. The higher the acidity, the greater the risk.

Researchers in Canada have discovered that oat bran reduces acidity and increases the action of the digestive system. A more active digestive system is actually thought to be the link between reduced acidity and reduced incidence of colon cancer.

So, do yourself and your colon a favor and talk to your doctor about adding oat bran to your diet.

MEDICAL SOURCE ─────────────────────────

Preventive Medicine (19,6:607)

The 'red' menace

Colon cancer — it can be caused by your diet or prevented by your diet, starting with your main entree. Eating beef, pork or lamb every day could be a great dietary mistake.

Although everyone seems to benefit from diets with less red meat, studies reveal that women in particular will benefit from substituting fish or skinless chicken for red meat in two to four main dishes weekly.

Regularly eating red meat greatly increases your risk of colon cancer, research suggests. In fact, those who eat beef, pork or lamb at least once a day have a two-and-a-half times greater risk of developing colon cancer than those who eat it less than once a month. And those who eat processed meats are in even greater danger. Weekly servings of processed meats increased the risk of colon cancer by 50 to 100 percent.

The good news is that women who eat fish or skinless chicken instead of red meat reduce their risk of colon cancer by 25 to 50 percent. Adding fruit fiber to your diet and substituting beans or lentils for red meat are other ways to reduce the risk of colon cancer, suggests the report.

MEDICAL SOURCES————————————————————

Science News (138,24:374)
The New England Journal of Medicine (323,24:1664)

Can a diet too low in fat raise your risk of colon cancer?

A low-fat diet is good for you, right?

And it helps lower your risk of colon cancer, right?

Well, not always.

Recent research suggests that a diet that is too low in fat could increase your risk of colon cancer. Researchers studied the effects of a low-fat diet on some people who were unable to eat because of neck surgery and were being fed through stomach tubes. The patients received a 1-percent-fat diet for 10 days. Two continued on that low-fat diet for another six weeks, while the others went to a 36-percent-fat diet.

The **36-percent-fat** diet is close to what everyday Americans eat.

Those who remained on the 1-percent-fat diet experienced a significant rise in cancer-risk markers, researchers report. That means that doctors tested them and found certain chemical compounds that are known to heighten chances of developing cancer.

The people on the 36-percent-fat diet did not experience the increase in colon cancer risk.

But, I thought a low-fat diet is good for me, you say.

It is, for most people, so long as it's done wisely. High-fat diets have repeatedly been linked to increased risks of colon cancer and breast cancer. And the National Research Council strongly recommends that you get no more than 30 percent of your daily calories from fat.

However, a diet that is almost completely lacking in fat (1-percent-fat diet) is as unhealthy as one too high in fats.

The best advice: Continue eating your low-fat diet, especially if your doctor recommended it for you. Keep your daily intake of fat below 30 percent of your daily calories, but don't go overboard.

Too little fat can be just as dangerous as too much fat.

MEDICAL SOURCE ————————————————

Medical Tribune (32,12:19)

Smokers — diet could help you avoid cancer

Smokers have two new enemies in the fight against cancer.

A 10-year study says that smokers who have a diet high in fat content and low in consumption of carrots, cabbage, cauliflower and other carotene-rich foods face increased risk of cancer of the larynx.

About 12,000 cases of cancer of the larynx are diagnosed each year. Smoking and drinking alcoholic beverages have long been recognized as contributing factors.

This study suggests diet might be a factor, as well, in cancer of the larynx and lung cancer, another smoking-related cancer.

Researchers found the cancer risk factor for smokers was higher if they had a diet loaded with milk products, donuts, veal and other fat-rich foods.

Smoking is by far the greatest risk factor for cancer of the larynx, but mom was right when she told us to eat all our vegetables!

MEDICAL SOURCE ————————————————

Nutrition and Cancer (17,1:33)

Help slow down certain form of leukemia with new treatment

A familiar substance may bring good news and quick healing to people with leukemia.

It is the same substance that is in Retin-A, which is used for acne and facial wrinkles. The substance is a cousin of vitamin A called tretinoin. It has helped control a form of leukemia, promyelocytic leukemia.

This type of leukemia causes white blood cells to "stick" at an immature stage of development and multiply quickly.

This cousin of vitamin A causes the cells to mature and stop dividing so the leukemia is slowed down or stopped. The tretinoin works best when used along with chemotherapy, the report says.

The tretinoin treatment has a few mild side effects, such as headache, chapped lips, nasal congestion and high-triglyceride count.

If you are currently under treatment for leukemia, check with your doctor about tretinoin.

MEDICAL SOURCE ————————————————

The New England Journal of Medicine (324,20:1385)

Power line static and cancer risk

Can that high-current electrical wire that goes across your yard cause you to develop cancer?

Some researchers believe it could. Exposure to electromagnetic fields could increase your chances of developing cancer.

The controversy began back in 1979 when Nancy Wertheimer and Ed Leeper found that children who lived near high-current electric power lines appeared to have twice the risk of leukemia as children who lived farther away from power lines.

The increase in cancer risk was caused by exposure to the electromagnetic fields produced as electricity ran through the wires, the studies concluded.

These discoveries lead to the beginning of bioelectromagnetics, which is the study of electricity and magnetism and their effects on life and people.

In 1986, researchers studied 500 homes in Denver. In half of the homes lived children with leukemia or other cancers. Results showed that those children who lived within 20 yards of lines carrying electricity from the substation to the neighborhood transformer had five times the risk of cancer as those who lived farther away.

High electromagnetic fields might be linked to brain cancer, breast cancer in males and females, and also leukemia in adults, further studies hinted.

Some researchers believe that electromagnetic fields disturb cell activity by agitating molecules in cell membranes potentially leading to cancer and increased health risks.

Other researchers are studying hormonal effects that would explain the link between electromagnetic fields and breast cancer.

Current research is ongoing to settle the issue.

MEDICAL SOURCES —————————————————————————

The Lancet (338,8781:1521)
Science News (140,1:15 and 140,13:202)

Reduce your risk of liver cancer — risk factors you can control

Current research confirms that there are important risk factors for liver cancer that we can control.

Researcher Mimi C. Yu says that all regular alcohol drinkers run an increased risk of developing liver cancer. And if you drink as much as six or more beers, glasses of wine or shots of alcohol daily, you are five times more likely to get this disease. Cigarette smoking is another risky activity.

Smokers are twice as likely to develop liver cancer, although that risk begins to decline as soon as you quit smoking, according to Dr. Yu.

Women who use birth control pills might also want to re-examine their method of contraception. Dr. Yu reports that oral contraceptives multiply the risk of liver cancer by three times. And if you have used the Pill for more than five years, you are more than five times as likely to develop liver cancer as other women who have not used birth control pills.

Giving up smoking and drinking alcohol are obviously wise choices to make if you want to reduce your risk of liver cancer. You should also discuss alternative means of birth control (other than the Pill) with your doctor.

MEDICAL SOURCE ——————————————————————
Journal of the National Cancer Institute (83,24:1820)

Secondhand smoke responsible for over 53,000 deaths each year

It's a cold, hard fact.

Secondhand smoke is hazardous to your health ... much more hazardous than was previously believed. Passive smoking is the third leading preventable cause of death in the United States today, right behind active smoking and alcohol.

Passive smoke is simply irritating to nonsmokers, too. Non-smokers are more sensitive to leftover smoke from cigarettes than the smokers who produce it. In other words, nonsmokers will probably be more uncomfortable in the nonsmoking area of the restaurant if the smoker's area is close by than the smoker who is also in the nonsmoking section.

But most importantly, secondhand smoke is harmful to nonsmokers. Since lung cancer was the first disease to be linked to active cigarette smoking, it was no surprise that lung cancer was also the first disease to be linked to passive smoking. Actually, passive smoking kills more people annually (53,000, according to the study) through heart disease than through lung cancer.

The researchers discovered that irritation from secondhand smoke reduces the nonsmoker's ability to exercise effectively. Lack of exercise makes you vulnerable to heart disease.

In addition, secondhand smoke makes your blood platelets abnormally "sticky" and more likely to clump together and form clots, evidence suggests.

Increased clumps of platelets are dangerous in another way, too. They form fatty deposits that stick to the coronary artery walls. Such fatty deposits often lead to heart attacks.

Researchers concluded that nonsmokers who live with smokers increase their risk of heart disease and heart attacks about 30 percent compared to nonsmokers who live and work in a nonsmoking environment.

And, you don't have to wait around for the bad effects of passive smoking to show themselves in your body. Your body starts feeling the effects right away.

For example, the transportation of oxygen by red blood cells is immediately hampered by the carbon monoxide in passive smoke, the study says. Carbon monoxide is a colorless, odorless gas found in cigarette smoke. It competes with oxygen in the body's red blood cells.

Therefore, if you increase the amount of carbon monoxide in the blood, you are limiting the amount of oxygen that will flow through the blood to the heart. The result is that the blood's ability to transport oxygen is impaired.

Coronary heart disease also limits the amount of oxygen getting to your heart muscle. So, for people who already have coronary heart disease, choking off yet more oxygen puts them in even more danger of a heart attack.

The lesson is that no matter where the smoker is, his trail of smoke can have deadly consequences for those who smell it or breathe it.

MEDICAL SOURCE ─────────────────────

Circulation (83,1:1)

Cancer from minty-fresh breath?

The quest for fresher breath could lead to some devastating results.

A recent study conducted by the National Cancer Institute revealed a possible link between oral cancer and mouthwashes made with a 25-percent or higher alcohol content.

Based on the study, men had a 1.6-fold increased risk of oral cancer and women had a 1.9-fold increased risk of oral cancer if they were regular users of any mouthwash with a high alcohol content. However, researchers found no increased risk for people who use mouthwash with an alcohol content of less than 25 percent.

Researchers surveyed 2,115 people about their dental habits. They found that 45 percent of all men and women surveyed used some type of mouthwash regularly at some time.

Of the men and women in the study who had oral cancer, about 49 percent of the men and about 58 percent of the women had used mouthwash regularly for more than one year before they were diagnosed with cancer.

The results of the study suggest that the risk of oral cancer increases with increased length, duration and frequency of mouthwash use.

Until scientists find more definite results, consider using a mouthwash with an alcohol content of less than 25 percent.

MEDICAL SOURCE ─────────────────────

Journal of the National Cancer Institute (83,11:751)

'C' this: 3-day sun-blocker being tested

Vitamin C.

You drink it every morning in your orange juice and eat it in various foods, but have you considered rubbing it all over your body? If you want to avoid sunburn and possible skin cancer, you might want to start considering it.

Rubbing vitamin C on the skin can help protect the skin from damage caused by the ultraviolet (UV) rays from the sun.

Vitamin C in the diet helps protect against cancer by working as an "antioxidant." An antioxidant functions by preventing the buildup of harmful products in the body known as free radicals. Free radicals have been linked to various forms of cancer in the body. Scientists now think that free radicals are also involved in UV damage to the skin.

Since vitamin C provides protection from free radicals inside the body, scientists think it will do the same outside the body.

The vitamin-C sunscreen comes in the form of a topical lotion known as L-ascorbic acid. And it has several advantages over traditional sunscreens.

First, the sunscreen effects of topical vitamin C last for about three days, and can't be rubbed, washed or sweated off. Many traditional sunscreens present problems because they are washed off so easily, especially in water at the pool or beach.

Also, the topical vitamin C helps protect the skin against UV rays of all wavelengths. Most other sunscreens protect only against certain wavelengths.

Some studies suggest that the topical vitamin C could also fight the effects of aging skin and possibly reduce wrinkle formation. Further testing is needed for the topical vitamin-C sunscreen before it will be sold in stores.

MEDICAL SOURCE ─────────────────────────

Medical Tribune (32,19:4)

Your tan isn't the only thing that is 'savage'

The quest for the savage tan is just what it says it is: savage.

In fact, your hours of sitting in the sun savage your skin, producing about 20 years of premature aging and possible skin cancer.

Despite hearing over and over again how dangerous the sun is, most people think that suntans and summertime just go together. You can't have one without the other. Beaches everywhere are covered with bronzed bodies. And if you choose not to get a tan during the summer, everyone thinks you've been sick because you're so pale.

Americans have been conned into believing that people with tans are healthier and more glamorous. The trouble is that most people never really understand exactly what a tan is. A good comparison to sunning is charring meat over a fire, says the FDA report.

Charring and tanning are both a cooking process. Rays from the sun kill skin cells with ultraviolet (UV) radiation, which damages two skin compounds, collagen and elastin. And even though you might not see or feel it right away, your skin has been damaged, and some of the damage is irreversible. The body has an enzyme that repairs some of the damage, but not all of it.

To really see just how much your skin has aged and been damaged, look at skin on your body that has never been exposed to the sun. You will find the unexposed skin wrinkle-free and healthy.

In some ways, getting brown from a tanning bed can be more dangerous than soaking up sunshine. The damage to the skin is the same or greater. Actually, there really is no such thing as a safe tan. Immediately after sun exposure, you see the changes in the form of a tan, sunburn, freckling, or all of these.

Sun exposure is one of the most common risk factors for skin cancer.

There are three types of skin cancer that can be linked to skin damage from the sun: melanoma, basal-cell carcinoma, and squamous-cell carcinoma.

Melanoma is the most fatal, but squamous-cell carcinoma is also deadly.

You increase your chances of getting skin cancer by spending long periods of time in the sun or receiving severe sunburns in your early childhood years. You should check your body regularly for signs of skin cancer.

Fortunately, not everyone who sunbathes gets skin cancer. However, everyone who sunbathes does get some degree of premature aging.

Although you can't stay out of the sun all the time, there are some precautions you can take if you know you're going to be outside.

Be sure to wear sunscreen and proper clothing, such as a hat or visor for protection. And some makeup manufacturers now have sunscreen added to their products to give you added protection from the sun.

All sun blocks will give you the protection stated on the bottle if you put it on according to the directions. And, most off-brand sunscreens should work as well as the better-known brands. Be sure to read the label for instructions on how to apply sunscreen properly. Reapply sunscreen as necessary after you have been in the water.

MEDICAL SOURCE ————————————————

FDA Consumer (25,4:16)

Skin cancer and sunshine — how can these things affect your life?

It's not a new fashion craze, yet over 600,000 Americans will get this in one year alone. And, sadly, some of that 600,000 will die from it. Skin cancer.

It kills people. And it can be caused by too much exposure to the sun. Yet people still stay out in the sun without proper protection.

Skin cancers that are linked to too much exposure to dangerous ultraviolet rays are the most common form of cancer. And most of those ultraviolet rays come from the sun. The sun sends out three kinds of UV rays, but one kind is absorbed by the ozone layer and never reaches our skin. Part of another kind — ultraviolet B rays — is absorbed by the ozone layer, but the rest of those rays reach the ground and our skin. The third kind, ultraviolet A rays, go straight through all ozone layers and reach the ground and us. It's the ultraviolet A and B rays that are hazardous.

The most common kind of skin cancer is known as "basal cell carcinoma." This kind of cancer makes up about 76 percent of all malignant skin tumors, and it affects whites much more often than it affects people with pigmented skin (Afro-Americans, Indians, etc.). This type of skin cancer grows very slowly, and it usually does not spread to other tissues in different places in the body. However, any cancer left untreated can be deadly. And basal cell carcinomas can cause serious disfigurements if not treated immediately. If you detect the basal cell carcinoma early and seek treatment right away, your chances of a complete cure are about 95 percent.

Another kind of skin cancer that has an even stronger link to being caused by the UV rays from the sun is known as "squamous cell carcinoma." This type of skin cancer makes up about 20 percent of all skin cancers, and these tumors are more common in dark-raced peoples than basal cell carcinoma.

The danger in squamous cell carcinoma is that these tumors grow quickly into large tumors, and this kind of cancer can (and does) spread to other parts of the body. The spread of cancer is called "metastasis," and any time a cancer metastasizes, it decreases your chances of a complete cure.

Squamous cell carcinomas occur most often on areas of the body that have gotten a lot of exposure to the sun—the neck, arms, face and legs. And people living in areas close to the equator where they get especially strong sun rays have increased rates of this dangerous cancer.

Although this is an especially dangerous cancer, if you detect it early and seek treatment right away, you have about a 95 percent chance of a complete cure.

A third, and by far the most dangerous, kind of skin cancer is known as "malignant melanoma." This kind of skin cancer makes up about five percent of all skin cancers.

But, even though the numbers seem smaller, the threat is greater. You see, malignant melanoma often spreads to other body parts quickly, and many people die from it. In America alone, the number of cases of malignant melanoma skin cancer has tripled in the past forty years, and many scientists estimate that this dangerous form of skin cancer will affect one in every 90 Americans by the year 2000.

Malignant melanoma appears most often on the upper back in men and on the legs in women. Scientists think that people with a history of many sunburns have a greater risk of getting malignant melanoma, and people with dark skin have a lower risk than those with light skin.

Obviously, the best way to deal with cancer is to avoid getting it in the first place. And the best way to minimize your chances of getting any type of skin cancer is to protect your skin from the dangerous rays from the sun. Some people have to go to greater measures to protect their skin because of their increased chances of damage from the sun. The following chart shows who has the greatest risk of damage:

Skin color	Skin type	Damage from sun	Needs sunscreen SPF
Very fair	I	Burns easily and often and never tans	15 or more
Fair	II	Burns easily and gets only very light tan	15
Light	III	Burns every now and then, tans evenly	10-15
Medium	IV	Burns only occasionally, always gets good tan	6-10
Dark	V	Hardly ever burns and always tans easily	4-6
Black	VI	Rarely, if ever, burns, tan turns skin even darker	0-4

The greater your risk of skin damage from the sun, the greater your risk of getting skin cancer. People with very fair skin and light-colored eyes are the greatest candidates for trouble from the sun. And although everyone should always protect their skin from the sun with sunscreen and protective clothing, people with light and fair complexions must take extra care.

The damaging effects of the sun add up in your skin. The sun and the sunburns you got as a kid and a foolish, sun-worshipping teen-ager are still adding up. So, the earlier in life you can begin protecting your skin, the better off you are in the long run.

Many people wait until they reach their mid-twenties or mid-thirties before they start taking proper care of their skin and stop getting too much sun. Starting at a younger age improves your chances of living skin-cancer-free. And, making sure your children are protected from the dangerous UV rays will help improve their chances as well.

Follow these simple tips to help protect yourself and your family members from the harmful rays of the sun, and help slash your risk of skin cancer:

❑ Use a sunscreen with an adequate SPF (sun protection factor) to provide the best protection. Make sure the sunscreen shields your skin from UV A and B rays. And look for some "waterproof" sunscreen to help maintain your protection even if you swim or sweat. However, even if you do use waterproof sunscreen, you should reapply the product every hour to ensure maximum protection.

❑ Use a sunscreen even on cloudy and overcast days — even in the winter. Ultraviolet rays come through the clouds, no matter how overcast it might be. Many times people are fooled into thinking they don't need sunscreen if it isn't hot and sunny — don't be that foolish.

❑ Wear a sunscreen even if you are going to sit in the shade. Sun rays reflect off water, sand, metal and concrete, and you can get just as sunburned in the shade. Also remember this concept in the winter — snow and ice reflect sun rays, so be careful to protect your skin even on cold days. Think of how many people come back from a skiing trip with sunburned faces, and try to avoid that for yourself.

❑ Apply sunscreen evenly to your whole body — even areas that you don't think will get much sun, like the insides of your arms. Remember that reflection often gives you as much sun as the actual direct rays. Use at least an ounce of sunscreen to cover your whole body. Many people use too little sunscreen, and they don't get the protection they think they are getting. Be generous and rub in plenty of protection. Also, apply it 15 to 30 minutes before going outside to give it enough time to absorb into your skin. And wait 10 to 15 minutes after putting on the sunscreen before you put on any makeup over it.

❏ Do not use sunscreen on infants that are six months of age or younger unless advised by your doctor. If you must take your baby out in the sun, cover his skin (and face) with protective clothing (including bonnets and blankets or umbrellas). Be sure to keep the sunscreen products out of the reach of children. And help your children apply their sunscreen to make sure they get it on properly, even in those hard-to-reach places.

❏ Learn how to examine your body (and your children's bodies) to check for possible evidence of cancer. Any unusual-looking freckle or mole should alert you, and any splotchy or discolored lesions on your skin should prompt you to see your doctor just to be safe. During a skin examination, be sure to look at the front and back of your body, using a mirror. Raise your arms and look at your sides and the insides of your arms. Bend your elbows and look carefully at your forearms, elbows and palms. Look carefully at your feet, including the soles and in between the toes. Look carefully at the backs of your legs and your buttocks. Use a hand mirror if needed. Also use a hand mirror to look at your ears, back of neck and scalp. Try to lift your hair and look at your scalp during the scalp exam. Report any unusual findings to your doctor immediately. Remember, early detection and prompt treatment helps to ensure a complete recovery.

MEDICAL SOURCE ——————————————————

U.S. Pharmacist (17,7:28)

Who has the greatest risk of melanoma?

Malignant melanoma is the most dangerous form of skin

cancer that you can get. While basal cell carcinoma and squamous cell carcinoma are both serious forms of skin cancer, they have a 95-percent cure rate if you catch them early and get treatment right away.

Malignant melanoma, however, often spreads to other parts of the body and is very difficult to treat. It is a dangerous and deadly form of cancer.

What are your risk factors, other than dangerous UV rays from the sun? Your family history might be the most dangerous risk factor.

To determine your risk, ask two questions:

1) Has anyone in my family ever developed malignant melanoma?
2) Has anyone in my family ever had a birthmark (nevus) that became cancerous?

If you answered "no" to both questions, you have no greater risk than the general population of getting melanoma. Have your doctor look at your skin when you go in for regular check-ups.

If you answered "yes" to one question, your risk just went up 10 to 100 times. Have your doctor or dermatologist check your skin every six months to a year.

If you answered "yes" to both questions, your risk just went through the roof, and you should see a dermatologist every three months for a general checkup. Your risk of getting malignant melanoma is so high that you cannot afford not to go to the dermatologist every three months.

The trick to treating all cancers, including malignant melanoma, is to catch it early. Give yourself a fighting chance if your risk is high, and see your dermatologist regularly.

MEDICAL SOURCE —————————————————

Emergency Medicine (24,4:288)

Monthly self-exams help check for skin cancer warning signs

❑ Examine your body, front and back, in the mirror, then the right and left sides with arms raised.

❑ Examine the back of your neck and scalp with the help of a hand mirror; part hair (or use blow dryer) to lift and give you a close look.

❑ Check your back and buttocks with a hand mirror.

❑ Bend your elbows and look carefully at your forearms, your upper underarms and palms.

❑ Look at the backs of your legs and feet including your soles and the spaces between your toes.

MEDICAL SOURCE ─────────────────────────

FDA Consumer (25,4:16)

Danger signs of skin cancer

Have your skin checked by a doctor once a year for any changes. If you notice any of the following changes in your skin, you should see a doctor immediately:

❑ Basal-cell or squamous-cell carcinomas are any new sores or growths that get bigger, change, bleed, become scabby, or that won't heal.

❑ Melanoma — Remember your ABCD's:
A = Asymmetry — One half of a mole or lesion doesn't look like the other half.
B = Border — A mole has an irregular, scalloped, or not clearly defined border.

C = Color — The color varies or is not uniform from one area of a mole or lesion to another, whether the color is tan, brown, black, white, red or blue.

D = Diameter — The sore or blotch is larger than 6 millimeters (larger than a pencil eraser).

❏ Actinic keratosis is a precancerous skin condition that is dry, scaly, reddish and slightly raised.

MEDICAL SOURCE —————————————————

FDA Consumer (25,4:20)

Turmeric might truly be the spice of life

A study reveals that a 1-percent turmeric diet decreased stomach and skin cancer in mice.

Turmeric is a member of the ginger family and has long been a standard of East Indian cuisine. Turmeric is already part of most of our diets.

It is a spice that is found in curry powders and is also used for yellow dye in some of our food. Aromatic roots from the plant native to India are finely ground to yield this common spice.

How and why turmeric battles cancer is largely unknown. This study suggests that it is a strong antioxidant — a free radical scavenger.

Not only did turmeric fight cancer in its beginning stages, but it also appears to be effective against cancer as it progresses.

Turmeric also makes a great vegetable dip mixed with yogurt and can be used in casseroles or dishes calling for curry powder.

MEDICAL SOURCE —————————————————

Nutrition and Cancer (17,1:77)

The soy story

Eating foods containing soy sauce can reduce your risk of cancer.

In a recent study, researchers fed 300 mice a diet laced with a chemical that produces or increases stomach cancer. For six months, half of the 300 mice received soy supplements, and the other half was given only extra water. Ninety-eight percent of the mice who had extra water in their diets developed stomach cancer. But, only 72 percent of the mice who had soy sauce in their diets developed stomach cancer.

In another test, half of the mice received nitrites in their diets. Nitrites interact with soy sauce and can cause stomach cancer. This experiment showed that even the nitrites didn't stop the cancer-fighting effects of the soy sauce.

All soy products from the soybean seem to have these cancer-reducing effects.

Soy is extracted from the bean after it has been cleaned, cracked and shelled. Then, moisture is added so the beans can be "flaked." Soybean oil and soy flour are products from the soybean that are often used in the food industry. They are sometimes added to foods such as cereals, chili and ground beef.

Talk to your doctor about soy products before changing your diet. Some people develop allergies to soy products.

MEDICAL SOURCE ————————————————————————

Science News (139,23:357)

Easy test detects stomach cancer culprit

Now there's a simple test of your stomach's health: A red dot means possible trouble; no dot means you can breathe — and digest — easy. The test tells you whether your digestive tract is infected with a germ known as Helicobacter pylori.

This is the germ that might cause chronic stomach irritation (gastritis). Lately, evidence is piling up linking the same common germ to stomach ulcers. And, doctors are beginning to suspect this bacteria in the development of deadly stomach cancer. With such a "criminal" record, the bacteria suddenly is high on everybody's "hit list."

The older you get, the greater the chances this villain is lurking in your stomach. For every year of your life, you have a 1-percent greater chance of being infected with Helicobacter pylori, researchers say.

In other words, about 20 percent of all 20-year-olds, 40 percent of all 40-year-olds and 60 percent of all 60-year-olds play host to Helicobacter pylori.

The office test is known as an enzyme-linked immunosorbent assay (ELISA) and can offer results in seven minutes. And the test is simple — if a little red dot appears on the slide, you have the infection. No dot means no infection.

Preliminary studies suggest that the test is up to 100-percent accurate. In fact, in a recent study, the ELISA test correctly gave positive results for 39 people who were known to have the infection and gave negative results for 23 people who were known to be infection-free.

Although doctors don't know how people become infected with the bacteria, it is a known health risk. The bacteria's link to the development of chronic gastritis is certain, and its link to gastric ulcers is virtually airtight.

The ulcers, which are generally notorious for coming back again, seem to heal permanently after successful treatment and elimination of Helicobacter pylori.

The stomach cancer link is more recent. One study suggests that between 35 and 55 percent of all cases of stomach cancer might be associated with a Helicobacter pylori infection. Another study showed that nearly 90 percent of all people in the study who underwent surgery for stomach cancer had the H. pylori infection. Once a person is infected, the germ lingers and rarely dies on its own without some form of treatment.

Fortunately, doctors have experienced success in treating the infection. Using a combination of two, and sometimes three, medications, doctors have been able to kill the bacteria.

One of the substances the researchers used in their tests is the same as that found in the over-the-counter medicine Pepto-Bismol.

It's called bismuth subsalicylate. Other researchers used another bismuth compound, bismuth subcitrate. However, either bismuth compound must be used with powerful antibiotics to clear up the infection.

Some of the antibiotics being tested with the bismuth compounds include tetracycline, metronidazole and amoxicillin.

Killing the bacteria allows the stomach to heal from cases of gastritis and gastric ulcers, the studies indicate. And, the elimination of gastritis and gastric ulcers helps reduce the risk of the development of stomach cancer, say some researchers.

Ask your doctor about testing for Helicobacter pylori.

MEDICAL SOURCES

Medical World News (32,2:20 and 32,6:58)
British Medical Journal (302,6788:1302)

Common bacteria linked to cancer?

Cancer caused by a bacterial infection?

If so, you could be at greater risk of stomach cancer than you think.

Scientists already know that bacteria called Helicobacter pylori may be responsible for a large number of peptic and duodenal ulcers. (The duodenum is the part of the small intestines directly connected to the stomach.) In fact, 90 percent of those ulcer cases carry the bacterial infection.

And now there is evidence linking this bacteria to stomach and intestinal cancer. Recent studies show that nine out of 10 people who have surgery for intestinal or stomach cancer also have H. pylori infection.

Scientists think that H. pylori might be linked to intestinal cancer because this is the only type of cancer associated with gastritis. The H. pylori bacterial infection causes chronic gastritis (stomach inflammation), which sometimes develops into hypertrophic gastritis. This is a more severe form of inflammation that is a known cancer risk factor.

H. pylori may also cause inflamed cells to release poisonous substances. And it seems to stimulate cell division, which makes the stomach cells more vulnerable to carcinogens (cancer-causing substances).

H. pylori infection is not considered to be the only cause or even the main cause of intestinal-type cancer. But its presence, along with other cancer risk factors, increases the risk of intestinal cancer.

Half of the U.S. population routinely has H. pylori present in the digestive tract, experts estimate. The good news is that H. pylori seems to be easily "killed" with a combination of antibiotics and Pepto-Bismol. In fact, this treatment is already used in some ulcer cases. Scientists are also testing the use of vitamin C and beta carotene as a possible way to kill H. pylori.

Researchers still have a long way to go, and it may be some time before they prove the association between H. pylori and stomach cancer.

Check with your doctor about this treatment.

MEDICAL SOURCE ———————————————————

Medical World News (32,2:20)

Is your flour 'bugging' you? Throw it away to avoid cancer

You open the canister and there they are — beetles in the flour.

Some people try to scoop around them, others laugh them off as "increased dietary protein," and still others toss the flour out. Which is best?

Beetles secrete a substance which when mixed with flour and fed to mice caused cancer in laboratory tests.

Although most of us would avoid contaminated foods like beetle-infested flour, in some Asian and African countries poor farmers do use beetle-ridden flour for making bread, cakes and biscuits.

So, next time you find bugs in your flour, you might want to toss it out and avoid the risk of cancer.

MEDICAL SOURCE ———————————————————

Nutrition and Cancer (17,1:97)

CARPAL TUNNEL SYNDROME

Take control of wrist pain

There's a "tunnel" in your wrist that can cause you problems.

The problem happens when you make the same series of movements hour after hour, day after day, for months at a time. The "tunnel" is the cavity formed by the carpal bones and ligaments just under the skin in your wrist.

Thousands of repetitive motions by your wrist and forearm can squeeze and irritate the nerves passing through this tunnel in the wrist. When that happens, you feel the symptoms of carpal tunnel syndrome.

You can suspect this is the problem when you experience numbness and tingling in the thumb and first two fingers. Sometimes the numbness and tingling spread to the rest of the hand. Gradually, the thumb becomes weaker and finally useless if there is no treatment.

The problem also occurs after a sudden weight gain or edema (fluid accumulation) puts pressure on the nerves in the carpal tunnel.

It's most apt to happen to middle-age women. It also occurs along with arthritis or other disorders that affect the bones and ligaments.

Managing carpal tunnel syndrome includes the following:

❏ If the symptoms are mild, use wrist splints to prevent pressure on the affected area.

❏ Lose excess weight.

❏ Control swelling caused by edema. To help control fluid accumulation, eliminate salt and salty foods from your diet.

❑ Get help for your arthritis flare-ups. Sometimes treating arthritis also eases carpal tunnel syndrome.

MEDICAL SOURCE ─────────────────────────

The Columbia University Complete Home Medical Guide, Crown Publishers, Inc., New York, 1985

CHOLESTEROL

Lowering total cholesterol — a mistake?

It's time to rethink the safety of lowering total cholesterol levels, say an increasing number of medical researchers.

Instead, say these doctors, we should concentrate on raising our levels of HDL cholesterol, the part that many call the "good" cholesterol.

This represents a big shift, since almost all food advertisements, consumer health organizations, and government health agencies currently preach the need to get your total cholesterol below 200 milligrams of cholesterol per deciliter of blood. Many people have to resort to prescription drugs to achieve a level of cholesterol that low.

But, if lowering your cholesterol is such a good idea, "why, in randomized trials, are cholesterol-lowering drugs and diets consistently associated with increased noncardiac mortality?" asks a group of doctors at the University of California at San Francisco.

In study after study, researchers have been shocked to discover a 7-percent net increase in total deaths from causes other than heart disease. They found this alarming increase in follow-up studies among people who use cholesterol-lowering drugs or who go on special cholesterol-lowering diets.

Even though the lowered cholesterol seemed to decrease deaths from heart disease, that decrease was more than wiped out by increased deaths from other causes.

The question more and more researchers are asking is this: Is the treatment itself or its result, long-term, worse than the disease for many people?

The same somber discovery was made in a large study of more than 17,000 male civil servants in London, England. The Whitehall Study began in 1967 with men ages 40 through 64 and followed them for 18 years.

The British study showed what many studies have reported: Deaths from heart disease rise with increased levels of cholesterol. It found no link between high cholesterol and increased strokes.

It also found that puzzling relationship between lowered cholesterol and higher rates of noncardiac deaths. The higher rates involved lung diseases, particularly lung cancer, and cancers of the pancreas and liver.

The British researchers found no evidence to support a theory that hidden or undiagnosed colon cancer is the reason behind the combination of lower cholesterol levels and higher death rates. It is known that colon cancer in particular causes lower cholesterol levels. But, the study found no significant increases in colon cancer cases over 18 years.

They speculate that people who had lower cholesterol levels at the time of death must have possessed "other characteristics that place them at an elevated risk of death." But, they don't speculate what the unknown "other characteristics" might be.

Another observational study of 9,021 Chinese men and women had a similar outcome. Most of the people in the study had total cholesterol levels on average below those of people in Western countries.

Again, "blood cholesterol concentration was directly related to mortality from coronary heart disease even in those with what was, by Western standards, a 'low' cholesterol concentration," according to the study.

And, they found some evidence of higher death rates from liver disease and liver cancer among those people with lower cholesterol, although the rates weren't enough to reach a degree of mathematical certainty called "statistical significance."

And then there's fat.
A small study found immediate jumps in blood fats after 13 Tarahumara Indians in northern Mexico ate a low-fiber, high-calorie, high-fat "affluent" diet for five weeks. The Indians had been used to living on a low-fat, mainly vegetarian diet of about 2,700 calories per day.

After five weeks of eating 4,100 calories a day, researchers found the Indians' total cholesterol had risen by 31 percent; their LDL "bad" cholesterol by 39 percent; their HDL "good" cholesterol by 31 percent; and their triglycerides by 18 percent. The Indians also gained an average of eight pounds each.

The researchers did no follow-up studies, so they couldn't say how the increases might affect the Indians' health.

As bad as the typical Western diet might be, simply lowering total fats and cholesterol might itself cause some harm.

Instead, say Harvard Medical School researchers, people with high-fat diets should try to adopt a "traditional Mediterranean diet," which is low in saturated fats and cholesterol.

People eating this diet get 30 to 40 percent of their calories from fat, but their rates of heart disease are as low as people eating very-low-fat diets, the editorial says. That might be because a major portion of this diet's energy comes from olive oil, a mostly monounsaturated fat.

"We believe that the majority of dietary fatty acids should be monounsaturated rather than polyunsaturated, because diets very high in polyunsaturated fats lower HDL levels," according to Drs. Frank M. Sacks and Walter W. Willett.

A 1991 analysis of several dietary studies said that lowering dietary fat intake to 30 percent of total calories would prolong life only about four months on average, and then mostly in people over 75.

That finding brought a barrage of complaints including one from Dr. Dean Ornish, a health newsletter publisher, worrying that such studies would lead people to shrug, "Why bother? Bring out the bacon and eggs!" Others argued there aren't enough data available to make any assumptions about the effects of diet on mortality.

"If not enough is known to estimate the likely impact of U.S. health policy about dietary fat, how confident should we be in that policy?" the authors of the controversial study fired back.

The same authors also urged the Food and Drug Administration to improve doctors' knowledge about the risks involved with cholesterol-lowering drugs.

"None of the drugs have been shown to decrease total mortality in primary prevention trials," argue the three researchers from the University of California at San Francisco. "Some have actually been shown to increase noncardiovascular mortality. ..." One drug reduced HDL "good" cholesterol and poisoned animals in test studies, the authors contend. And, there haven't been any studies done to show the effects of the most popular cholesterol-lowering drug on the outcome of heart disease. All we know is the drug lowers cholesterol.

Still another analysis of several drugs used to lower cholesterol concluded that their effectiveness was only modest at best, and that they were especially weak at preventing disease.

Two other drugs, gemfibrozil (brand name Lopid) and cholestyramine (brand name Questran), also seem to have limited effectiveness. Use of the drugs would prevent only one heart attack among 50 middle-age men over a 10-year period.

The nutrient niacin, in prescription quantities, does a little better. It would prevent one heart attack among 10 to 15 men over 10 years.

The implication is that the drugs, including niacin, would have no benefits at all for the rest of the men.

The author recommends saving such drugs for people with the greatest risks for first or second heart attacks. Overall, the shift in attitudes among leading researchers is striking. More and more are growing uneasy about the fierce war being waged to lower total cholesterol.

With growing evidence that lowering cholesterol can be harmful, even fatal, to some people, and that HDL cholesterol might be the real key to better heart and blood-vessel health, some researchers are beginning to wonder out loud whether we have picked the wrong enemy to war against.

MEDICAL SOURCES ————————————————

Journal of the American Medical Association (265,24:3285 and 267,3:361)
British Medical Journal (303,6797:276)
The New England Journal of Medicine (325,24:1704)

How to raise your HDL levels

Many researchers agree that raising your blood levels of HDL cholesterol can help your heart and arteries. Besides the total amount of HDL (expressed in milligrams per deciliter of blood volume), another measurement is considered important. That's the ratio of HDL to LDL cholesterol, or the amount of HDL compared with the amount of LDL. Here are some ways to raise your HDL level and your HDL to LDL ratio.

Pectin — this soluble fiber, found mainly in fruits and some vegetables, lowers LDL.

Psyllium — another soluble fiber that lowers LDL, this is the main ingredient of several natural laxatives like Metamucil.

Oat bran — lowers LDL, mainly because of a high concentration of a soluble-fiber component called beta-glucan.

Rice bran oil — the most popular cooking oil in Japan, it lowers LDL.

Olive oil — contains mostly monounsaturated fat and lowers LDL

Omega-3 oil — known as "fish oil," it raises HDL. Also available from several vegetable sources.

Garlic — in pill form, has been shown to lower LDL and raise HDL in some studies.

Exercise combined with weight loss — raises HDL.

Prescription-level doses of niacin — lowers LDL, but has some side effects, including potentially fatal reactions involving megadoses of one gram and higher per day. The timed-release kind seems to be the most dangerous.

Estrogen-replacement therapy (for women) — lowers LDL,

raises HDL.

Starchy foods — known these days as complex carbohydrates, starches raise HDL levels, while sugary diets lower the good-cholesterol ratio.

Chromium — this trace nutrient raises HDL and has few side effects, even in large doses.

MEDICAL SOURCES ───────────────────────────────

Annals of Internal Medicine (115,12:917)
Journal of the American Medical Association (267,24:3317)
Heartstyle (1,3:17)
The Edell Health Letter (9,7:6)
Harvard Health Letter (17,8:6)

HDL low? Check out chromium

The nutrient chromium appears to cause long-lasting increases in HDL cholesterol levels. This big jump occurs even in men who take powerful blood-pressure medicines that normally decrease the "good" form of cholesterol.

In one study, men who took 600 micrograms per day of biologically active chromium showed a 16-percent increase in HDL levels after two months, compared to the men who took only a placebo (a fake pill). That lowered their heart-attack risk by up to 17 percent.

Most of the 72 men were taking propranolol. About three out of 10 were taking another beta-blocker, atenolol. In addition, nearly six out of 10 were also taking another powerful nutrient-drainer, thiazide diuretics or "water pills." The men who took the fake pill showed a net decrease in their HDL levels during the study.

But the group taking chromium supplements seemed to beat

the nutrient drain and helped their chances for healthier hearts, suggest the researchers.

The supplements contained glucose-tolerance-factor chromium, known as GTF-chromium, the report says. The men received the high-chromium brewer's yeast supplement in six gelatin capsules divided into three doses taken before meals. The capsules are available in health stores for less than $5 per month, the researchers say.

The study strongly recommends chromium supplements since the nutrient is "low in cost ..., is easily administered in the form of gelatin capsules, and is associated with no known risk."

No specific Recommended Dietary Allowance exists for chromium. A range of 50 to 200 micrograms per day for adults is "tentatively recommended." There are no known bad effects from chromium doses several times the RDA.

Approximately half to 90 percent of all Americans take in less than the minimum recommended amount daily. A lot of what we do take in is poorly absorbed. In addition, the report says, chromium levels drop with increasing age, infections, pregnancy, high-glucose intake and stress.

Besides high-chromium brewer's yeast, chromium picolinate is another biologically available form of the nutrient. Good natural sources of bioavailable chromium include calf's liver, American cheese and wheat germ.

MEDICAL SOURCE ─────────────────────────

Annals of Internal Medicine (115,12:917)

Putting the squeeze on cholesterol

Your doctor glares at you after looking at your cholesterol test results.

"Your cholesterol is high," he scowls.

Just what exactly is "high?" you ask yourself.

Doctors always seem to use those nondescriptive words. You don't know if your cholesterol level is dangerously high or just mildly elevated.

And just that little bit of knowledge will probably make a difference in how drastically you change your diet.

To get a better idea of what many doctors currently consider high and mildly elevated, look at the table below.

Risk	Total cholesterol	HDL (good)	LDL (bad)
High	above 240	less than 35	above 160
Borderline	200-239	35-45	130-159
Good	below 200	above 45	below 130

Too much cholesterol in your blood greatly increases your risk of heart disease and strokes, according to many doctors. So, if your cholesterol levels fall in the "High" or "Borderline" categories, it might be time to change your diet.

Cutting out some of the fat and cholesterol in your diet can reduce your blood cholesterol by as much as 15 percent, which will cut your risk of heart disease by as much as 30 percent, say some studies.

Follow these simple cooking tips to lower the amount of fat and cholesterol in your diet:

Cut down on the "bad" fats in your diet — saturated fats.

❑ Take the skin off your poultry before cooking, and trim the fat off beef and pork.

❑ Drink skim milk or low-fat milk.

❑ Eat low-fat cheeses.

❑ Carefully read labels on cream substitutes. Sometimes they are made with palm oils or coconut oils, which are high in saturated fats.

❑ Cut down on the amount of high-fat meat products that you eat, such as bacon, sausage and hamburger.

❑ Avoid candy, nuts and chips when snacking. Eat pretzels, fruits and air-popped popcorn instead.

❑ Check your labels for saturated fats. These include coconut and palm oils, beef fat, lard and hydrogenated vegetable oils. Increase the amount of "good" fats in your diet — unsaturated fats.

❑ Use soft margarines that are high in unsaturated or dehydrogenated fats.

❑ Make your own sauces and dressings using oils that are high in unsaturated fats and low in saturated fats.

❑ Cook, fry and bake with oils that are high in unsaturated fats and low in saturated fats, such as safflower oil, sunflower seed oil and corn oil.

❑ Cut back on the amount of cholesterol in your diet.

❑ Eat less organ meats such as liver, kidneys and brains.

❑ Where possible, cook only with the egg whites and not the whole egg (the yolk is high in cholesterol).

❑ Avoid fast foods and other retail baked goods that are high in cholesterol.

❑ Eat more water-soluble fiber such as fruit, legumes and bran.

MEDICAL SOURCE ───────────────────────────────

Postgraduate Medicine (87,2:63)

Simple tips to help you lower the amount of fat in your diet

You can make a big change in your blood cholesterol levels just by changing your eating habits. Eating a well-balanced diet is the easiest and least expensive method to reduce cholesterol.

Consider the wisdom of lower saturated fat intake, which accounts for up to 40 percent of our daily calorie count. But be careful to keep on getting proper nutrients.

Lower your dietary cholesterol, found in meats, dairy products and animal fats, and count calories. Overweight people are more likely to have higher cholesterol levels.

Dairy products: Choose skim milk instead of whole milk; low-fat, plain yogurt instead of fruit yogurts made with whole milk; low-fat cheeses (farmer's, mozzarella), and ice milk or sherbet instead of ice cream. Limit egg yolks to less than three per week; use egg whites in place of whole eggs in recipes.

Meats and seafood: Think lean. Choose chicken, turkey and well-trimmed cuts of lean beef. Eat at least two servings of fish per week. Fish from deep, cold waters are best because they're high in essential omega-3 oils. Fresh or frozen fish are better than canned. But if you eat canned fish, choose fish packed in water, not oil.

Fruits and vegetables: Eat three servings of fresh fruits daily (except coconuts). Avoid fruit canned in heavy syrup. Read the labels on jams and jellies and choose a low-sugar product. Most vegetables and preparation methods are fine, but avoid avocados, olives, cheese, cream and butter sauces. Restrict starchy vegetables, such as potatoes.

Cereals, nuts, breads: Most hot and cold packaged cereals are fine, but watch the sugar and salt content. Also check the labels and buy those that are highest in dietary fiber, vitamins and minerals (remember that dietary fiber is not the same thing as crude fiber). Use pecans, walnuts and peanuts sparingly. Avoid hydrogenated peanut butter. Choose whole-grain breads, and avoid commercially baked goods, such as cakes and pastries, which are loaded with fat. Instead of egg noodles, choose pastas and rice.

The above guidelines are based on recommendations from the American Heart Association and the National Cholesterol Education Program Expert Panel.

How you prepare food will also affect your cholesterol levels. You may freely use vinegar, soy sauce (but watch the sodium) and most spices and herbs.

Cooking oils are another matter. Choose polyunsaturated vegetable oils, such as safflower, corn and sesame oils. Avoid lard altogether. Instead of butter, try polyunsaturated margarine.

MEDICAL SOURCE ───────────────────────────────

Postgraduate Medicine (87,2:63)

Lower cholesterol levels — Eat smaller meals more frequently

Lowering your cholesterol might no longer be a question of what you eat, but of when and how often you eat.

And, surprisingly, the more often you eat, the lower your cholesterol might be.

Scientists tested a sample of 2,034 white men and women between the ages of 50 and 89 years. They asked the volunteers how much they drank and smoked, how often they exercised, and when they ate meals and snacks.

For nearly three years, researchers measured total cholesterol, LDL (low-density lipoproteins) cholesterol, HDL (high-density lipoproteins) cholesterol and triglyceride levels in the study participants.

Seven out of 10 people in the sample reported eating three meals a day. One out of 10 reported eating one or two meals each day, and two out of 10 reported eating more than four meals each day.

Total cholesterol levels among those people who ate four or more meals each day were an average of 2.5 percent lower than the cholesterol levels of those eating only once or twice a day.

Those people eating four meals daily also experienced a lower LDL cholesterol level than those eating once or twice a day.

Researchers discovered a surprise: The lower total cholesterol and lower LDL cholesterol levels seen with increased meals occurred even though frequent eaters ate more calories, more total fat and more cholesterol than infrequent eaters.

But, don't just eat more meals or snacks throughout the day. Instead, eat smaller meals more frequently. Stretch out your normal daily food intake over four or more meals instead of over two or three meals, these results suggest.

A rule of thumb is that for every 1-percent reduction in your total cholesterol, you experience a 2-percent reduction in coronary heart disease risk. Eating smaller, more frequent meals each day might translate to lower cholesterol levels and lower risk of heart disease.

MEDICAL SOURCE ———————————————

The American Journal of Clinical Nutrition (55,3:664)

Right breakfast menu could lead to lower cholesterol levels

Are you rushed in the mornings? And all you have time to eat is a bowl of cereal?

You might be doing yourself a favor.

Not by rushing — but by having a bowl of cereal. Especially if it contains one of two fibers recently shown to lower cholesterol. The kind of fiber that helps lower cholesterol is known as soluble fiber.

Here is a partial list of soluble-fiber foods: oats, oat bran, guar gum, acacia gum, locust bean gum, karaya gum, psyllium and pectin.

It seems that psyllium and pectin are most efficient in lowering LDL cholesterol. And lowering your cholesterol might lower your risk of coronary artery disease (CAD), according to many studies. Pectin seems to be more effective if cholesterol levels in the blood are fairly high.

If you are suffering from high cholesterol, there is an easy way to help lower your LDL level and reduce your risk of CAD.

How? Every day, eat two ounces of cereal which is high in soluble fiber.

A recent study reports that including soluble fiber in your diet also helps reduce triglycerides, another kind of troublesome substance in your blood. Pectin seems to do the best job of lowering triglyceride levels.

Here is some more good news — if you eat cold cereal with skim milk, you might also lower your cholesterol even more.

MEDICAL SOURCE ——————————————————

The American Journal of Clinical Nutrition (52,6:1020)

Garlic lowers cholesterol by up to 15 percent

Any way you press or powder it, new studies show that garlic may reduce your cholesterol levels by up to 15 percent.

And it's available as a garlic "pill," without the odor.

The new garlic pill developed by German scientists is coated to prevent foul breath and skin odors usually associated with people who eat lots of garlic.

Researchers hope that using the garlic pill as a dietary supplement could soon eliminate the need for some cholesterol-lowering drugs.

MEDICAL SOURCE —————————————————————

Modern Medicine (58,11:17)

New cooking oil helps lower cholesterol

The Japanese are masters at "lowering." They lowered the production costs of televisions. They lowered the costs of VCRs. And now they may have found a new way to lower cholesterol, too.

U.S. researchers suggest that Japan's most popular cooking oil, rice bran oil, can lower your cholesterol by up to 30 percent. Until now, scientists have overlooked rice bran oil because they thought it was high in saturated fats.

But now, researchers have found that the type of fat in rice bran oil is able to "lower the bad cholesterol without lowering the good cholesterol," according to Dr. Robert Nicolosi, Director of Heart Research at the University of Lowell in Massachusetts.

But don't throw out your olive and canola oils, Dr. Nicolosi cautioned.

Instead, consumers should consider combining rice bran oil with other oils considered part of a healthy diet.

MEDICAL SOURCE —————————————————————

Heartstyle (Spring/Summer 1991:17)

Oat bran is back in the cholesterol-lowering business

A recent study suggests that two to three ounces of oat bran added to the diet every day for about six weeks could reduce your cholesterol levels by 7 to 10 percent.

Funded by a grant from the Quaker Oats Company, a group of Chicago scientists tested the effects of oat bran on cholesterol levels in 140 volunteers, all of whom had high cholesterol.

The volunteers were divided into seven groups. All groups started eating a low-fat diet. Group one, the control group, ate one ounce of a wheat cereal each day, in addition to their low-fat diet. Groups two, three and four added one, two and three ounces of oatmeal to their low-fat diet. And groups five, six and seven added one, two and three ounces of oat bran to their low-fat diets.

The seven groups stayed on these diets for six weeks. At the end of the six weeks, the volunteers tested their total cholesterol levels and their LDL cholesterol levels. (LDL cholesterol is the "bad" form of cholesterol that contributes to clogged arteries.)

Group one, the control group that ate wheat cereal, showed no drop in cholesterol levels. In fact, the group experienced a slight rise in cholesterol.

The group that ate two ounces of oatmeal daily experienced a drop of 2.7 percent in total cholesterol and a 3.5 percent drop in LDL cholesterol. The group that ate two ounces of oat bran daily experienced a 9.5 percent drop in total cholesterol and a 15.9 percent drop in LDL cholesterol.

The oat bran had a greater reducing effect on the cholesterol levels than the oatmeal due to the oat bran's higher concentration of a kind of fiber known as beta-glucan fiber. The study demonstrates that this type of water-soluble fiber, beta-glucan fiber found in oat bran and oat cereals, is effective in lowering cholesterol levels.

The cholesterol-lowering effect is probably most effective when the oat fiber is combined with a low-fat diet, as in the study.

The study concludes that it requires three ounces of oatmeal to achieve the same cholesterol-lowering effects as two ounces of oat bran due to the higher content of beta-glucan fiber in the oat bran. Anything less than two to three ounces daily results in fewer benefits, and anything more doesn't do any more good.

Talk with your doctor about a safe, low-fat diet and daily servings of oat bran or oat cereals to help lower your cholesterol levels.

MEDICAL SOURCE ─────────────────────

Journal of the American Medical Association (265,14:1833)

Barley, soy and prunes: New ways to lower cholesterol

Researchers added prunes, which contain pectin (a type of soluble dietary fiber), to the diets of men with mild high cholesterol. Eating 12 prunes daily lowered "bad" LDL cholesterol in just four weeks. Fruits like apples and grapefruit, and vegetables such as carrots and cabbage, are also good sources of pectin.

Italian researchers tested families with a tendency toward high cholesterol by substituting soy for animal protein in another study. There was a dramatic drop of over 20 percent in the total cholesterol level after only four weeks of eating soy protein instead of animal protein.

At the same time, Australian researchers compared the effects of barley fiber and wheat fiber on lowering blood cholesterol in a third study. When the men in this study switched over to eating products that were made from barley flour instead of wheat, LDL cholesterol and total cholesterol levels both went down.

If cholesterol is a problem for you, you might want to make

some of these changes a part of your diet.

But be sure to check with your doctor or nutritionist before making big changes in your diet.

MEDICAL SOURCE ────────────────────────

The American Journal of Clinical Nutrition (53,5:1191, 1205 and 1259)

Coffee filter helps in the cholesterol fight

Worried about that morning cup of coffee jacking up your cholesterol levels? Now, you can remove all doubt.

Studies show that using a simple paper filter when making your coffee can remove its cholesterol-raising effects. Scandinavian-style coffee, made by boiling ground coffee beans and water without a filter, seems to raise cholesterol levels, according to researchers. Drip-filtered coffee, on the other hand, seems to have no bad effects on cholesterol levels.

Dutch scientists conclude that separating coffee grounds through a paper filter is crucial in determining how coffee affects cholesterol levels. They discovered a fat-rich component of boiled coffee. A tiny fraction of your brewed coffee contains fatty compounds from the coffee bean. Apparently, within that fatty fraction is something that triggers a rise in blood cholesterol levels.

If you brew your coffee through a filter, you filter out most of that compound, researchers found.

Coffee appears to lose both its lipids (fatty substances) and its cholesterol-raising properties when a paper filter is used. The filter catches the suspect fats, Dutch scientists report.

The study involved 64 healthy people (33 men and 31 women) and lasted for 14 weeks. During the first 17 days, everyone drank six cups of boiled-and-filtered coffee a day. Over the next 79 days, they drank either six cups of boiled-unfiltered coffee, six cups of boiled-and-filtered coffee, or no coffee at all. They were then divided into three groups. Everyone maintained their usual diets and activity levels.

In the group drinking boiled-unfiltered coffee, cholesterol levels (including the LDL "bad" form) rose by an average of 16 milligrams per deciliter, according to researchers. But there was only a small and insignificant increase in total and LDL cholesterol levels among those who drank coffee that was both boiled and filtered.

The no-coffee group drank one glass of orange or apple juice, one glass of mineral water and four cups of herbal tea each day. Those in the no-coffee group who normally used milk in their coffee ate special fatty-acid-enriched cookies to compensate for the missing milk.

According to researchers, the cholesterol concentrations in the no-coffee group stayed the same as those in the boiled-and-filtered-coffee group. The "good" HDL cholesterol levels stayed about the same in all groups. The changes in cholesterol levels were basically the same for men as well as women.

MEDICAL SOURCES ——————————————————
> American Heart Association news release (June 5, 1991)
> *The Lancet* (335, 8700:1235)

Bathe your beef to lower the cholesterol

For all you cholesterol watchers, red meat may no longer be a forbidden fruit or a thing of the past. Researchers have come up with a "safe" way to eat it.

So, if drenching your hamburger in oil before browning it and then rinsing it afterwards in boiling water seem an odd way to cut cholesterol, it's time for you to rethink your kitchen chemistry.

The challenge was to find a practical diet containing less than 30 percent of its calories in the form of fat, less than 10 percent in saturated fat and fewer than 300 milligrams of cholesterol. The kitchen chemists were also charged with using flavorful foods that are standard American fare.

In other words, the challenge was to come up with healthy hamburger, rather than tasty tofu.

In the past, cholesterol-conscious cooks bought lean meat, trimmed off the fat and ground it into hamburger. The hamburger was traditionally browned, removed from the skillet and then drained on absorbent toweling before it was used. But, because of where the unwanted cholesterol is located in the meat's chemical structure, it is difficult to extract the cholesterol by trimming, browning and draining.

What was needed, the chemist-cooks decided, was a method that would take away a large amount of the saturated fat, as well as at least half of the undesirable cholesterol.

To achieve the goals, the chemist-cooks took away the fat and cholesterol from the meat by heating it in vegetable oil. Next, they rinsed the meat with either boiling water or steam. Then, they separated the oil and water (broth) and returned the broth to the meat.

Presto, the reconstituted hamburger becomes a low-fat, low cholesterol, flavorful ground beef that can be used in chili, spaghetti sauce, casseroles or a wide variety of other dishes.

Cooking ground meat in this fashion has the added advantage that it is something any home cook, regardless of culinary ability, can do with very little effort.

Begin with about two pounds of ground meat (beef, pork,

lamb or even poultry). Place meat in Dutch oven or large saucepan and add three cups of vegetable oil.

Mix and cook over medium heat until the temperature reaches 185 degrees. (Use a candy thermometer attached to the side of the pan, being careful not to allow the bottom of the thermometer to touch the bottom of the pan. Otherwise, you will get a false reading.)

Heat and stir for another five minutes so the oil will permeate the meat. This will allow the replacement of saturated fat with unsaturated fat and the partial removal of some of the undesirable cholesterol. Heat mixture to about 220 degrees and continue cooking about five minutes to brown meat, boil off excess water, and extract additional cholesterol.

Next, pour meat and oil into a fine-mesh strainer attached to a medium-size bowl.

Pour one and a half cups of boiling water over the meat. The water will extract even more oil. Cool bowl of water/oil and then chill until fat solidifies on the surface. Remove the fat.

Mix as much of the remaining broth with the meat as you desire and proceed with your recipe. After you have used this method of preparing meat several times, you will be able to gauge your heat well enough that you probably won't need a thermometer.

The purpose of the thermometer is to give you an idea of what your meat and oil should look like. It also wouldn't be too difficult to cook up several pounds of fat-free ground meat at once and freeze or refrigerate it until you're ready to use it.

In any case, you don't have to say "goodbye" to spaghetti and chili when you say "goodbye" to unwanted fat and cholesterol.

MEDICAL SOURCE ————————————————————

The New England Journal of Medicine (324,2:73)

Job may raise cholesterol level and increase risk of heart disease

You've heard about all the risk factors that can raise cholesterol levels and increase your risk of heart disease—too many fats in the diet, lack of exercise and so on.

But have you heard that your job could be influencing your cholesterol levels?

Scientists warn that the risk of unemployment increases serum cholesterol concentration in middle-aged men.

So, men who work in companies or factories that are in danger of closing down or laying off workers have an increased risk of heart disease.

Apparently, stress seems to be one of the culprits behind the increased level of cholesterol in the blood.

Sleep disturbances also contribute to increases in serum cholesterol levels and a greater risk of cardiovascular disease.

Men who are in danger of losing their jobs usually experience higher stress levels and have difficulty sleeping.

These two factors increase the cholesterol in their blood and increase their chances of heart disease.

Men who may be in danger of losing their jobs should consider visiting their doctor.

The stress associated with unemployment often puts them at greater risk of heart disease, and the regular checkups may be helpful in monitoring their health.

MEDICAL SOURCE ———————————————————

British Medical Journal (301,6750:461)

CHRONIC FATIGUE SYNDROME

Symptoms of chronic fatigue syndrome

- Confusion and difficulty in concentrating and difficulty in finishing mental tasks.
- Reduced short-term memory.
- Unexplained neurological impairments such as loss of balance or trouble adding and subtracting.
- Localized muscle pains and aching joints.
- Headaches, depression, ringing in the ears.
- Prickling, tingling or creeping sensations on the skin.
- Difficulty in sleeping that lasts for more than six months.
- Enlarged lymph nodes.
- Sore throat or pharyngitis.

MEDICAL SOURCE ——————————————————

The Lancet (337,8744:757)

Magnesium might relieve fatigue symptoms

Feeling tired and weak lately, but your doctor can't figure out what is wrong with you?

You may be suffering from what is called chronic fatigue syndrome, and magnesium may be just what you need to put the spring back in your step.

Chronic fatigue syndrome seems to have been around for centuries, in some form or another, and the cause is unknown. Doctors aren't too sure about it, either. Some say that it doesn't even exist. Some doctors don't consider CFS to be a very serious condition, but many people suffer from the disease without knowing exactly what is wrong.

Diagnosis of CFS is difficult, and patients are often stressed and anxious because their friends and family can sometimes be unsympathetic, dismissing it simply as tiredness or even laziness.

Among those who have been diagnosed as having chronic fatigue syndrome, researchers have found abnormally low levels of magnesium in their red blood cells. Some factors that may lead to this deficiency of magnesium are low physical activity, nervousness and stress.

According to a recent study, 32 people with CFS received 15 magnesium sulphate injections into the muscles each week for six weeks, while the remaining 17 people took a placebo (fake pill).

Those treated with magnesium seemed to have improved levels of energy, a better emotional state and less pain.

Some natural sources of magnesium are almonds and other nuts, wheat germ, flounder, shrimp, leafy-green vegetables and soybeans. The recommended daily allowance of magnesium for males is 350 milligrams; and for females, it is 280 milligrams.

Be sure to check with your doctor before beginning supplements of magnesium.

MEDICAL SOURCE ——————————————————————
The Lancet (337,8744:757)

New link between sinusitis and chronic fatigue syndrome

If you can't seem to find relief for your constant fatigue, the solution might be right under your nose.

Chronic fatigue syndrome might be linked to nose, throat and ear problems.

Apparently, many people who suffer from unexplained chronic fatigue also suffer from nose, throat and ear problems that are commonly associated with sinusitis.

Doctors commonly fail to diagnose sinusitis in people because the sinuses are difficult to visualize with X-rays.

However, once diagnosed, sinusitis is easy to treat.

Dr. Alexander Chester from Georgetown University in Washington, D.C., recognized the link between chronic fatigue and nose, throat and ear problems. After treating people for sinusitis, he found that the fatigue seemed to disappear in about half of the treated people.

In other words, the chronic fatigue responded to the sinusitis therapy.

If you are suffering from severe fatigue and suspect you have chronic fatigue syndrome, ask your doctor to examine your nose, throat and ears for the signs of sinusitis.

Relief from your fatigue could be right there under your nose.

MEDICAL SOURCE ───────────────────────

Modern Medicine (59,8:13)

Chronic fatigue syndrome from a simple virus?

Could a simple virus be to blame for the so-called "Yuppie flu"?

Researchers have been trying to find out more about this "mystical illness" called chronic fatigue syndrome (CFS) that is often difficult to diagnose. Doctors have often blamed the symptoms of CFS on psychological problems.

Researchers now suggest the culprit is a virus that can cause immune system disorders. Some studies show that people with severe chronic fatigue symptoms suffer from immune system irregularities that might provoke many of the characteristics of the illness.

CFS sufferers have abnormal immune systems that might fail to clear invading viruses from the body, according to Nancy Klimas, an immunologist at the University of Miami School of Medicine.

Dr. John Martin, chief of molecular pathology at USC Medical Center in Los Angeles, has found evidence of a spumavirus in about half of the people diagnosed with CFS. Although the spumavirus appears to be linked to chronic fatigue syndrome in some cases, researchers aren't ready to say for sure that this virus is the cause of CFS.

Scientists agree that if they can pinpoint the viral cause of CFS they can launch efforts to find a treatment against the virus. For now, experimental treatment efforts for chronic fatigue syndrome have focused on trying to regulate the immune system.

MEDICAL SOURCES————————————————————

The Wall Street Journal (Sept. 23, 1991, B6D)
The Lancet (338,8769:707)

COLD SORES

Cold-sore sufferer? You don't have to dodge the sun anymore!

They are irritating, painful and socially embarrassing—cold sores.

If you suffer from them, you are not alone. About 150 million Americans occasionally have flare-ups from a virus known as herpes simplex type 1. That leads to over 100 million recurrences of herpes cold sores each year.

Once you've been infected, you can't get rid of it. All you can do is treat the cold sores when they surface. (Although the virus has the same first name, it's not the same virus as the sexually transmitted disease.)

The cold sores occur on or around the lips and gums. And, some of the factors that seem to trigger the onset include stress, hot beverages and direct sunlight.

Until now, most people who suffer from cold sores have been told to avoid sunlight. However, scientists suggest that might not be necessary anymore. Using sunscreen on and around your lips can help prevent the recurrence of cold sores caused by the herpes virus.

Scientists conducted a study in which they applied sunscreen (with a sun protection factor of 15) to the lips of 38 people who suffered from herpes cold sores. When they were exposed to ultraviolet light (sunlight), none of the people developed cold sores.

Two months later, the scientists repeated the trial, but instead of using sunscreen, they applied a lotion that did not contain sunscreen. After being exposed to the ultraviolet light, 71 percent of the people developed cold sores.

The results of this trial indicate that the sunscreen filtered out the irritating ultraviolet light from the sun that seems to trigger cold sores.

Herpes simplex type 1 virus can be transmitted by kissing, touching or drinking after someone who has a herpes cold sore. Avoiding contact with the open sore will prevent the transmission.

If you suffer from cold sores, using sunscreen might be the answer for you.

MEDICAL SOURCES —————————————————————————

Medical Tribune (32,26:20)
The Lancet (338,8780:1419)

COLDS AND FLU

How to tell if you've got a cold or something else

It just doesn't matter, you say.

No matter how much orange juice you drink, how well you bundle up when you go outside, or how hard you try to avoid sick co-workers, you always manage to come down with at least one cold each year.

The common cold — it's a fact of life for most people. But even though it is so common, many people still aren't quite sure what to do when they've got one or when one of the kids has one.

The first thing to do is figure out whether your "cold" is really a cold. It could be the flu or allergies. Look for your symptoms in the accompanying chart to help decide if you really have a case of the common cold.

For example, let's say you have a combination of symptoms.

You have a runny nose; that could be any one of the three conditions. But you also have a fever; that rules out an allergy. And your third symptom is sneezing. That cinches it: You have a common cold. Flu is never associated with sneezing, according to the following chart.

Now that you have determined that you have a cold, what can you do about it?

The first thing to remember is that your doctor cannot give you a drug to make your cold go away, because that kind of drug doesn't exist. The only thing your doctor can do is recommend medicines that will act only on your symptoms and make you feel a little better until the cold runs its course — usually about three days.

Symptoms	Flu	Cold	Allergy
Fever	often	occasional	never
Headaches	usual	usual	sometimes
Runny nose	occasional	often	usual
Dry cough	often	rare	sometimes
Sore throat	often	often	never
Sneezing	never	usual	rare
Muscle aches	usual	rare	never
Dizziness	often	rare	rare
Hoarse voice	often	rare	never
Coughing up sputum	rare	rare	rare
Tired and weak	often	rare	never

MEDICAL SOURCE ————————————————

Gilbert A. Friday, M.D.; Department of Asthma, Allergies and Immunology; Children's Hospital of Pittsburg (Penn.)

Follow these simple tips to help relieve the discomfort of the common cold:

❑ Drink eight to 10 glasses of nonalcoholic liquids each day. Warm or hot beverages (hot cocoa, herbal tea, etc.) are often more soothing than cold beverages, but try to drink as much water as you can in addition to your other liquids.

❑ Do not smoke. Your body is trying to get rid of your cold, and smoking only slows down that process. Smoking decreases the ability of the cells in the lungs to keep the air passages clear and clean.

❑ Avoid touching your eyes, nose and mouth. Most colds are spread through hand-to-hand contact. Touching your eyes, nose and mouth increases your chances of spreading the cold to someone else.

❑ Wash your hands often to reduce the chances of spreading your cold.

❑ If you have a runny nose, try to just put up with it. Grab a box of tissues and try not to take any medicines that will stop your nose from running. A runny nose is your body's natural way of flushing out the virus that caused your cold in the first place. So let your body do its job.

❑ If your nose is "stuffed-up" instead of runny, try an over-the-counter nasal decongestant to "unstuff" your nose. This will help you sleep a little easier at night.

❑ The best way to treat a fever is to drink lots of fluids and get plenty of rest. A fever is another one of your body's natural ways of fighting off sickness. Unfortunately, a high fever can do more harm than good. So, if you need to bring your fever down, take some aspirin or acetaminophen (Anacin or Tylenol are two examples).

❑ If your fever goes over 103 degrees, call your doctor. High fevers can be dangerous.

❑ If you have a fever of 100 degrees or more for more than four straight days, call your doctor. You could be dealing with something more serious than a common cold.

❑ Do not give aspirin to children, teen-agers or young adults for fever if they have the flu or chicken pox. Taking aspirin with the flu or chicken pox increases their risk of getting Reye's syndrome. This is a rare but serious illness that can cause lifelong troubles. If you are not sure whether your child has a cold or the flu, give him acetaminophen for his fever, just to be safe.

❑ If you have a "productive" cough (you are coughing up phlegm), try to let it take its course. A productive cough is your body's way of cleaning out any fluids, mucus or other unwanted substances in the lungs caused by the cold.

❑ Expectorant cough medicines will help speed up the process of coughing up the phlegm and mucus. Drinking warm liquids or eating warm soup also helps your lungs do their job — the warm moisture "loosens" the mucus and makes it easier for your lungs to cough it up. (Do not confuse an expectorant cough medicine with an antitussive cough medicine — the expectorant "helps" you cough, and an antitussive stops any coughing.)

❑ Standing in a hot shower, sitting in a steamy room (the bathroom during a hot shower), or using a humidifier will also help loosen the mucus in your lungs.

❑ If the mucus or phlegm that you cough up is green, yellowish or smells bad, you need to see your doctor. That signals another infection, something other than the common cold.

❏ Also call your doctor if coughing or taking deep breaths causes sharp pains in your chest. Shortness of breath is another signal to call your doctor.

❏ If you have a "dry" cough — that is, a cough that doesn't bring up any mucus — you might need to use an over-the-counter cough suppressant (also known as an antitussive) to help stop the coughing. Cough suppressants can be in liquid form or in lozenge form. Find the one that works best for you, and be sure to follow the instructions carefully. Also, drink plenty of liquids to keep your lungs and throat from becoming dry and irritated.

❏ For sore throats, try drinking warm liquids or warm soup broth for soothing relief. Try to keep the air moist with a humidifier to keep your throat from drying out and becoming even more irritated.

❏ Throat lozenges are helpful in keeping your throat moist to avoid any additional irritation. Aspirin or acetaminophen can also help ease the pain of a sore throat.

Following these commonsense tips will help ease the discomfort of the common cold while the cold runs its course.

Unfortunately, what many people think is just a case of the common cold sometimes turns out to be strep throat. This is an illness that needs to be treated with antibiotics from the doctor. If you have the following strep throat symptoms, see your doctor:

❏ Pus on your throat or tonsils. This looks like white or yellow spots on the back of your throat.

❏ Contact with someone who has strep throat — it is contagious.

❏ Fever higher than 101 degrees

❏ An unusual rash that came with the sore throat.

If you suspect that you have more than a common cold, you should act on that feeling and see your doctor. You should also see your doctor if any of the following happens:

❏ Sharp pains in your chest when you take a deep breath or cough.

❏ Coughing up blood.

❏ A high fever (greater than 101 degrees) with shaking chills and coughing up thick phlegm.

❏ Any significant, unusual or severe throat pain.

❏ Swollen or painful glands or bumps in the front of your neck or under your jawbone along with a sore throat.

MEDICAL SOURCES ————————————————————

British Medical Journal (298,6683:1265)
Health Letter (6,2:1)
Medical World News (32,4:24)

T-shirt helps unstuff your head

Suffering from a stuffy nose, but don't have time to sit with your head over a pot of hot water?

The solution is probably in your bottom drawer. If you have an old T-shirt, you have a ready-made remedy.

Cut a strip from the old T-shirt and soak it in hot water. Tie the wet strip around your head, covering up your nose, then take a deep breath.

The T-shirt material has a good balance between water retention and breathability.

This gives you the same effect as sitting over hot water in a pot, but it allows you the freedom to read, work, cook or continue any other activity.

This simple remedy provides quick relief without slowing you down, according to a medical journal report.

MEDICAL SOURCE ————————————————————————

The Lancet (338,8765:522)

Breathe easier with steaming vaporizer or cool humidifier

The cold, dry air of winter might be a relief after a hot and humid summer. But that invigorating air can cause respiratory problems including coughing, hoarseness, and a dry, sore throat. It might also dry and crack your skin, making it vulnerable to germs.

The problem with cold air is that it holds less moisture than warm air. For example, when the weather reporter says the temperature is 40 degrees and the relative humidity is 35 percent, this means that the air contains only 35 percent of the water it can hold at 40 degrees.

And when that cold air is heated inside your home, the air gets even drier. People breathe easiest when relative humidity is 100 percent at body temperature. That's why breathing is best for most people in a warm shower.

So, many people turn to humidifiers or vaporizers to put some of the moisture back into dry air to keep skin and breathing passages moist.

But which method is better? Each seems to offer advantages.

Vaporizers work by boiling water to release steam into the air. Because a vaporizer depends on the minerals in water to complete an electric circuit that heats the water, too many or too few minerals interfere with the effectiveness of a vaporizer.

Too many minerals in the water can make the water foam or spill out of the vaporizer. It can cause your lights to flicker or blow a fuse. The simple solution to this problem is to use distilled water in the bowl of the vaporizer. If there are too few minerals in the water, the vaporizer won't produce any steam. In this case, you can solve the problem by adding a pinch of borax or baking soda to the water.

You should clean your vaporizer after you use it for three to five days. Take it apart and soak it in a vinegar solution overnight.

A humidifier, on the other hand, releases a cool mist as the motorized top siphons water from the bottom reservoir and spins out tiny droplets of water into a room.

You can use regular tap water in a humidifier, and there is no problem when the water in the reservoir runs out. Another advantage to using a humidifier is that they use about one-sixth the electricity used by vaporizers.

A potential health problem from using humidifiers is that bacteria and molds can grow in the cool, damp insides of the unit. This can cause respiratory problems. To kill these molds and bacteria, clean your humidifier weekly with hot, soapy water, and rinse it with clear water.

An even better cleaning method is to add half a cup of bleach to the water in the reservoir, plug the spray outlet with a towel and run the unit for 30 to 90 minutes. Then empty the reservoir, rinse it out, and run clear water through the machine for a few minutes.

The newest kind of humidifier on the market is the ultrasonic humidifier. In these models, a small part vibrates so fast that it produces a very fine vapor. A fan then blows this mist out into a room.

There are several advantages to ultrasonic humidifiers. They are quiet, they kill molds and bacteria, and many have a humidistat that shuts the unit off when the room is humid enough. Ultrasonic humidifiers should not be run dry.

Humidifiers or vaporizers can improve the quality of indoor air in the winter. Talk to your doctor or pharmacist about which is best for you.

MEDICAL SOURCE ────────────────────────────────

U.S. Pharmacist (16,11:28)

Guidelines for safe, effective use of vaporizers and humidifiers

No matter which type of unit you choose to humidify your room, follow these precautions for safe, effective use.

❏ Place the unit on the floor, not on furniture.

❏ Protect the floor under the unit with a plastic sheet and folded towel.

❏ Place your humidifier well away from sensitive electronic equipment, such as VCRs and computers.

❏ Direct steam or vapor flow toward an open area, not toward a person, drapery or other material that you don't want to get damp.

❏ Don't insert your finger into the water supply to see if a vaporizer is working.

❏ Unplug any unit before working on it, filling it or cleaning it.

❏ Before buying any unit, check for an Underwriters Laboratory seal of approval sticker.

❑ Never leave a unit operating unattended.

❑ Most modern vaporizers include a solid base so they won't tip over even when turned at a 30-degree angle.

❑ Make sure the cord is out of the way so no one can trip on it.

❑ Aromatic substances work only in vaporizers. They should be placed in the small cup below the steam port.

MEDICAL SOURCE ————————————————————————

U.S. Pharmacist (16,11:33)

Avoid flu, cold? Stay away from people

To avoid catching a cold or the flu, just staying away from those who are infected may not be adequate protection.

Even though it's easy to confuse a cold with the flu, the two viruses have nothing in common — except their ability to inflict misery, say scientists. Colds come wrapped in sneezes, coughs, occasional fever, congestion and a general listlessness.

When cold sufferers wheeze, sneeze or cough, they spray fine droplets of virus-bearing mucus and saliva into the environment. Until those tiny droplets dry, which can take several hours or even days, they are capable of infecting others with the cold virus.

According to some experts, "It's usually the people who are considerate enough to cough or sneeze into a tissue or handkerchief who spread the infection." The mucus, say the experts, leaks through the paper onto their hands, taking the virus along with it. As a result, you can catch a cold virus from a telephone receiver, computer keyboard, coffee utensils or by shaking hands with your germy friend or co-worker.

Influenza is characterized by fatigue, chills, body aches, a sudden fever, runny nose, congestion, headache and coughing. Less common symptoms include nausea, vomiting and diarrhea.

One of the most discouraging aspects of the flu is how long it takes to recover. Even though the acute symptoms will probably go away in a week or so, the general weakness and fatigue can hang on for weeks.

For healthy, young adults, the flu is a casual misery that seems to accompany the dreariness of late winter. But, for the very young; those over age 65; or anyone with heart disease, diabetes, kidney disease, asthma or any chronic respiratory condition, the flu could be life-threatening. If you fall into one of these categories, you should treat your bout of influenza with respect.

There are two distinct problems with the flu.

The first is that it is highly contagious. Somewhat like a cold, the flu is transmitted through respiratory droplets exhaled, coughed or sneezed into the air.

The second problem with the flu virus is that it has an incubation period of 24 to 72 hours; so you can spread it before you even start to feel sick. Even worse, many victims remain asymptomatic — meaning they can spread the virus, but never exhibit its symptoms.

It's not too late to get a flu vaccination, says Dr. Walter Gunn of the Centers for Disease Control in Atlanta, Ga. Dr. Gunn says it takes about two weeks for the vaccination to become effective. In young, healthy adults, the vaccination is about 70- to 90-percent effective.

It may take longer for the vaccination to kick in if you're over

65, and when it does, its effectiveness rate of preventing the virus drops to 40 to 50 percent, Dr. Gunn says.

But, he adds, if you get the flu after your vaccination, the chances of death or hospitalization are far less likely than if you hadn't been immunized. Also, your bout with the flu will be less severe than if you had not been vaccinated.

There is one cautionary note, however. Those who are allergic to eggs or chicken feathers should not be immunized because the vaccination includes elements of both.

If you get the flu, there are ways to relieve your misery.

❑ Consider taking more vitamin C. Studies show that people taking vitamin C have fewer and milder symptoms and seem to recover from the flu faster. But check with your doctor before taking vitamin supplements.

❑ No one who has the flu has to be told twice to get plenty of bed rest, since fatigue is one of the symptoms. Also, drink plenty of liquids.

❑ Don't take antibiotics because they kill bacteria, not flu viruses. Bathing in warm water and taking aspirin (if you're an adult), acetaminophen or ibuprofen will help ease your fever and aches.

❑ Sore throats respond well to hot liquids laced with honey. Some doctors also recommend gargling with aspirin dissolved in a glass of warm water (or an aspirin-like product) or salt water.

❑ Sore throats also respond well to chewing on cloves (no more than four a day for adults and three for children).

❑ Hot tea with a little honey has long been the home cure for a stuffy nose, and many say chicken soup works even better.

❏ There's also some evidence that hot, spicy foods will clear up your sinuses, your nose and your lungs. A stuffy nose can also be relieved by inhaling steam.

❏ A good, healthy diet won't ward off the flu, but it will help your body fight the virus more effectively.

❏ High levels of mental stress have been linked to respiratory infections and can, therefore, increase your susceptibility to colds and flu. Try to avoid things that might upset or aggravate you.

❏ Try to get adequate amounts of rest and sleep.

Naturally, if you suspect you have the flu — and particularly if you are in a high-risk category — you should talk with your doctor right away.

MEDICAL SOURCES ───────────────────────────
Medical World News (32,4:30)
Science News (140,9:132)

Low stress, clean hands and winter kill cold viruses

Colds account for more absences from work and school and are the cause of more visits to doctors' offices than all other diseases.

So far we have no sure way to protect ourselves from getting colds. Experts disagree on whether cold-causing viruses are transmitted by hand or through the air.

And since there are more than 200 cold-causing viruses, it's almost impossible to track every one.

Airborne cold viruses seem to thrive in cool fall and spring air and then die off in the winter.

But you can't go wrong by washing your hands frequently,

since many of the viruses do live for hours on hard surfaces such as pens, glasses and even towels.

Another cold question revolves around the effect of stress on our immune systems. Stress seems to suppress the body's immune system, which weakens the body's ability to fight off common cold viruses.

Researchers from the National Institute of Allergy and Infectious Disease in Bethesda, Maryland, tested some volunteers for stress and then gave them nose drops loaded with cold viruses.

Of the volunteers who received the virus nose drops, nine out of 10 who were under stress came down with a cold. Only 74 percent of those who were not under stress got a cold from the viral nose drops.

The stressed-out subjects had a higher rate of infection and developed symptoms more often than those who had lower stress levels.

Researchers cautioned, however, that it might be the way people cope with life's troubles that lowers their resistance.

In reaction to stress, people might drink more alcohol, smoke more and might not sleep as well, all of which could make them more susceptible to cold-causing viruses.

The lesson: If you are experiencing stress in your life, stay away from friends who are sick with colds — your chances of catching one just went up.

No matter how careful you are, you probably won't be able to avoid colds altogether.

Studies reveal that young children have about six colds a year. However, as we age, we build up immunity to cold viruses, so that by the time we reach 60, we average less than one cold a year.

Elderly cold sufferers may have genuine symptoms for an

average of 18 days, although they can sometimes last up to 46 days.

MEDICAL SOURCES————————————————————

Medical World News (32,4:24)
The New England Journal of Medicine (325,9:606)
Pharmacy Times (57,2:108)

Stuffy nose, aching head and fever — is it safe to exercise?

Is it safe to exercise when you have a cold?

Exercising with a cold can be fine in some cases, yet leads to more severe illnesses in others.

According to Dr. Edward R. Eichner, professor of medicine and chief of hematology at the University of Oklahoma, you should not work out if you have a fever, aching muscles, a bad cough or other cold symptoms below the neck.

Doing so could increase your chances of turning a simple cold into something more severe while the cold is still in the incubation stage.

Dr. Eichner suggests that exercise is usually safe when your symptoms are above the neck, including sneezing, runny nose and scratchy throat.

Even then, he advises that you take a "test drive" and exercise for a few minutes at about half-speed.

If your head clears and you feel okay, it's probably safe to continue with your exercise routine. But, if each step you take is painful and makes your head pound, then there's probably no point in continuing.

Dr. Eichner also suggests that you should not exercise when symptoms are below the neck, such as fever, aching muscles, loss of appetite and bad cough.

Use your best judgment on how you feel and ask yourself if a workout would benefit you when you're not feeling well—listen to your body.

MEDICAL SOURCE —————————————

The Physician and Sportsmedicine (18,6:120)

Zinc helps zap infections?

Running on empty? You might want to add some natural zinc-containing foods to your diet.

Research has shown that during strenuous exercise, cell-damaging superoxides build up in the body. Over a period of time these superoxides can increase your risk of infection.

Zinc appears to combat superoxides. In one study, runners who took zinc had more active immune systems and fewer upper respiratory infections.

Some natural sources of zinc include meat, liver, eggs and seafood.

The recommended dietary allowance for zinc is 15 milligrams for men ages 25 and older, and 12 milligrams for women 25 and older.

MEDICAL SOURCE —————————————

Medical Tribune (33,9:25)

The future of cold prevention

Not only are there over 200 cold-causing viruses, these tricky viruses are survival experts, changing so rapidly that scientists have found it hard to formulate one medicine that will block all forms.

Here are some new treatments being tested:

❏ A nasal spray that keeps cold viruses from locking into your system. The drawback of this spray is that it must be used six to seven times daily to prevent colds.

❏ Tissues medicated with a cold-killing mixture. They do prevent the spread of cold viruses, but when they were test-marketed, the high cost discouraged buyers.

❏ Virus-proof lotion that can be rubbed on the hands. Prolonged use of this lotion during testing has caused skin irritation.

Until some of these methods are perfected, focus on treating your symptoms when you do get a cold.

MEDICAL SOURCE ———————————————————
Medical World News (32,4:24)

Colic

Coping with colic

Colic or sharp pains in the intestine occurs in many newborns and mysteriously seems to run its course by the time the baby is three months old. Usually, colic begins when the baby is two to four weeks old.

His tummy becomes distended with gas. As a result, he frequently pulls his legs up, screams and passes gas through the rectum.

This is similar to the newborn who is just irritable and cries for several hours a day, usually at about the same time each day.

The two conditions are similar in that it doesn't seem to make any difference what the parents do; the result is the same. Sometimes changing formula or feeding times helps for a while. But, ultimately, time is the cure. Almost all babies outgrow colic, most by the time they're three months old and even in severe cases, by the time they're six months old.

Pediatricians don't know what causes colic or irritable crying, only that it's far harder on the parents than the baby.

Interestingly, colicky babies tend to thrive in other areas. They gain weight well and usually experience overall robust health. The doctors speculate that part of the problem may be the baby's immature nervous system.

The two most important things for the parents to remember are that the condition will pass and that they haven't done anything to make this baby unhappy.

The following suggestions sometimes help:

❏ Some colicky babies seem to do better in quiet surroundings.

❏ A pacifier is often effective.

❏ A baby with colic is usually more comfortable on her tummy than on her back.

❏ Some colicky babies get relief with a hot-water bottle or by being placed across the mother's or father's knees.

❏ Sometimes, the steady motion of a car or a baby carriage will put the baby to sleep.

❏ It's important for the parents to get some relief from the colicky baby, so don't hesitate to hire a babysitter for a few hours each week.

Naturally, the parents should keep in close contact with their baby's doctor to rule out other problems.

MEDICAL SOURCE ——————————————————————
Dr. Spock's Baby and Child Care, Pocket Books, New York, 1992

CONSTIPATION

Simple tips to help improve constipation

It's not a life-threatening illness, but it is extremely uncomfortable, and at this moment, it's affecting over 4.5 million Americans.

Constipation is an uncomfortable, and sometimes painful, condition that people of all ages and from all walks of life suffer from occasionally. Doctors report that constipation causes over 2.5 million doctor visits each year — people just want relief.

The most common cause of constipation is an improper diet and the overuse of laxatives. People don't get enough fiber and liquids in their diets, so they become constipated. Then, they begin taking too many laxatives, which often cause the symptoms to get worse.

However, constipation can occasionally be caused by other health problems. People with colon problems often suffer from constipation because the colon muscles don't work together to manage normal bowel movements. The feces stay in the colon too long and become stiff and hardened, as in constipation.

Other people suffering from dehydration, stroke and Parkinson's disease might also experience delayed colon activity and the resulting constipation. Other illnesses that sometimes cause constipation include hypothyroidism, irritable bowel syndrome, diabetes and kidney diseases.

Constipation can even be a warning sign of colon cancer, if it is present with the following symptoms: anorexia (loss of appetite), weight loss, blood in the stool, extreme fatigue and abdominal discomfort. If you have these symptoms, see your doctor right away. Trying to treat your constipation with laxatives or dietary changes will only delay the treatment of a possible cancerous tumor.

Most people, however, can use simple home remedies to get rid of their constipation.

❑ Add more fiber to your diet. Bran cereals are good sources of natural fiber. If you don't want to add more natural bran to your diet, try a commercial product, such as Metamucil or FiberCon. These products can also provide the fiber that you need to soften your stools and help you avoid constipation. When you add more fiber to your diet, do it slowly. Adding too much fiber to your diet too quickly can backfire and cause more constipation until your body gets used to the new addition. So, to avoid this, add a little fiber at a time, and build up to a larger daily amount. Always follow the instructions on the labels of the commercial fiber products.

❑ Drink at least eight glasses of nonalcoholic, noncaffeinated drinks each day. Often, people become constipated because they don't have enough liquid in their system to soften the stools. Drinking plenty of liquids (especially water) will help you avoid that problem.

❑ Avoid the use of laxatives. The concept of laxatives is good, but, unfortunately, they are addicting and overused. Using laxatives too often damages your colon and eventually makes your constipation problems worse. Stay away from remedies in a bottle, and go for some simple dietary changes instead.

❑ Understand what constipated really means. Some people think that if they don't have three bowel movements a day, they are constipated. That is incorrect. Many doctors say that bowel movements from three times a day to three times a week can be considered normal. Unless you are having difficulty defecating when you feel the urge because your stools are too small and too hard, you probably aren't constipated. Allow your body to maintain its own bowel movement schedule — if your body naturally needs just three a week, don't force it to do more.

❏ Get plenty of exercise. Constipation is sometimes caused (and often aggravated) by too little activity. Spend at least 20 to 30 minutes three times a week walking or exercising in some other way. This helps keep your abdominal muscles healthy and toned, and it will improve your constipation problems. Elderly people and pregnant mothers, who often don't get enough exercise, should remember to exercise regularly. Getting too little exercise can cause or worsen their constipation symptoms.

❏ Use enemas and suppositories carefully and infrequently. Sometimes, for extremely hardened stools, an enema or a glycerin suppository is necessary to help relieve the constipation. However, these methods should be used as a last resort. Using enemas and stool-softening suppositories too often will make your colon "lazy," and it will stop doing its job. This will cause you to be constipated more often. Avoid this dangerous cycle by avoiding enemas and suppositories unless absolutely necessary, and don't start using them regularly.

❏ Do not suppress the urge to have a bowel movement. Many times we ignore the urge because of inconvenient timing. Soon the urge goes away, and the stools become just a little hardened. Constantly ignoring the urge leads to hardened stools and constipation. If you feel the urge, go. Waiting too long can lead to problems later.

❏ Try to manage your body's "clock" and put your bowels on a regular schedule. Eating meals (especially breakfast) often triggers your body's need for a bowel movement. Listen to these urges, and soon your body will signal you regularly. Establishing a daily "schedule" helps avoid constipation. Most people find that right after breakfast is the most convenient time.

❏ Do not strain. Straining often causes hemorrhoids and other problems. The pain from the hemorrhoids is enough to make you avoid bowel movements for a while — which just makes your problem worse. Let your body do the work. The muscles in your colon can pass the stools effectively without you having to strain.

❏ Ask your doctor or pharmacist if any of the medications you are taking cause constipation as a side effect. If so, ask your doctor if she can change your prescription.

MEDICAL SOURCE ─────────────────

U.S. Pharmacist (17,7:21)

Sugar, cream or laxative in your coffee?

Eggs, toast, bacon and a nice cup of . . . laxative?
Laxative it is, if you're drinking coffee.
Recent studies show that both regular and decaffeinated coffee can act as laxatives. One such study involved 14 healthy men and women who drank regular or decaffeinated coffee. Most reported that the coffee stimulated an urge for a bowel movement. And the laxative effect only took about four minutes after drinking the coffee.
 Scientists suspect that the coffee somehow sends a message to the large intestines and stimulates the bowel movement. Women are said to be more affected by the laxative abilities of coffee.

MEDICAL SOURCE ─────────────────

The Atlanta Journal and Constitution (March 28,1991,W22)

Depression

Underactive thyroid gland might be a hidden cause of depression

If you've got a bad case of the blues that you can't seem to shake, you might need to have your thyroid gland checked.

People who suffer from hypothyroidism often experience mental and physical sluggishness and depression.

Hypothyroidism is a condition in which the thyroid gland does not produce enough of its hormone.

In this case, antidepressant medication won't help the true problem.

So, if your antidepressant medications don't seem to be helping, ask your doctor about the possibility of hypothyroidism.

He can help you determine the best course of action to restore proper thyroid function and help you shake the blues.

MEDICAL SOURCE————————————————

U.S. Pharmacist (15,12:78)

Diabetes

Take charge of your diabetes with the diet that is right for you!

Approximately 12 million people in the U.S. are believed to have diabetes.

Over half have been diagnosed and are being treated for the disease. Only a fraction of the six million people who are being treated have been taught basic self-care skills.

An element that is very essential to successfully treating diabetes, yet is the most difficult to manage is — yes, you guessed it — diet. Diabetics can reduce their risk of complications like heart, kidney and eye disease by learning one essential skill: how to eat properly.

Your doctor should teach you how to balance your medicine, exercise and food to maintain the right blood sugar level.

Diabetics need these things:

- The right amount of calories to maintain a reasonable weight.
- Enough high-fiber carbohydrates, such as whole-grain cereals and breads, to provide about 55 to 60 percent of calories.
- Enough protein (eggs, milk, meat and fish) to provide about 12 to 22 percent of calories.
- Fats to provide less than 30 percent of calories; in addition, less than 10 percent from saturated fats like eggs, butter, cheese, meats and organ meats.

If your doctor says that you are a Type-I diabetic, that means that you must eat right and have insulin shots daily to control your diabetes.

But, Type-II diabetics might be able to keep the right balance of blood sugar just by eating properly, without having to take daily insulin.

To coordinate your diet with your insulin shots, your doctor or nutritionist will probably recommend that you eat three small meals and three snacks each day.

Meals that contain a mixture of carbohydrates and a small amount of protein and fat are more satisfying and stabilize blood sugar better than meals that contain just fats, carbohydrates or protein.

The best way for Type-I diabetics to control blood sugar is by eating the right amounts of carbohydrates on a regular schedule every day. Type-I diabetics must take insulin every day.

Another name for Type-II diabetes is noninsulin-dependent diabetes. One of the biggest factors in Type-II diabetics is excess body fat. And since about eight out of every 10 Type-II diabetics are overweight when they develop diabetes, losing weight is the best way to control the disease. In fact, a loss of from 10 to 15 pounds seems to help most Type-II diabetics dramatically.

The main goal is for you and your doctor to design a diet plan that you feel comfortable with and that will fit your lifestyle.

Diet can also help diabetics avoid many of the complications associated with diabetes.

For example, the danger of heart disease for diabetics is two to three times higher than for people without diabetes. This risk makes it necessary for diabetics to maintain healthy levels of blood cholesterol and blood pressure.

High blood pressure also contributes to kidney disease and a form of eye disease called diabetic retinopathy. A diet low in fat and high in carbohydrates and fiber helped diabetics lower their weight, cholesterol and blood pressure.

MEDICAL SOURCES ————————————————————————

U.S. Pharmacist (16,11:22 Supplement)
The American Journal of Clinical Nutrition (54,5:936)

'Work up a sweat' to help prevent this form of diabetes

Vigorous exercise might help prevent Type-II diabetes, a new study says.

Women who engage in vigorous exercise at least once a week have a reduced risk of developing Type-II diabetes, also known as noninsulin-dependent diabetes.

Noninsulin-dependent diabetes affects almost 12 million Americans over age 20.

It is characterized by an increase in blood sugar levels without destruction of the body's insulin-making capacity. In other words, the pancreas turns out normal amounts of insulin, but blood sugar levels keep going up anyway.

Physical exercise appears to lower glucose (blood sugar) levels and enhance the effects of insulin. In addition to reducing your risk of developing this form of diabetes, researchers go as far as to say that physical activity might prevent its onset.

Researchers studied over 87,000 women 34 to 59 years of age for eight years. They found that physical activity can help your body maintain the proper glucose level as well as help transform glucose into energy.

Regular exercise seems to be effective in reducing the risk regardless of weight and age, the study shows.

Another study shows that highly active lifestyles can cut your risk of Type-II diabetes by 41 percent. Doctors in the study analyzed nearly 6,000 nondiabetic male students at the University of

Pennsylvania between 1928 and 1947. The students later responded to follow-up questionnaires in 1962 and 1976.

The risk of developing this form of diabetes increased threefold for men whose parents had diabetes, doubled for men with high blood pressure, and was also doubled for men 55 years of age or older. There was a steady decline in the risk with increasing levels of exercise. The study suggests that people at high risk of developing mid-life diabetes should use regular exercise and proper diet to combat the risk.

Some of the strongest factors for developing Type-II diabetes are obesity, a family history of diabetes, high blood pressure and increasing age over 40 years. According to the study, 80 percent of people with Type-II diabetes are obese.

Rena Wing, a diabetes researcher at the University of Pittsburgh, says that even though you can't modify your age or family history, you can increase your activity. Talk to your doctor about what kind of exercise is best for you.

MEDICAL SOURCES ——————————————————————

The Lancet (338,8770:774)
The New England Journal of Medicine (325,3:147)

If you have high blood sugar, high blood pressure could be right around the corner

As early as 1968, researchers reported that men with high blood sugar, or glucose intolerance, had a greater chance of having high blood pressure.

High blood sugar is a condition in which the body doesn't use sugar efficiently. This results in an abnormally high amount of sugar in the bloodstream.

Dr. V. V. Salomas and his colleagues studied 945 men from the middle 1960s to the late 1980s.

The researchers found that the men in the study with high blood sugar went on to develop high blood pressure. The study confirmed that men who develop high blood pressure often experience glucose intolerance first.

Dr. Norman Kaplan suggests that testing now done for diabetes should also give early warnings for high blood pressure. Dr. Kaplan says that you should be especially concerned if you are overweight in the upper half of the body.

Being overweight is a major cause of diabetes and high blood pressure.

If you are a diabetic, be sure to keep a close watch on your blood pressure by regular visits to your doctor.

If you have high blood pressure, have your blood tested to make sure your blood sugar level is normal.

MEDICAL SOURCE —————————————————————
Medical Tribune (32,6:9)

Spare tire could signal diabetes

Although your car's spare tire is considered a safety feature, the spare tire around your waist could signal that trouble lies ahead.

People who carry fat around the middle are more prone to noninsulin-dependent diabetes than lean people or those whose fat is distributed more evenly.

This is especially true for women, according to researchers, although they are not sure why.

MEDICAL SOURCE —————————————————————
The American Journal of Clinical Nutrition (53,5:1312)

Diabetic retinopathy

Q. What is diabetic retinopathy?

A. It is a disorder in which the small blood vessels on the retina of the eye might die or leak blood into the eyeball. Some people develop retinopathy as a result of diabetes.

Q. How will I know if I have diabetic retinopathy?

A. You might see floating spots, streaks, lines or a hazy cloud in your vision. You might feel pressure in your eyes and have problems seeing color and light.

Q. Can retinopathy be prevented?

A. No medical treatment can prevent diabetic retinopathy, and about 60 percent of people who have diabetes for at least 15 years develop retinopathy. It is now the leading cause of new cases of blindness among people 24 to 74 years of age.

Q. What is the treatment for diabetic retinopathy?

A. For about 20 years, ophthalmologists and retinal specialists have successfully used laser surgery to halt the progress of retinopathy. In some cases, laser treatment can restore sight to people who have lost some vision to diabetic retinopathy.

Q. Can my family doctor check my eyes for retinopathy?

A. It is best to have your eyes dilated and tested by a retinal specialist or an ophthalmologist who specializes in retinopathy.

Q. When should diabetic people have a test for diabetic retinopathy?

A. If you are below the age of 31, see your ophthalmologist five years after you develop diabetes, then yearly after that. If you are 31 or older, see your ophthalmologist when you are diagnosed with diabetes, then on a yearly basis. If you are diabetic and you become pregnant, see your ophthalmologist within the first three months of your pregnancy.

Q. Can I do anything to prevent the development of retinopathy?

A. You might be able to prevent retinopathy by keeping your blood sugar and blood pressure under strict control. You might also want to sleep with your head elevated by an extra pillow to relieve pressure on your eyes. Diabetic retinopathy develops more often in older people, those who have been diabetic for a long time, and people who must take insulin.

Diabetics are also in danger of developing cataracts and glaucoma. If you have diabetes, ask your doctor to refer you to an ophthalmologist or retinal specialist for regular checkups.

MEDICAL SOURCE ————————————————

U.S. Pharmacist (16,11:36, Supplement)

Change in time zone? Adjust insulin dosage

Flying across several time zones means more than just jet lag for diabetics.

Doctors suggest that people with diabetes should increase their insulin doses when traveling west and decrease the doses when traveling east. For westward travel, the time zone shift should be covered by one or two injections of short-acting insulin while on the plane. However, don't try a "do-it-yourself" adjustment of your insulin schedule. If you're planning a long plane trip, talk to your doctor before you leave about dosage changes.

MEDICAL SOURCE ————————————————

British Medical Journal (301,6749:421)

Relief in sight for diabetics suffering from aching feet

The age-old complaint, "Oh, my aching feet!" takes on a new meaning when people suffering from diabetes experience foot problems.

But a recent invention promises relief for the 12 million diabetes sufferers in the United States.

A new kind of sock with extra, high-density padding in the common pressure areas of the foot offers relief from the blisters, lesions and severe foot pain that plague most diabetics.

The yarn used in these socks helps reduce the amount of moisture next to the skin. This helps prevent blistering and other skin problems, such as athlete's foot.

The new "diabetic sock" received the Seal of Acceptance from the American Podiatric Medical Association.

For more information on the sock, contact the Thorneburg Hosiery Co., Inc., 2210 Newton Drive, Statesville, NC 28677, or call (800) 476-0209.

MEDICAL SOURCE ——————————————————

Thor•Lo, a news release published by Thorneburg Hosiery Co., Statesville, N.C., Dec. 13, 1990

Diabetics have greater risk of dental disease

Diabetes sufferers, take special care to keep your pearly whites in pearly condition.

Studies reveal that people with noninsulin-dependent (Type II) diabetes have a great risk of developing periodontal disease.

Periodontal disease is the inflammation or degeneration of the tissue that surrounds and supports the teeth, and it is a major cause of tooth loss in adults.

Apparently, periodontal disease is more common in people

with diabetes.

So, diabetics should take extra care to brush and floss their teeth regularly as well as maintain routine dental exams.

MEDICAL SOURCE ————————————————————

Pharmacy Times (56,10:92)

Put that insulin up your nose?

Would you rather sniff your insulin than inject it?

That might be one of your options in the near future: an insulin nose spray.

A new, "intranasal" insulin spray seems to be more effective in controlling blood-sugar levels than injected insulin. The latest study included 10 Type II diabetics, ages 20 to 50.

They were given an injection of insulin or an equivalent dose of insulin nose spray 30 minutes before breakfast.

Among those who used insulin nose spray, their blood-insulin levels returned to normal ranges much more quickly than those who used hypodermic injections.

Scientists speculate that using a nose spray form of insulin might remove a diabetic's need to snack throughout the day.

For diabetics, frequent snacking is now necessary to offset low-blood-sugar levels experienced with injected insulin.

The only reported side effect associated with the intranasal insulin spray was temporary irritation of the nasal passages.

The intranasal insulin spray is expected to give more flexibility and control in adjusting insulin doses.

Scientists hope this will greatly improve a diabetic's quality of life.

MEDICAL SOURCE ————————————————————

Medical Tribune (32,13:1)

DIAPER RASH

Diaper downers — how to get rid of diaper rash

Diaper dermatitis (diaper rash) is one of the most common irritations in a baby's (and mother's) young life. And while the rash is certainly irritating and distracting, it is usually not serious. A few simple remedies will restore peace and quietness to your happy home.

There are four different kinds of diaper rash that commonly affect your children. The most common kind is known as chafing dermatitis. Children suffering from this kind of diaper rash have a mild redness and scaliness around the buttocks, waist and thigh areas where the diaper comes into contact with the skin.

The second type of diaper rash causes well-defined areas of redness only in the skin folds.

A third type of diaper rash causes shallow "ulcers" or blisters over the whole area where the diaper touches the skin.

The fourth kind causes a beefy redness over the diaper area and oval sores filled with pus around the outer edges of the diaper area.

What causes the rash? Well, many doctors think that the skin irritation comes from too much contact with urine or the baby's bowel movements. Doctors also think that the physical rubbing of the diaper against the baby's skin can irritate the skin and set up the right conditions for a rash. The tighter the diaper, the greater your chances of the baby getting a rash. And, some babies are just more likely to get them because of sensitive skin.

Follow these simple tips to help rid your home of this diaper disorder:

❑ Change your baby's diaper regularly. Don't allow your baby to wear a dirty diaper any longer than necessary. And even if it isn't dirty, it is a good idea to change the diaper on a regular schedule (once every few hours or so). If you use child care, make sure the workers know to change your child's diaper regularly.

❑ If your baby has a tendency to get diaper rashes easily, try switching to a more absorbent diaper that pulls moisture away from her skin.

❑ Try letting your baby go diaperless for a little while. Place the baby on her stomach in her crib on top of some towels and a liquid-proof mattress liner, and let her bottom "air out" for a bit. This will cool off the skin and help cut down on irritation. But don't leave her bottomless for too long — that's a messy accident just waiting to happen!

❑ When you are bathing your baby or cleaning her after changing the diaper, try to avoid rubbing the skin in the diaper area with a towel. Rubbing with a towel can irritate the tender skin. Instead, blot the skin gently, or use a blow dryer set on its coolest temperature. If you use a blow dryer, don't hold it too close to your baby's skin. Hold it far away enough that you can just feel the air against your baby's skin.

❑ Zinc oxide, petroleum jelly, calamine and cocoa butter are each examples of skin protectants that you can use on your baby's skin before putting on the diaper.

❑ If your baby is at least 2 years old, you can use an over-the-counter cortisone cream to help clear up the rash. But never use the cream for longer than a week at a time to avoid any possible side effects in the baby.

❑ Don't use boric acid on diaper rash. Boric acid can be absorbed into the blood through irritated skin and can make your baby very ill.

❏ Don't use anti-rash creams or powders on your baby unless you need to. Many babies don't get diaper rash, so don't use them "just in case" unless your baby begins to suffer from rashes.

❏ If you notice isolated areas of dermatitis or unusual sores on your baby's skin, see your pediatrician. That could be a yeast infection or a bacterial infection that needs medication to clear up.

❏ If your baby is drinking juices, try giving her some watered-down cranberry juice. The cranberry juice changes the makeup of the urine just a bit, and that little change might be all your baby needs to avoid skin irritation from urine.

❏ Don't put the diapers on so tightly. And get larger diapers as your baby grows. If the legs or waist are too tight, it will irritate or chafe the skin and increase the baby's chances of getting a rash.

MEDICAL SOURCE ——————————————————

U.S. Pharmacist (17,6:26 Supplement)

DIARRHEA

How to undo diarrhea

Although runny bowel movements can be an unpleasant inconvenience for most folks, it can turn into a serious problem. In fact, almost 30,000 people die each year in the United States from diarrhea.

But, for most cases, treatment for diarrhea is fairly simple: Discontinue food and substitute clear liquids, such as apple and other fruit juices or carbonated beverages.

Unfortunately, these liquids are high in carbohydrates, which give you energy, but they don't replace the sodium that your body needs. Diarrhea drains a lot of fluid electrolytes from your body, a loss that can cause serious problems. This makes these fruit juices and carbonated beverages insufficient in severe cases of diarrhea.

Consider the benefits of adding commercial rehydrating products. Rehydrating means restoring fluids to a person who has been dehydrated. These pre-mixed solutions are a balance of glucose, electrolytes (different salts needed by the body) and water.

Small, regular feedings of these liquids have proven to be helpful in treating mild, moderate and severe dehydration.

Another suggestion is to start solid foods within 24 hours of the initial diarrhea. The rehydration fluid can be continued, but solid food should not be ignored.

Begin with a diet rich in carbohydrates, but lactose-free. Bananas and rice cereal are good choices. Start with small amounts and gradually increase your intake and variety of foods until you are back to normal.

Check with your doctor if this doesn't help you — it could be something more serious.

MEDICAL SOURCE ————————————————————

American Family Physician (43,3:991)

DRUG REACTIONS

Tips on how to avoid possible negative side effects from your prescription medications

❑ Ask your doctor to prescribe the least expensive type of drug that will do the job.

❑ Try to deal with one pharmacy. Saving a little might cost a lot later.

❑ See as few doctors as possible.

❑ Ask your doctor to prescribe as simple a schedule as possible, yet still be effective.

❑ When you get a new prescription, be sure to remind your doctor about medication you are already taking. Some medications work against each other.

❑ Take your medication even if you don't "feel" it working. The effects of some medications are not noticeable early on.

❑ Ask your doctor or pharmacist for the prescription data sheet for your drug. It has all of the information you should need.

❏ Review your medication schedule often enough to keep it fresh in your mind.

MEDICAL SOURCE ─────────────────────

Drug Therapy (19,11:45)

What you and your doctor should know about your medications

Before you take a prescription or nonprescription drug, ask a few basic questions that might shorten your illness and prevent side effects for you.

You should ask the following:

> • The name of the drug, and what it is supposed to do.
> • When and how to take the drug, and for how long.
> • Whether you should avoid any foods, drinks, activities or other drugs while taking the drug.
> • What are the side effects and what you should do if side effects occur.

You should tell your doctor the following:

> • The names of all prescription drugs you are now taking.
> • If you are allergic to any medications.
> • If any medicine gives you side effects.
> • Whether you are pregnant or trying to become pregnant.

MEDICAL SOURCE ─────────────────────

FDA Consumer (24,9:27)

Dangerous side effects from diuretics can easily be avoided

Suffering from high blood pressure? Taking diuretics to help control your high blood pressure?

Then you might want to check your dosage.

Diuretics, sometimes called "water pills" because they increase the body's output of urine, have a proven track record of controlling high blood pressure. Unfortunately, they sometimes have potentially dangerous side effects as well.

New reports indicate, however, that some diuretics may not deserve a bad reputation after all. Usually, the problems occur only when people take a higher dosage than necessary to control blood pressure.

The correct dosage can mean the difference between safe blood pressure control and serious side effects.

So if you're taking a diuretic for high blood pressure control, ask your doctor to double-check the dosage and make sure you're taking the smallest dosage that will control your blood pressure without increasing your risk of bad side effects.

Don't stop taking your diuretic or change the dosage without your doctor's advice.

MEDICAL SOURCE ————————————————

Medical World News (31,18:13)

Nagging cough that just won't go away? It could be your medicine

Suffering from a dry, hacking cough, and you can't seem to get rid of it? It could be your high-blood-pressure medicine.

Researchers have discovered a new, unpleasant side effect of ACE inhibitors (a group of medicines used to treat high blood pressure). These drugs might lower your blood pressure, but they can also cause harsh, dry coughing.

In one study, 20 people complained of a persistent, hacking cough that worsened at night. They had all been suffering for weeks, with no idea why. Some coughs became so severe that they caused other serious problems, such as urinary incontinence, and rectal and vaginal muscle strain. Within about five days of discontinuing the ACE inhibitors, everyone's cough had gone.

Scientists think that the ACE inhibitors might cause coughing because they restrict the action of some inflammatory enzymes in the body.

If you are taking ACE inhibitors for your blood pressure, and you develop some unexplained coughing, check with your doctor to find out if your medication is to blame.

Common ACE inhibitors include the following:

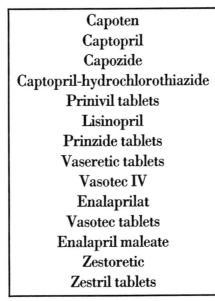

Capoten
Captopril
Capozide
Captopril-hydrochlorothiazide
Prinivil tablets
Lisinopril
Prinzide tablets
Vaseretic tablets
Vasotec IV
Enalaprilat
Vasotec tablets
Enalapril maleate
Zestoretic
Zestril tablets

MEDICAL SOURCE ——————————————————

American Family Physician (42,5:1357)

Allergic reactions to medications can occur even after years of use

Taking medication for high blood pressure is a necessary way of life for many people, but it isn't totally risk-free.

Doctors are warning consumers about the possibilities of potentially fatal reactions associated with ACE inhibitors occurring several years after the beginning of the treatment.

Allergic reactions are most common in the first few months of treatment.

But don't be lulled into thinking your tolerance of the drug is "guaranteed" just because you've taken it for a number of months or even years.

You can develop a sensitivity to a drug after years of use and suddenly experience an allergic reaction.

Allergic reactions can take the form of severe tongue swelling, airway obstruction and inability to swallow.

Check with your doctor or pharmacist to learn what allergic reaction symptoms are most common for the medications you use.

If you are taking ACE inhibitors for regulation of your blood pressure, make sure you report any strange reactions — even a mild reaction, such as tongue swelling that goes away on its own — to your doctor immediately.

MEDICAL SOURCE ─────────────────────────

Emergency Medicine (22,21:11)

Age + medication can sometimes = danger for elderly people

For the elderly, forgetting important information about their drugs can be dangerous.

Aging is an independent risk factor for the development of

negative side effects from drugs.

This might be due in part to the fact that older people tend to have more illnesses and consume more drugs than younger people, the report says.

Who most often forgot?

Older people who live alone, use two or more medications at the same time, and use two or more pharmacies tend to forget important information about their medication.

People who use more than one physician also have a greater chance of misusing prescription drugs, as do people who are able to remember only part of their prescription instructions.

Which drugs? The drugs which were most often the cause for hospitalization due to failure to follow directions are: furosemide, theophylline, warfarin, prednisone and others, including aspirin, insulin, nitroglycerin, methyldopa, and verapamil.

MEDICAL SOURCES

Annals of Internal Medicine (114,11:956)
Archives of Internal Medicine (150,4:841)

Lupus-like symptoms from your cholesterol medication?

Can your medication cause symptoms of lupus?

It did for some people who were taking the drug lovastatin.

Two new case studies show that lovastatin is a potential cause of drug-induced lupus syndrome.

Lovastatin usually is prescribed for high cholesterol levels. Now, it has joined the ranks of nearly 50 other drugs considered to be potential causes of this syndrome.

Symptoms of the lupus syndrome include joint pain, mild jaundice, fatigue, fever and swollen joints.

Those people who had drug-induced lupus syndrome from the

lovastatin got relief after they stopped taking the drug.

If you are taking lovastatin and have any lupus-like symptoms, talk to your doctor right away.

MEDICAL SOURCE —————————————————

Archives of Internal Medicine (151,8:1667)

EAR PROBLEMS

Simple tips for healthier ears:

❑ Don't insert any object into your ear canal.

❑ Avoid forceful nose blowing.

❑ Stay away from extremely loud music and loud firearms. They can cause loss of hearing.

❑ Wear earplugs when your ears are exposed to prolonged environmental noises and as needed in water sports and swimming.

❑ If you think that there is a live insect in your ear, don't try to lure it out with a bright light. This can make it crawl deeper into the ear. Instead, try dropping in a bland oil (like mineral oil) and floating the insect out.

❑ If something solid gets down into the ear canal, don't use oil or water. It can cause the foreign body to go deeper or cause the ear to swell.

MEDICAL SOURCES ———————————————————

Taber's Cyclopedic Medical Dictionary, Edition 16, F.A. Davis Co., Philadelphia, 1989
The Merck Manual, Sixteenth Edition, Merck Research Laboratories, Rahway, N.J., 1992

Earwax: What it is and what to do about it

Most people don't understand the purpose of earwax and consider it to be something dirty that has to be cleaned out. Others feel that wax buildup causes infections. But, according to researchers, earwax has gotten a bad rap over the years.

Earwax is a friend, not a foe. Earwax is a natural product that your body makes to help keep foreign particles from getting to and damaging your fragile eardrum. It protects your ears from infection. It traps dust, sand, insects and other particles and keeps them from getting into the ears.

In most cases, earwax gets rid of itself by traveling outward, drying up and flaking away. Unfortunately, many people have earwax-producing cells in their ear canals that work overtime. You end up with too much wax.

Apparently, you can run into some problems when you attempt to clean your ears out yourself.

The softer wax can get pushed back into the ear, block the canal and get trapped. The wax can become impacted and then you've got trouble.

Other reasons why wax can become impacted in your ears are an increase in the number of hairs in your ears as you age, producing an unusual amount of wax, or abnormally shaped ear canals. Lack of chewing your food properly can also keep the wax from migrating out.

Devices that fit into the ears such as hearing aids, stethoscopes or molded earpieces can also create problems leading to excessive earwax.

Too much wax in your ears can cause hearing problems, ringing in the ear and just simple problems with personal hygiene. Symptoms of wax buildup can range from slight annoyance to severe pain in the ear. It can sometimes cause hearing loss, dizziness and vertigo.

To help treat an overabundance of earwax, use an eyedropper and put two to three drops of mineral oil into each ear, one or two times a day. Use a piece of cotton to hold the oil in your ear.

If you have a lot of wax in your ear, do this oil treatment for seven to 10 days. Then after your ears clear up, use the mineral oil once or twice a week to keep your ears from building up too much wax again.

If this doesn't work, your doctor might recommend an over-the-counter product, a prescription medication or an ear syringe.

Most drug stores or pharmacies sell over-the-counter ear cleansing kits. The kits include some eardrops that will soften the hardened wax buildup. After the wax is softened, you can use the syringe from the kit to gently cleanse your ear with clean, warm water. The wax should flow right out of your ears into the sink or shower.

If you still notice a ringing noise, try some more drops and repeat the cleansing process.

If your ears become red and irritated, put the kit away and try it again the following day. Your ears aren't used to so much attention and might need a rest from the cleaning.

Removing normal amounts of wax from your ears can cause problems.

Taking away the fluid and its normal function can sometimes lead to dry ears. Your ears can become itchy due to the dryness.

It can also lead to conditions such as swimmer's ear, because earwax helps to waterproof your ears. When you remove the oily coating, it can leave your ears unprotected.

Your doctor can clean the wax out of your ears if you have difficulty doing it yourself. Your doctor will also clean out your children's ears — special care should be taken with children because their ear canals are shorter than adults, and it is easy to damage the tender eardrum.

Never use your finger, a hairpin, a pencil, tweezers, sharp objects or even cotton swabs to clean your ears. Putting these things in your ear could push the wax deeper into your ear and even damage your eardrum.

MEDICAL SOURCES ————————————————————

Postgraduate Medicine (91,8:58)
U.S. Pharmacist (17,4:20)

Temporary deafness a side effect from a common antibiotic drug

Are you taking a drug that can cause hearing loss? You might have used it many times without even thinking about it. Your friends and family have used it.

But for one woman, using it resulted in temporary deafness.

The culprit: erythromycin — one of the most commonly pre-scribed antibiotics in America.

This 77-year-old woman had been coughing and suffering with a fever for about two weeks. Her doctor prescribed a common treatment, the antibiotic erythromycin for nine days.

One day after she started taking the medicine, she noticed her hearing began to deteriorate rapidly . A hearing test revealed serious hearing loss.

After nine days, she stopped taking the erythromycin, and her hearing improved about two days later.

Another hearing test showed complete recovery of her ability to hear.

Apparently, the temporary deafness was caused by the buildup of the drug in her body, leading to ototoxicity, an extremely rare side effect.

If you think you might be experiencing side effects from your medicines, be sure to talk to your doctor right away.

MEDICAL SOURCE —————————————————————

British Medical Journal (302,6788:1341)

EPILEPSY

Blue sunglasses help prevent epileptic seizures

Sunglasses with mirrored blue lenses might be more than a summer fashion craze. They might be a new way to help prevent epileptic seizures.

Epilepsy is a complex disorder of the nervous system. A person with epilepsy experiences irregular nerve impulses in the brain that can cause seizures. These seizures range from the person seeming to "drift off" for a moment (as if in deep thought) to the person falling on the floor and going into convulsions.

Epileptic seizures sometimes are triggered by things outside the body. Flashing lights, flickering lights or flickering geometric shapes (as seen on television) are common triggers in people who have "light-sensitive" epilepsy. That's where the blue sunglasses come in.

Investigators recently did a study on the effects of blue sunglasses (and other colored lenses) on epileptic seizures that were triggered by different kinds of light. Eight volunteers (ages 13 to 31) who suffered from epilepsy participated in the study.

They asked volunteers to wear different types of sunglasses: blue lenses, smoky lenses and brown lenses. Then the scientists exposed the volunteers to different kinds of light impulses while they measured the nerve impulse activities in the volunteers' brains.

The studies showed that the light impulses that would normally cause increased nerve activity did not produce the same effects when the volunteers wore the blue sunglasses. Apparently, the blue lenses filter out different wavelengths of light that seem to trigger the seizures.

The brown lenses and the smoky lenses were helpful with a few of the different light wavelengths, but the blue sunglasses seemed to have the most remarkable effects.

Researchers recommend that people with "light-sensitive" epilepsy wear sunglasses with blue lenses, even when they watch television, to help reduce the risk of epileptic seizures.

MEDICAL SOURCE ————————————————————

Epilepsia (33,3:517)

EYE PROBLEMS

Eye problems you can handle

"She's got Bette Davis eyes . . ."

"Don't it make my brown eyes blue . . ."

"When Sunny gets blue, her eyes get gray and cloudy . . ."

It seems that songs and singers throughout the ages have praised the mysteries of the eyes. But when your eyes start giving you problems, there's not a whole lot you want to sing about.

Irritating eye problems usually feel much worse than they really are because the eye tissues are so delicate. And the eyes often need special attention to help clear up the problems. But, fortunately, the special attention can come in the form of simple home remedies.

❑ **A small, swollen nodule** on the eyelid is known as a "chalazion." The nodule comes and goes from time to time and usually is not inflamed, but it can be a little unsightly. Getting rid of small chalazions is as simple as applying hot-cloth compresses to the eyelid in the morning and evening until the swelling goes down. Chalazions that don't go away might need a small dose of medicine from the eye doctor.

❑ **"Blepharitis"** is the inflammation of the edges of the eyelids. The lids look red and inflamed, sometimes covered with scaly skin. Sometimes the lids are swollen and the edges look greasy and infected. This eye disease is not dangerous or blinding, but it is irritating and embarrassing. The best thing to do for this eye disorder is to hold a hot-cloth compress to the infected eyelid for five minutes a couple of times a day. This helps soften the scaly skin and soothe the irritated glands in the eyelid. You can use a mild, nonirritating baby shampoo to wash the eyelid clean of any loose scales, eyelashes or pus. If the disorder does not clear up, your eye doctor can prescribe an eye ointment that will help soothe and relieve any inflammation and infection.

❑ **Allergic reactions** from seasonal allergies are common eye complaints. Red, itchy, irritated eyes can be found everywhere during pollen season. The best thing to do is to wash the eyes out with artificial tears (an over-the-counter saline solution) to get rid of any irritants and the natural chemical histamine that causes the symptoms of hay fever. Taking antihistamine tablets will also help your body cut down on the amount of histamine it releases, and this will help relieve your irritated eyes.

❑ **Keratoconjunctivitis** is an eye disorder that sounds more threatening than it really is. This disorder is the inflammation of the conjunctiva, the thin covering on your eyeball. The main symptom of this disorder is dry eyes. Artificial tears, eye drops which are sold over-the-counter, will help keep your eyes moist and clean from any dust and debris.

❏ **Red, irritated eyes** are something that everyone is familiar with. Eye redness can be caused by many different things, including cigarette smoke and air conditioning. Lack of sleep is a common culprit behind red eyes, as is too many hours straining at a computer screen or book. The thing to remember about common eye redness is to stay away from medicated eye drops. These drops cause the swollen blood vessels in your eyes to shrink and disappear, and your eyes look white again. But the drops really haven't relieved the irritation. As soon as the drops wear off, your eyes turn red again. Instead, use artificial tears (they are just like natural tears) to soothe your tired eyes, and try placing cool compresses on your closed eyes for some quick relief. Try to get more sleep. Use a humidifier to keep the air from being so dry and irritating. And take breaks from your computer or books during the day to keep your eyes from straining for long periods of time.

If you have trouble with your eyes, see your eye doctor right away. But remember that some of the more simple eye irritations can be treated just as well with home remedies.

MEDICAL SOURCE ───────────────────────────

Emergency Medicine (24,7:33)

Sunglasses key to better vision

Sunglasses can be more than a fashion statement.
For some people, they are the key to better vision.
Sunglasses with a yellow tint are a common sight among people who live in areas with lots of sunlight glare, and the reason is

simple: The yellow tint helps improve vision.

Yellow filters in lenses for sunglasses cut out the short (ultraviolet and blue) light wavelengths. These wavelengths are damaging and also cause a blurring effect.

Wearing glasses with the yellow filter improves several aspects of vision, including the contrast sensitivity and apparent brightness under daylight conditions.

To test the positive effects of the yellow filter, researchers studied 20 children who suffered from a visual disorder known as binocular amblyopia. In addition to other tests, each child attempted to read normal print through four colored overlays presented in random order: yellow, red, blue and green.

All of the children agreed that the yellow overlay improved their vision greatly. None preferred any other color. The researchers then gave the children yellow-tinted glasses to wear for three months.

When they were retested three months later, their vision was remarkably better. Six of the children had permanent improvement, even when they weren't wearing yellow-tinted glasses.

The yellow tint seems to cut out the effects of the blue wavelengths of light that cause a blurring known as chromatic aberration.

Wearing the yellow-tinted glasses helped the children develop the mechanisms for coping with chromatic aberration that apparently hadn't developed normally in them.

If your vision seems blurred or hazy in sunlight, consider talking to your eye doctor about yellow-tinted sunglasses.

MEDICAL SOURCE ————————————————

The Lancet (338,8775:1109)

Another smoking danger: It could cause you to go blind!

Smokers, if you still need another reason to quit, here it is.

People who smoke run a higher risk of going blind.

Smoking reduces the blood supply to the optic nerve. Smoking also tends to increase production of fibrinogen, which causes blood to clot and platelets to stick together, says Dr. Sofia Chung of the department of ophthalmology and neurology, St. Louis University Medical Center.

The blockage of blood flow to the eye can cause partial or complete blindness if prolonged, due to a condition called anterior ischemic optic neuropathy (AION).

Some symptoms of AION include blurring, clouding or loss of the upper or lower half of your vision in one eye.

Scientists have not found a cure for the disease, but blood thinning with aspirin seems to help, the article states.

Smokers are at a higher risk for the disease and usually contract it at an earlier age than nonsmokers. The average age for smokers who contract AION is 57, while the age for nonsmokers is 64.

The good news is if you quit smoking now, you can lower your risk of getting the disease. In those people who stopped smoking, the age of onset of AION was the same as that of nonsmokers, says Dr. Chung.

MEDICAL SOURCE ———————————————————

Medical Tribune (32,23:16)

Lower your risk of eye infection; use hard lenses

Soft contact lens wearers alert: The convenience of extended-wear lenses might not be worth the risk of keratitis (inflammation of the cornea).

Eye injuries used to be the main cause of this potentially blinding disease. But, now, it has been reported that soft contact lenses cause over half the new cases of keratitis.

Researchers compared the risk from hard contact lens use, daily soft contact use, and extended-wear soft contact use, and then assessed the way people cleaned and disinfected their lenses.

Poor hygiene is not the reason that people get keratitis, according to John K. G. Dart of the Moorfields Eye Hospital.

Instead, leaving soft contact lenses in your eyes for an extended period of time starts to break down your eyes' resistance to infection. The result can be that you are more vulnerable to keratitis.

If you wear contact lenses and are concerned about getting keratitis, you might consider trying hard contact lenses. The chances that you will get keratitis from hard contact use are only one in 10,000.

The risk is four times greater for daily-wear soft contact lens users, and 21 times greater for extended-wear soft contact lens users.

Researchers recommend that the only times you should choose extended-wear soft contact lenses are when you have to work for 24 hours at a time, or if you have an eye disease like herpes that requires your eyes be covered at all times.

If you are concerned about getting keratitis from soft contact lens use, talk to your doctor.

MEDICAL SOURCES ──────────────────────

The Lancet (338,8768:650)
Medical Tribune (32,20:2)

Avoid 'egg on your face' — Microwaving eggs is no 'yolk'

Exploding eggs? Two women who microwaved eggs and received painful eye damage aren't laughing.

Both women cracked an unbeaten egg into a dish and then microwaved it at full power for a minute. They pierced the yolk of the egg immediately after removing it from the microwave.

In both cases, the eggs exploded in the women's faces and caused temporary eye injuries and severe pain.

The explosion burned the first woman's eyelid and damaged her left cornea. She was in severe pain and had temporary blurred vision. The vision in her left eye was temporarily reduced from 20/20 to 20/200.

The second woman also had severe pain, became teary-eyed and sensitive to light in her left eye. Her vision was also temporarily reduced to 20/200.

Both women were treated with an antibiotic ointment and eye padding. In about a week, their eyes healed and their eyesight returned to normal. Eggs can also explode if you microwave them in their shells. The contents of an egg cooked in the microwave are under pressure and very hot.

To avoid an explosion, be sure to take the eggs out of their shells and pierce the yolks before you cook them in the microwave.

MEDICAL SOURCE ———————————————————
The New England Journal of Medicine (325,24:1749)

Detect this eye disease early with simple test

Looking at the lines on a wall calendar could save your vision. If the lines look broken, distorted or wavy, you might have a condition called macular degeneration.

If doctors are able to catch macular degeneration in time, it could save your eyesight.

Age-related macular degeneration (ARMD) is the most common cause of vision loss in people over 50.

The macula is the area of your eye that is most sensitive to light and is located at the back of your eye in the center of the retina.

If the macula deteriorates, the middle of your field of vision becomes blurred or dark.

Blurred vision is the most obvious sign of macular degeneration.

Or, you might see a "spot" in the center of your vision that moves as you move your eyes.

Another symptom might be that you need more light in order to read clearly and that it takes longer for your eyes to adjust when you come in from being outside in bright sunlight.

The most simple way to test for this disease is to use an Amsler grid. The Amsler grid tests your visual sharpness.

Your doctor can give you an Amsler grid that looks much like a calendar to use when checking your vision.

To check your eyes, cover one eye and look at the Amsler grid or a calendar to see if the area on which you are focusing is clear or distorted.

Then cover the other eye and check it.

If the center of the grid pattern looks broken, distorted, wavy or any of it appears to be missing, visit your doctor right away.

Detecting changes in your vision early could help save your eyesight.

There are two types of age-related macular degeneration: atrophic or "dry" and neovascular or "wet."

Wet ARMD occurs when tiny blood vessels at the back of the

eye begin to leak, causing scarring and loss of central vision.

The neovascular or "wet" kind is most dangerous and can cause permanent vision loss.

Another type of macular disease is called diabetic macular edema. This disease occurs in noninsulin-dependent diabetics.

Diabetics are 25 times more likely to become blind than those people who do not have diabetes, according to the American Academy of Ophthalmology.

Diabetic macular edema occurs more frequently in those people who develop adult diabetes and require insulin.

To minimize your risk of developing age-related macular degeneration, keep your blood pressure under control, stop smoking, wear protective sunglasses and stay out of the sun during the brightest times of the day.

Be sure to see your eye doctor every year, and check your eyes regularly with a calendar or Amsler grid. It could save you from serious vision loss.

For information on poor-vision devices, such as high-powered reading glasses, write to: American Foundation for the Blind, Consumer Products Division, 15 West 16th Street, New York, NY 10011.

MEDICAL SOURCE ———————————————————————

Senior Patient (2,9:39)

FOOD AND DRUG INTERACTIONS

Avoid these foods when you're taking medications

You saw your doctor, got your prescription filled, and now you're set. At least you think you are.

Millions of Americans across the nation often make the mistake of thinking that once you get your medicine, everything will be all right.

But it's not as simple as just popping a pill.

To get the best results from the medications your doctor prescribed, you need to know how to take the drug.

For example, some drugs should be taken with lots of water, others on a full stomach, and still others on an empty stomach.

Following the directions carefully will often determine whether the drug helps you the way it should. Taking medications improperly can reduce the effectiveness of the medication, and is sometimes like not taking the drugs at all.

An important part of getting the most out of your medications is knowing which foods to avoid while taking the medicine. Listed below are some commonly prescribed drugs and the foods you should avoid while taking them.

❏ **Antacids.** These drugs are used to help relieve acid indigestion, heartburn and other mild digestion problems. Some of the more well-known brands of antacids include Alka-Seltzer, Maalox, Mylanta, Gaviscon, Soda Mints and Riopan. While taking antacids, you need to avoid foods or drinks that are very acidic, like fruit juices, sodas and wines. Also cut back on how much caffeine you're drinking. And watch your chocolate intake.

❑ **Anti-gout drugs.** These drugs are used to relieve the buildup of urate crystals in the joints — the situation that causes gouty arthritis. The drugs also help reduce the amount of uric acid in the blood. Too much uric acid causes the urate crystals to form in the first place.

A brand name anti-gout drug is Probenecid. Try to avoid coffee, tea (including herbal tea), sodas and alcoholic drinks while taking anti-gout drugs. Also stay away from sardines, liver, kidney, meat extracts and anchovies.

❑ **Antihistamines.** You take them every winter and spring to help get rid of your cold and allergy symptoms. Some common examples are Benadryl, Nytol and Actifed.

Stay away from drinking a lot of milk or buttermilk when you take antihistamines. Go easy on all vegetables except corn and lentils. And avoid fruits except for cranberries, plums and prunes.

❑ **Aspirin.** Aspirin is probably the most commonly used drug when it comes to relieving headaches, fever, and pain or inflammation. Different brands of aspirin include Bufferin, Anacin, Excedrin and Midol. Don't avoid food when you're taking aspirin products. Just remember to drink a glass of milk or eat a small snack when you take aspirin. Having something in your stomach will help avoid any stomach irritation from the aspirin.

❑ **Bronchodilators.** People who suffer from asthma use these drugs to help clear out their airways. People suffering from emphysema or other lung diseases also use bronchodilators to help make breathing a little easier.

Some name-brand examples include Albuterol, Ephedrine, Epinephrine and Terbutaline. Bronchodilators act by stimulating or exciting your nervous system, so you need to avoid foods or drinks that do the same thing, like caffeine and chocolate.

❑ **Cimetidine.** These drugs are used to treat stomach ulcers. The most well-known is Tagamet. You already know some of the foods to avoid: pepper, chili powder and caffeinated drinks. Also stay away from cocoa and alcoholic drinks.

❑ **Codeine.** This is a drug found in many different types of drugs. It is usually prescribed as a pain reliever or to help control coughing. Your doctor can prescribe different forms of aspirin with codeine or different cough syrups with codeine. Remember to avoid charcoal-broiled meats, brussels sprouts and cabbage while you are taking any medications that contain codeine.

❑ **Corticosteroids.** These drugs are used for a number of things, but mainly for the relief of the pain, swelling and tenderness that comes with any kind of inflammation. One of the best-known corticosteroid drugs is Prednisone. If you are taking Prednisone or other corticosteroid drugs, try to avoid all processed cheeses and cold cuts. Also stay away from TV dinners, canned soups and vegetables, dill pickles and sardines.

❑ **Digoxin.** This is an important drug that is used to help keep your heartbeat regular. These heart medications include Inderal and Lanoxin. Take care to avoid large amounts of caffeinated drinks if you are taking these heart drugs, and stay away from dairy products for at least two hours before and two hours after taking them.

❑ **Diuretics.** Also known as "water pills," diuretics are used to help your body get rid of any excess fluid (swollen ankles, bloated stomach, etc.). Many people with high blood pressure take diuretics to help lower their blood pressure. Some examples of common diuretics are Lasix, Naturetin, Exna, Diuril, Hygroton, Anhydron, HydroDIURIL, Esidrix, Oretic, Saluron, Lozol, Enduron, Zaroxolyn, Diulo, Mykrox, Renese, Hydromox and Naqua.

When you take these drugs, you might need to eat foods that are high in potassium, such as tomato juice, bananas, peanut butter, almonds, milk, asparagus, other fresh fruits and vegetables, dried peas and beans, fresh meats and sunflower seeds. Your doctor might also prescribe potassium supplements. Check with your doctor about your need for potassium. There is a special class of diuretics called potassium-sparing diuretics. Some examples include Midamor, Aldactone and Dyrenium. When you are taking these kinds of diuretics, it is not necessary to add extra potassium to your diet. In fact, if you add extra potassium, you might develop a condition known as hyperkalemia, which is excessive amounts of potassium in the blood.

Ask your doctor about what kind of diuretic you are taking, and whether you need to add extra potassium or avoid extra potassium.

❑ **Erythromycin.** This is one of the most commonly prescribed antibiotic drugs and is used to treat bacterial infections. Avoid drinking any acidic drinks for one hour after taking erythromycin. Acidic drinks include fruit juices, sodas, colas and wines. The acidic liquids reduce the effectiveness of the antibiotic.

❑ **Estrogen.** This hormone-replacement drug offers relief from hot flashes and night sweats that come with menopause. It also helps prevent the dangerous bone loss, known as osteoporosis. A common source of estrogen is the drug Premarin. Women taking estrogen should avoid eating too much salt. Smoking cigarettes is also a big no-no for women on these drugs.

❏ **Laxatives.** These common medications are used to help relieve constipation. You can purchase most over-the-counter laxatives, such as Ex-Lax or Correctol, at your local drug store or supermarket. The important tip to remember about laxatives is this: Don't overuse them. Taking too many laxatives day after day can lead to vitamin and mineral deficiencies. When taking them, stay away from milk products or antacids for at least an hour.

❏ **Nitroglycerins.** These are the well-known drugs that people take to relieve chest pain or angina. People who take nitroglycerin medication should avoid salty foods like chips, processed cheeses, luncheon meats and many canned foods. Also try to limit your alcoholic beverages.

❏ **Thyroid hormones.** These hormone-replacement drugs are given to people who suffer from hypothyroidism (under-activity of the thyroid gland). Avoid eating large amounts of cabbage, cauliflower, kale, turnips, rutabagas, spinach, carrots, brussels sprouts, peaches, beans and soybean products.

MEDICAL SOURCES ———————————————————

Healthline (7,12:12)
Postgraduate Medicine (85,6:87)

Grapefruit juice doubles effects of some blood pressure drugs

Grapefruit. No matter how you slice it, when you hear that word you think of dieting. Soon grapefruit could have a whole new reputation.

In addition to taking those numbers off the scales, it's also helping unexpectedly in taking numbers off the blood pressure gauge. Drinking grapefruit juice with some blood pressure medications seems to double the drug's effect on high blood pressure.

Dr. David Bailey from the University of Western Ontario conducted a study with six people with slightly high blood pressure.

All six were given the blood pressure medication felodipine with either water, orange or grapefruit juice. The results were amazing.

The grapefruit-juice drinkers with the felodipine lowered their diastolic blood pressure by 20 percent, while the subjects drinking water with the medication experienced only a 10-percent drop in diastolic blood pressure. (Diastolic blood pressure refers to the second number in the blood pressure reading.)

The orange juice had no effect and really made no difference in blood pressure readings.

Somehow, the grapefruit juice seemed to increase the availability of the drug in the body and allowed the body to absorb the drug more efficiently.

A few of the volunteers experienced some normal side effects associated with blood pressure medicine. Common complaints were headaches, flushing and light-headedness. The side effects were more common with the grapefruit juice than the water.

Researchers then tested the effect of grapefruit juice on another blood pressure medication.

This time six people were given the drug nifedipine, which also helps lower blood pressure.

Neither the grapefruit juice nor the water had much effect. Orange juice was not tested. This means not all blood pressure medications will react with, or are affected by, grapefruit juice.

However, the study indicates the effectiveness of some blood pressure medications could be influenced by grapefruit juice.

Make sure you ask if there are any known substances (food or drink) that will alter the effectiveness of drugs you take.

MEDICAL SOURCE ———————————————————

Medical Tribune (32,4:9)

Ulcer medicine raises blood-alcohol levels

Enjoy an occasional social drink? If so, the side effects of two commonly prescribed ulcer medications might leave you with some intoxicating side effects.

Recent studies suggest that the ulcer medications cimetidine (Tagamet) and ranitidine (Zantac) can greatly boost blood-alcohol concentrations, even after just one drink.

Cimetidine and ranitidine belong to a class of drugs that inhibits the action of a stomach acid known as gastric alcohol dehydrogenase. Decreasing the activity of this acid helps in the treatment of ulcers.

However, it also increases the amount of alcohol that reaches the bloodstream.

To test the effects of these two drugs on alcohol levels in the blood, scientists gave 20 healthy men (ages 24 to 46) breakfast with orange juice spiked with enough alcohol to equal one-and-a-half glasses of wine.

The scientists measured the blood-alcohol concentrations of the men to establish the baseline level without any drug influence.

Then for the next week, eight men took 300 milligrams of ranitidine per day, six men took 1,000 milligrams of cimetidine per day, and six men took a third, different medication each day. At the end of the week, each of the men received another glass of orange juice spiked with the same amount of alcohol as they had received in the baseline trial.

Compared to the baseline, the men taking the drug ranitidine experienced a 34-percent increase in blood-alcohol concentration. The men receiving cimetidine experienced an amazing 92-percent increase in blood-alcohol concentration. The third drug had no effect on blood-alcohol concentration.

These amounts of alcohol are well within the range of what most people consider moderate social drinking.

The test results indicate that taking the ulcer medications ranitidine and cimetidine lead to significant increases in blood-alcohol levels after drinking a small to moderate amount of alcohol.

Increased blood-alcohol levels cause significant impairment in mental attention and coordination.

So people who are taking either of the two ulcer medications could experience unexpected impairment after drinking only a small amount of alcohol.

In some states, this increased alcohol level might exceed the legal limit set for driving.

Researchers suggest taking extra care when driving or operating machinery for those people who are taking ranitidine or cimetidine along with alcoholic beverages.

MEDICAL SOURCES —————————————————————

Journal of the American Medical Association (267,1:83)
Science News (141,2:28)

FOOD POISONING

How to keep what you eat from making you sick

The familiar groan, "It must be something I ate," is often the explanation people give for an upset stomach, diarrhea or abdominal cramping.

And, unfortunately, your meal is often the source of those symptoms, commonly caused by food-borne illnesses.

In fact, as much as 30 percent of all food-borne illnesses are caused by improper handling of food in the home. These food-borne illnesses are caused by a variety of bacteria that can infect foods you eat every day.

Common symptoms of food-borne illnesses include upset stomach, abdominal cramping, diarrhea, vomiting, headache, fever, fatigue and sometimes blood or pus in the stools. Victims often refer to their illness as "stomach flu," but the influenza virus has nothing to do with most such cases.

Symptoms can occur as soon as 30 minutes after you eat, or they might not show up until days or weeks after you have eaten the contaminated food. The symptoms usually last for a day or two, but sometimes they can last for up to 10 days.

For most healthy people, these food-borne illnesses are not life-threatening. However, they can be very dangerous in children, the elderly or those who are already sick or who have weak immune systems. People who experience severe symptoms should see their doctor right away.

However, the best way to fight food-borne illnesses is to prevent them from occurring. And you don't need to prepare your food in a sterilized laboratory to prevent the spread of bacteria. You just need to follow a few simple safety tips.

Preventing food-borne illnesses starts on your trip to the supermarket.

❑ Always pick up your packaged and canned foods first, and never buy food in cans that are bulging or dented, or in jars that are cracked or have loose or bulging lids.

❑ Look for expiration dates on the food you buy and never buy outdated food, especially among the dairy products such as milk and cheese. Instead, pick the ones that will stay freshest the longest.

❑ Buy eggs that are Grade A or better, and always open the package to make sure none of the eggs is cracked and leaking.

❑ Pick up your frozen foods and meats last, just before going to the checkout counter. And always put these foods in separate plastic bags to keep them from dripping on other foods in your shopping cart.

❑ Another tip: Check for cleanliness in your supermarket. If the place is dirty, especially around the meat and fish counters, it might not be the best place to shop.

❑ Finally, take the food straight home and store properly. If it will take you more than one hour to get home, take an ice chest to help keep frozen and perishable foods cold.

❑ Once you get home, put away the frozen and perishable foods first.

❑ If you are going to store your meat or poultry in the refrigerator, wrap it loosely. Foods that will be stored in the freezer should be wrapped tightly.

❑ Store eggs in their carton on the inside of the refrigerator rather than in the door of the refrigerator where the temperature is warmer.

❑ Here's a tip most people don't know: Don't crowd food in the refrigerator or freezer. Too much food prevents the cold air from circulating properly, and the food will go bad more quickly.

❑ Also, make sure you check any leftovers in the refrigerator each day. You should throw away anything that looks or smells odd.

❑ And, make sure you store any leftovers in tight containers to help prevent spoilage.

Now that you're ready for the food preparation, the first rule is: Keep everything clean.

❑ When cooking, you should always wash your hands thoroughly before starting a meal and after handling any raw meat or poultry.

❑ Keep your work area and countertops clean and uncluttered.

❑ Always keep your utensils clean, and wash them between handling different foods.

❑ Be sure to keep your cutting board clean by washing it thoroughly after each use. And, by the way, untreated, wooden cutting boards are your best barrier against bacteria. While bacteria left in the knife-cut grooves of a plastic board actually breed and multiply, wooden cutting boards appear either to kill or absorb bacteria. They seem to just disappear in a few hours. Glass is also a good alternative.

❑ Never put cooked meat on the same plate that held the uncooked meat unless you first wash the plate. This is very common among people who cook on the outdoor grill.

❏ Always wash fresh fruits and vegetables thoroughly, but don't use soap or detergents on them. Wash only with water.

The second major rule of safe food preparation is this: Keep cold foods cold and hot foods hot.

❏ If a dish is supposed to be served hot, then get it from the stove to the table as quickly as possible. Keep your cold foods in the refrigerator or on a bed of ice until you serve them.

❏ After a meal, put up your leftovers as soon as possible. Never leave food at room temperature for longer than two hours. If you are going to store leftovers, be sure to do it as soon after the meal as possible.

❏ Cut large pieces of meat into slices of three inches or less to help promote cooling and store them in small, shallow containers.

❏ Be sure to remove all stuffing, rice or giblets from your turkey or chicken before storing, and store them separately.

Remember that many kinds of food-borne bacteria can't be seen, smelled or tasted. So after three days, even if the leftovers look fine, it would be better to throw them away.

MEDICAL SOURCE ——————————————————

FDA Consumer (25,1:18)

Deli dangers — what to avoid

If you recently had a deli-prepared sandwich, and you've come down with some flu-like symptoms, you might not be dealing with the flu. You could be suffering from a kind of food poisoning that you got from the deli food.

Food from delicatessen counters, some kinds of soft cheese, undercooked meats and some ready-to-eat foods are the culprits behind a group of illnesses caused by the bacterium Listeria monocytogenes.

Listeria is not a new bacteria. It is found in many types of foods, but it is usually killed when the food is cooked. The problem comes in when foods are not properly cooked (meats) or when you eat "uncooked" foods that are contaminated with the bacteria, like cheeses, deli meats, etc.

Different types of cheeses that have been found to contain the organism include feta, Brie, Roquefort, Queso Blanco and Queso Fresco. These are all soft, white cheeses. So far, scientists have not found problems with hard cheeses, processed cheeses, cottage cheese or yogurt.

If you have eaten some food contaminated with Listeria, chances are, you never knew it, because you never got sick. Most healthy people never notice any symptoms of food poisoning. The people who are in danger are the elderly, pregnant women (and the unborn baby), and people with compromised immune systems, like those with long-term illnesses (cancer, bronchitis, AIDS, diabetes, cirrhosis, etc.).

People who do get sick experience symptoms that include fever, nausea and vomiting, diarrhea and fatigue. These symptoms can progress to a more serious illness, such as meningitis (infection of the brain) or septicemia (bacterial infection of the blood). Pregnant women can experience these symptoms, but they are also at risk for miscarriages, stillbirths or serious illnesses in the newborn (including meningitis).

Elderly people and children have an increased risk of developing pneumonia and heart problems from the infection. And sometimes, just handling food that is contaminated with Listeria can result in skin rashes and lesions.

In most cases, it takes anywhere from one to six weeks for the full-blown infection to show up. But many people suffer from flu-like symptoms a day after they ate the contaminated food.

Although most people can eat contaminated food and not get sick, those who do get sick are in serious danger. In fact, in a recent study, scientists reported that out of 301 cases of listeriosis (infection with Listeria) in the states of California, Tennessee, Oklahoma and Georgia, 23 percent of the people died from the sickness. This can be a dangerous illness.

The Centers for Disease Control speculates that listeriosis infects about 1,850 people and causes 425 deaths each year.

Researchers studied 165 people infected with listeriosis and 376 healthy people. Studies revealed that those with the infection were more likely to have eaten some kind of soft cheese (feta, Brie, or some types of Mexican cheese) or to have bought foods from a deli counter.

The best way to deal with Listeria infections is to do all that you can to avoid getting one. Follow these tips on safe food handling to reduce your risk of food poisoning:

❑ Don't eat raw meats or drink unpasteurized milk products.

❑ Wash your hands and any knives, plates or cutting boards you used when handling raw meat. Never place cooked meat back on the same unwashed plate you used for the raw meat.

❑ Keep raw foods and cooked foods separate from each other when cooking, storing or preparing the foods. If the foods come into contact with one another, the bacteria from the uncooked foods (especially raw meat) could contaminate the cooked foods.

❑ Make sure you thoroughly cook any meat products, including chicken, fish and eggs. Cook raw meat and fish until its internal temperature reaches 160 degrees Fahrenheit. Chicken or other forms of poultry should reach an internal temperature of 180 degrees Fahrenheit before you take it out of the oven.

❑ When eating leftovers, make sure you heat them thoroughly.

❑ When preparing meals, plan your menu so that all the foods are ready about the same time. Don't prepare a dish and then let it sit out for two hours or more while waiting for another dish to finish cooking. If the food is to be eaten hot, keep it hot while it is out. If your dinner is going to be delayed, refrigerate it and reheat it closer to the time of your meal. Leaving the food out at room temperature for two or more hours can encourage the growth of bacteria.

❑ Don't allow any cold foods to sit out at room temperature for longer than two hours. Refrigerate the food until you need to serve it.

❑ Read the labels of your foods. Always refrigerate the foods that require it as soon as you get home from the supermarket. Watch out for expiration dates, and try to use the foods before those dates. The safest rule to use when dealing with old food is this: "When in doubt, throw it out." It's better to be safe and throw away some food than to risk the chance of a bacterial infection.

❑ When storing leftovers, put them in small, shallow, covered containers before refrigerating. This helps the food to cool quickly and evenly.

❑ Keep your refrigerator and freezer clean, and always keep the temperature down to the recommended level.

MEDICAL SOURCES————————————————

FDA Consumer (26,6:9)
Journal of the American Medical Association (267,15:2041)
Science News (141,16:247)

Food packaging leaves bad taste in your mouth?

Have you ever opened a package of food to eat and noticed that the food tasted something like the plastic wrap it was packaged in? If you have, you probably stopped briefly and wondered whether that food was contaminated and unsafe to eat.

The question arises: Am I eating more than just the food?

That's a question that the Food and Drug Administration (FDA) has to answer.

The FDA monitors all packaging that comes into contact with food, whether it is used for transport from the food processor to the grocery to the home, or while it is being stored in the pantry or cooked in the microwave.

And all manufacturers of food packaging are required by law to obtain approval from the FDA for all the material used in food packages before they can be marketed.

Any component of the package that is dangerous or causes cancer in humans or animals cannot be used in the packaging. So, all packages on the market today have been approved by the FDA as safe to use.

Food tasting like the package it came in is annoying, but it isn't dangerous. The problem is known as "off-taste." It is the same thing that happens when you wash out a plastic orange juice jug with soap and water but find that the jug still smells like orange juice — the opposite happens with the food when the food tastes like the package.

Although the problem presents no danger to consumers, food manufacturers know that the problem is irritating, and they are trying to come up with ways to avoid it.

The serious dangers involved with food packaging come in when people use packages for purposes other than FDA-regulated uses.

Bread bags are an example. Some people turn bread bags inside out to pack sandwiches or homemade bread. The ink used on the outside of the plastic bag contains lead, and when this lead-based ink comes into contact with the food, the food can become contaminated with the lead. (Right-side out, the lead-based ink doesn't come in contact with the food.)

A recent study showed that some foods could extract as much as 5 percent of the lead from the ink in as little as 10 minutes. Lead poisoning is a serious condition and can even lead to brain damage if the lead content in the blood is high enough.

Scientists state that the risk of serious lead poisoning from a bread bag is very low. However, they strongly recommend against such use of bread bags.

Food packaging is a big business in the United States with 55 percent of all packaging made in the U.S. going to food packaging. If you have questions about any food packaging, contact the local office of the FDA in your area.

MEDICAL SOURCE ————————————————————

FDA Consumer (25,9:9)

FOOT PROBLEMS

Walk away from aching feet — steps to help with your foot problems

When they're healthy and pain-free, they're ignored and given little care or attention.

But when they start to hurt, it's almost impossible to ignore them. Each step can bring discomfort and irritating pain. And although foot ailments are irritating and inconvenient, they're not uncommon.

Almost 90 percent of Americans suffer from some sort of foot problem from time to time, whether it be as simple as too many hours on your feet at work or as serious as bunions that need corrective surgery.

Common foot problems include the following:

❑ Corns and calluses. These develop much like calluses on your hand develop when you overdo your yard work — from nonstop rubbing of the skin against a hard surface. The skin on your feet (usually around bony areas of the foot) often rubs too much against your ill-fitting shoes, resulting in hard, thickened areas of skin made up of dead skin cells. Calluses are usually flat and found on the bottom of the foot. Corns are raised and are most often found on the toes.

❑ Ingrown toenails are nuisances that develop when the corner of the toenail (usually on the big toe) grows into the neighboring skin. The skin and surrounding tissue become swollen, red and tender. Poor fitting shoes can trigger ingrown toenails. Think comfort, not style, when buying a new pair of shoes.

❑ Bunions are deformities of the joint of the big toe. In this case, the joint of the toe seems to jut outward and rub against the shoe. The tip of the big toe points in the other direction — towards the other toes. Some cases of bunions are inherited; however, bunions can also be caused by shoes that are narrow or pointed in the toe area.

❑ A hammertoe is often more of a cosmetic embarrassment than a painful problem. A hammertoe is a toe that generally is longer than the others (often the second toe) and bends over in a claw-like manner. Although most people just dislike the way their toes look, other people with hammertoes suffer from pain and problems with walking comfortably. It might be hard for some people to find comfortably fitting shoes.

❑ Athlete's foot is also known as "tinea pedis" and is actually caused by a ringworm infection. The infection usually starts in the spaces between the outer three toes and occasionally spreads over the bottom of the whole foot. The skin on the soles of the feet becomes thickened and scaly, and occasionally the toenails get infected and become thickened and distorted.

❑ Smelly feet are really more of an embarrassment than a true problem. Although some people simply inherited a tendency to have a strong body or foot odor, other cases of smelly feet might arise from socks that don't absorb sweat or from shoes that don't allow proper ventilation. In other words, your feet get hot and sweaty, and some shoes and socks won't let them "breathe" and cool off.

If you have ever suffered from any of those foot problems, you know how tired and grouchy sore feet can make you feel. Below are some tips on how to avoid foot problems, and some tips on what to do if you already have some foot problems:

First, buy the right shoes.

❑ Wear shoes that have low heels, wide toes and firm, supportive soles. A well-trained shoe salesperson can help you pick shoes that fit you properly.

❑ When buying new shoes, make sure you buy shoes that don't need to be "broken in." Your shoes should be comfortable from the minute you walk out of that store. Again, a good salesperson will know which shoes don't fit you as they should.

❑ When you try on new shoes, make sure your foot doesn't move around in the shoe, especially around the heel area. The shoe should fit your heel snugly. Also, make sure the ball of your foot rests on the widest part of the shoe.

❑ When buying new shoes, select a pair that is comfortable and well designed. Look for features such as soft leather tops, closed toes, low heels and flexible soles. Try to avoid shoes that have thick seams that will irritate your feet.

Second, wear your shoes correctly.

❑ Wear clean socks or stockings each day. If possible, wear seamless socks, and ask your shoe salesman which socks are most absorbent and will help keep your feet cool and sweat-free. White or light-colored socks and stockings are usually cooler than darker colors.

❑ Always look into your shoes before you put them on. A small pebble or stick could rub against your foot and cause an ulcer before you even realize it.

❑ Avoid wearing the same pair of shoes every day.

❑ Try alternating wearing high and low heeled shoes on different days to help avoid rubbing calluses and to avoid stress on any one muscle group or set of joints in your feet.

❑ Women especially need to choose "sensible" shoes as often as possible. If high heels are necessary at work, try wearing a pair of sneakers with good arch support around the house. If possible, save the high heels for special occasions and use low heels or flats for everyday office wear.

❑ Try using insoles in your shoes to give your feet more cushion and support.

❑ Pain from bunions and hammertoes is occasionally relieved by better fitting shoes or shoe inserts. However, if your bunions or hammertoes cause you pain and discomfort that cannot be relieved by these tips, contact your doctor. Waiting to treat painful foot ailments may make them worse and the treatment more difficult.

Third, take care of your feet properly.

❑ Wash your feet each day with warm water and a mild soap, then dry them thoroughly with a towel. Try to stay away from simple perfumed soaps and instead use soaps that help kill bacteria.

❑ After each bath, use moisturizing cream on your feet after drying them.

❑ Trim your toenails about once a week right after a bath. Trim the nails straight across, without curving them at the edges.

❑ Take care when walking around barefoot, especially outside. Many bacteria, molds, fungi and worms live in dirt, and walking around barefoot exposes you to infection. If you do walk around barefoot, be sure to clean your feet afterwards with a strong disinfectant soap.

❑ Make exercise part of your regular routine. Walking is great for building tone and strength in your feet. Healthy, toned feet don't suffer from fatigue and aches as often as lazy, sedentary feet.

❑ If you suffer from athlete's foot or other fungal infections, clean your bathroom floor and bathtub with a disinfectant. The bathroom is a place where most people go barefoot, and the moist environment is a good place for molds, fungus and bacteria to grow. Walking barefoot there can expose you to infections.

❑ Although athlete's foot will occasionally go away without medication, you will probably need to buy an over-the-counter medication to treat your infection. Follow the instructions on the label, and if the infection does not go away, you might need to call your doctor for some antibiotics to get rid of the infection.

❑ Exercise your feet when they start to ache. Try tapping your toes, flexing your ankles and toes, or writing out the alphabet on the floor with your feet. The exercise helps circulation, which is often all you need to relieve that tired, aching feeling.

❑ For aching feet, try a contrast bath. Soak your feet in very cold water for about one minute. Then move them into hot water and soak them there for a minute. Continue to switch back and forth. This helps increase blood circulation in the feet and relieves foot fatigue.

❑ If you have callused feet, soak them in warm, watered-down chamomile tea or plain warm water for about 10 minutes. Then use a soft brush or a pumice stone on the callused areas.

❑ A moleskin patch might help relieve the pain associated with corns or calluses during the day until the soaking and pumice stone help remove them.

❑ Treat yourself to a foot massage. Use your fingers on the bottoms of your feet and your thumbs on the top. Work up your foot from your toes to your ankles.

❑ If your feet smell bad, try spraying foot deodorant directly on your feet and in your shoes. Underarm deodorant can often be used on your feet for the same effect. Sprinkling powder in your shoes might help absorb any extra moisture and odor.

If you suffer from diabetes, you have to take extra special care of your feet. To keep your feet healthy and free from infection or injury, add these additional safety steps to your list of proper foot care tips:

❑ Keep your blood sugar level within the proper limits. Work closely with your doctor or nurse to learn how you can control your blood sugar level. If your blood sugar gets too high, your diabetes can become dangerous.

❑ Carefully inspect your feet each day. Look and feel all over your feet for signs of injury or infection. Warning signs include the following: blisters, cuts, bruises; signs of infection, such as redness, warmth, swelling, pain, drainage or red streaks; signs of fungal infection, such as itching, scaly skin, cracking, peeling or wrinkling of the skin; or changes in color of the skin on your feet.

❑ If you have lost feeling in your feet due to your diabetes or had foot infections in the past, check your feet more than once a day. Use a hand-held mirror to look at hard-to-see places, or ask a family member to help you inspect your feet.

MEDICAL SOURCES ─────────────────────────

Postgraduate Medicine (89,5:183)
The Merck Manual, Sixteenth Edition, Merck Research Laboratories, Rahway, N.J., 1992
Solutions for Better Health (9:26)

How to tell if your shoes are too small

Doctors are always telling you that your feet will stop aching if you'll buy a pair of shoes that fit your feet. Unfortunately, many people purchase shoes that are too small simply because they think that it's fashionable.

And many other people can't really tell if the shoe is too small or if it is just stiff because it is new.

For a quick and easy way to tell if the shoes you want to buy are too small, get a piece of paper and pencil. Put the paper on the floor and put one bare foot on it. Trace the outline of your bare foot.

Then put the shoe you want to buy on top of that drawing and trace the outline of the shoe on the same paper. If the outline of your foot is larger than (or even the exact same size, in some cases) the outline of the shoe, then the shoe is too small. Go to the next size or half size.

MEDICAL SOURCE ───────────────────────

Emergency Medicine (24,2:141)

These exercises produce healthier feet

You do exercises for your legs, your arms, your stomach, your back and even your hands. But do you ever do any exercises for your toes?

Sounds crazy, but it is not such a bad idea. In fact, if you have trouble with claw toes or hammertoes, these exercises can bring you some much-wanted relief from tired, aching feet.

A claw toe is exactly what it sounds like — the toe is bent over in a claw-like shape. A hammertoe is when the first bone in the toe is fixed in an elevated position, and the second bone is fixed in a bent position. That causes the shape of the whole toe to look like a hammer.

Foot disorders of this kind are occasionally hereditary (you get them from your parents), but sometimes they're caused by ill-fitting shoes, socks that are too tight, high-heeled shoes with pointed toes, and even the covers on your bed.

Yes, the covers on your bed. You see, the pressure from your bed covers can push your toes into unnatural positions if you sleep on your back.

If you suffer from foot disorders, or just tired and aching feet, doing a few simple foot exercises will help bring you some relief.

❏ One of the best things you can do to keep your feet healthy and pain-free is to go barefoot as often as possible. This gives your toes a chance to stretch out, especially if you wear ill-fitting or pointed-toe shoes.

❏ Help relax the muscles in your feet by stretching them. First, extend your toes as far as you can (lift them up and back toward your shins). Then curl them under and hold. Do this several times. Then rotate your whole foot at your ankle joint, as if you were drawing a circle in the air with your toes.

❏ Massage your feet with your hands. Also try soaking them in warm water to relieve the aches of a long day on your feet.

❏ Allow your toes to relax. If your toe knuckles are white when you stand, your toes are probably not relaxed.

❏ Practice proper standing. Your feet are made to support your weight evenly. If you put too much weight on one foot, instead of evenly distributing your weight on both feet, you could begin to notice foot problems. To test your weight distribution, stand barefoot on an uncarpeted floor with your feet shoulder-width apart. If your weight is more on one foot than the other, or more on your heels than your toes or vice versa, you don't have an even distribution of weight. Try to shift your weight so that it is centered, with an even amount of weight on each foot. Practice standing this way for several minutes each morning and evening.

❏ To stretch your toes, place the fingers of one of your hands in between the toes of the opposite foot. Spread your fingers gently to stretch your toes.

❏ Stand up and spread your toes apart so that none are touching each other and you can see space between them. Try to hold your toes spread apart for about 30 seconds. Practice this exercise often (while in the shower, drying your hair, cooking supper, washing dishes, etc.).

❏ If your big toes point inwards towards your other toes, reach down and pull the big toe into its normal position with your hand, and then try to hold it there for 45 to 60 seconds without the help of your hand. Practice this exercise everyday.

❏ If you sleep on your back, and the covers are forcing your toes into unnatural positions, try sleeping on your side to relieve that pressure on your toes.

MEDICAL SOURCE ─────────────────────────

The Physician and Sportsmedicine (20,7:107)

Get back on your feet — how to deal with toenail trauma

Have you ever had to stop playing a game of tennis or basketball before you wanted to because your big toe was killing you?

And when you took off your shoes and socks, you noticed that the toenail of your big toe was black — it looked as if you had dropped a heavy brick on it three days ago.

What you were suffering from is known as an acute subungual

hematoma. What that really means is that you have blood trapped under your toenail. The excess blood puts pressure on the nerves in your toe, and that causes your toe to ache.

This kind of injury can result when you drop something heavy on your toenail. But it can also happen during sports activities. Contact sports and sports that have rapid start-stop motions (tennis, basketball or racquetball) cause repetitive pressure and trauma on the toes.

The continuous trauma and pressure rips and tears the delicate blood vessels underneath your nail. The blood seeps out from the damaged vessels and collects in the space just beneath the nail. The resultant pressure causes the pain you experience.

To relieve the pain and pressure, you do the same thing that you would do for a smashed fingernail that has turned black. You relieve the pressure by letting out the trapped blood.

Many people prefer to go to the doctor's office for this procedure. The doctor can give you a local anesthetic to make your toe numb. Then, he will drill a small hole in the center of the nail with a small medical drill, a hot needle point or an injection needle point. Occasionally two or more holes in the nail are necessary to get rid of all the collected blood.

You can do the same thing at home using a heated paper clip or needle. Just be sure to clean your toe (before and after the procedure) and the needle or paper clip with some antiseptic soap to cut down on the chance of infection.

If your toe continues to ache a day or two after you removed the blood, you could be suffering from a small fracture or break. Check with your doctor to see if you should have the injury X-rayed.

MEDICAL SOURCE ——————————————————————

The Physician and Sportsmedicine (20,7:107)

Take off your shoes for your feet's sake

Remember those long summer days of your childhood when you used to run and play barefooted? And, think about how good it feels to take off your shoes after a long day at work. Ever wonder why being barefoot just feels so good?

Some scientists suggest it's because shoes are not good for your feet.

Apparently, people who live in countries where going barefoot is common (Africa, Philippines and China, for example) have healthier feet than do we shoe-wearing Americans.

The people in those countries seem to have better arch development and fewer foot complaints than shoe wearers, claims the report.

A surprising four out of five adults in America suffer from some type of foot pain from time to time. And, if left untreated, foot problems can get worse and eventually lead to pain in the ankles, legs, knees, hips and lower back.

But until American fashion trends allow barefoot businessmen, a few simple guidelines will allow you to properly care for your feet and help decrease any problems you might have from going barefoot when you can:

❑ Wash your feet daily in warm water, and dry them by blotting with a towel instead of harsh rubbing.

❑ Look closely for any abnormal red spots, sores or ulcers on your feet. If you find anything abnormal, ask your doctor about it right away.

❑ When you trim your toenails, do it soon after a bath or shower when your toenails are softer. Always cut straight across with a toenail clipper, and don't cut your toenails too short.

❑ If your feet sweat a lot, dust your feet lightly with foot powder or plain talc. But don't use cornstarch; it can lead to fungal infections.

Consider going barefoot around the house. It might be better for your feet, and it just plain feels good.

MEDICAL SOURCE ─────────────────────────────

Modern Medicine (59,11:29)

GOUT

Out with gout — how to help prevent future attacks of gout

You swing your legs out of bed in the morning, ready for a full day — only to double over from the searing pain in your big toe.

You've just had your first attack of gout.

Gout is a disease that causes pain and stiffness because of the buildup of crystals in the joints. The crystals are known as monosodium urate crystals, and they develop when there is too much of a substance known as uric acid in the blood.

Urate crystals form much like rock candy forms on a string in a glass of sugar water. The crystals attach to the string because there is too much sugar in the water for the sugar to stay dissolved.

When there is too much uric acid in the blood, the uric acid forms crystals, and the crystals attach to joints and cause pain and tenderness.

According to investigators, too much uric acid in the blood can be caused by a number of things. Some people are born with the tendency to have too much uric acid in their blood — these people are usually treated with medication.

However, other perfectly normal people often develop gout from too much uric acid for two reasons: high-protein diets and weight gain.

Researchers have found that a gain of 12 pounds or more between the ages of 22 and 35 results in a two-fold increase in your risk of developing gout.

What does weight gain have to do with it?

Well, when you gain weight, it shifts your metabolism a bit. Certain functions of the body do not work as well as they did before you gained weight. Getting rid of excess uric acid is one of those functions — gaining weight cuts down on how well your body gets rid of uric acid. That results in too much uric acid in the blood, then gout.

People who have never experienced an attack of gout can prevent it from developing by avoiding weight gain. Those people who are overweight should lose weight to prevent gout from developing.

If you have already experienced an attack of gout, you can prevent future attacks by slimming down. A sensible diet that is low in protein, fat and salt will help decrease the amount of uric acid in your blood and prevent future attacks of gout.

MEDICAL SOURCE ——————————————————

Arthritis Today (5,5:8)

GUM PROBLEMS

How you can give your gums help

Gingivitis is when the gums (what the scientists call the gingiva) swell and become inflamed due to bacteria in plaque, a thin transparent film that sticks to the teeth. If plaque is not removed, it forms tartar, a process that promotes tooth decay.

You can suspect gingivitis if your swollen gums bleed easily when pressed or when you brush your teeth. Left untreated, gingivitis soon progresses to periodontitis, a more serious condition that eventually leads to tooth loss.

The primary cause of gingivitis is poor dental hygiene aggravated by rough tooth surfaces or fillings. Smoking or grinding the teeth also speeds up the process of gingivitis.

To prevent or to treat gingivitis:

- Floss regularly. Have your dentist or hygienist show you how to floss most efficiently.
- Brush your teeth at least twice a day. Your dentist can show you the most effective ways to brush your teeth.
- Massage your gum tissue daily.
- Use an interproximal brush, which is designed to brush between the teeth.
- Have your teeth professionally cleaned regularly.

MEDICAL SOURCES

The Columbia University Complete Home Medical Guide, Crown Publishers, Inc., New York, 1985
Taber's Cyclopedic Medical Dictionary, Edition 16, F.A. Davis Co., Philadelphia, 1989

HAIR PROBLEMS

Hair today, gone tomorrow

See that hair in the wash basin, the steady daily shedding of hair that your combing produces? Don't mourn. That strand has had a normal, hairy life span of about three to five years.

It grew continuously for that long, then rested for about three months. At the end of its rest, it turned loose and came out with your comb.

Give that naked hair follicle just beneath the scalp another three months, and it will grow another strand to start the cycle all over again.

For every 10 of your scalp hairs, nine are growing at about one-third of a millimeter each day (about one inch every two or three months), and one is resting just before shedding. (Eyebrows are different. They have a 10-week growth phase before shedding.) To calm your fears, a normal person loses about 50 to 100 scalp hairs each day just as part of the typical cycle of hair growth.

You lose more hair in certain situations: during severe emotional stress, during rapid-weight-loss diets of under 800 calories per day, after a high fever, after major surgery, after blood loss, and three to four months after childbirth. It may come out by the handful in these cases, but it almost always grows right back within six months or so.

Another cause of hair loss might be medicines you're taking. Blood thinners like warfarin and heparin increase hair loss in about one out of every two people taking them.

Other hair-loss-causing drugs include amphetamines, the blood pressure medicine propranolol, the arthritis medicine oral gold, and L-dopa.

There's one drug that actually causes some hair growth — minoxidil. Originally used as a drug to lower blood pressure, researchers noticed that it seemed to reverse the balding process in some people.

The problem is that it works best in those whose hair loss has just begun. It doesn't help people who've been bald for more than 10 years or whose bald spot is larger than four inches across. And it works only as long as you apply it to your scalp twice a day. If you stop, the new hair growth stops, and your bald spot enlarges again. It ain't cheap, either: the prescription drug costs $20 to $30 per week.

MEDICAL SOURCE ─────────────────────────

   Your Good Health, Harvard University Press, Cambridge, Mass., 1987

The best anti-dandruff shampoos

When your scalp goes into overdrive and starts shedding too much dead skin, you have dandruff. Nobody has come up with a cure for the flaky stuff yet, but some medicated shampoos can help put the brakes on the rate of shedding.

The best against dandruff snow are shampoos containing zinc pyrithione (Head and Shoulders, Danex, and Zincon, for example).

Next best are shampoos containing sulfur and salicylic acid (Sebulex, Ionil and Vanseb).

Third in line are those with so-called tar (Ionil, Zetar, Sebutone and Pentrax).

Last in effectiveness are standard, nonmedicated shampoos that contain detergents. But these must be used at least every other day to keep the dandruff shower under control.

MEDICAL SOURCE ————————————————

Your Good Health, Harvard University Press, Cambridge, Mass., 1987

Out with oily hair

Top fashion models usually are not born with shiny, bouncy, beautiful hair. It takes a little effort to maintain gorgeous tresses, they say.

First, even though healthy hair needs some oil, too much leaves hair looking limp, stringy and flat. To prevent oily hair, do what the models do:

- Wash hair daily, preferably in the mornings.
- Use a shampoo formulated for oily hair.
- Leave the suds on the hair for several minutes.
- Keep your comb and brush squeaky clean.
- Choose a simple hair style.
- Set your dryer on a medium or cool temperature. (High heat might activate sweat or oil glands.)
- Rinse hair with lemon juice or vinegar diluted with water and poured over the hair during the final rinse.
- Blend two egg yolks with a couple of drops of lemon juice; work into the wet hair and leave on for several minutes before rinsing.
- Don't wear tight hats or bands.
- Comb your hair; don't brush it.
- Since perms and coloring are well-known drying agents, they are sometimes used as treatments for overly oily hair.

MEDICAL SOURCE ————————————————

The Ford Models' Crash Course in Looking Great, Simon and Schuster, New York, 1985

Dealing with ingrown hair

Ingrown hair is a feature of two conditions, pilonidal sinus and pseudofolliculitis barbae.

In the former — pilonidal sinus — one or more hairs become trapped in the skin between the buttocks, causing a painful swelling or an ulcer from which fluid and pus may leak. The condition is most likely to occur in young, overweight men who have a lot of body hair.

Often in the early stages, the fluid and the hairs can be removed. In all stages it's important to keep the infected area dry and clean.

Pseudofolliculitis barbae is when the facial hairs become trapped and small swellings, often filled with pus, occur. The condition occurs most commonly among black males. The easiest way to deal with it is to grow a beard.

MEDICAL SOURCE ──────────────────────────────

The American Medical Association Family Medical Guide, Random House, New York, 1987

HANGOVER

Hang the hangover

In the movies, hangover symptoms — headache, fatigue, nausea, vomiting, no appetite, raging thirst, sweating, poor vision, depression, giddiness — often seem amusing. But in real life, they are the unfunny and painful result of too much alcohol in the system, causing an unbalanced biochemistry in the body. The feeling of dehydration occurs because alcohol is a diuretic.

The first and best way to avoid a hangover is not to drink. The second best way is not to drink to excess. For many people, excess means when they "get a buzz." Other ways to avoid a hangover include the following:

- Set reasonable limits for yourself and learn to say no.
- Drink slowly.
- Dilute your drinks with water or other nonalcoholic beverages.
- Don't drink by yourself.
- Smoking makes the hangover worse.
- Eat a full meal before drinking; fatty foods are good choices because the fat seems to coat the stomach and cut down absorption of alcohol.
- Drink plenty of nonalcoholic liquids.

Most alcoholic drinks contain added coloring and flavoring substances. Different substances in different combinations combined with the alcohol are an almost certain formula for a hangover, say medical experts. The alcoholic beverages with the highest amount of these headache-producing substances are brandy, bourbon and red wine.

Although there is little evidence that one alcoholic beverage causes less severe hangover symptoms than another, drinking several different kinds of alcoholic beverages during a bout does seem to produce more severe hangovers.

Should you have a hangover, the following might help:

❏ Two aspirin or buffered aspirin, or antacid for stomach upset.

❏ Lots of nonalcoholic beverages, particularly fruit juices loaded with vitamin C.

❏ Sweet, bland foods.

There is no evidence that a "hair from the dog that bit you" will do anything but make the situation worse. Obviously, if your hangover is caused by too much alcohol in the blood stream, having more will not help.

The only "cure" for a hangover is aspirin, (nonalcoholic) liquids, sleep and time.

MEDICAL SOURCE ——————————————————————

The American Medical Association Family Medical Guide, Random House, New York, 1987

Headaches

Heading off the pain in your head

It can be mildly bothersome to horribly incapacitating. It affects men, women and children alike, and it can spring up at any time without a moment's notice and ruin the rest of your day. And it affects at least 30 percent of the American population each year.

"It" is a headache, and it has become a complaint that almost everyone can sympathize with because of personal experience with one.

There are several different types of headaches, each having different causes or triggers, and different headaches require different remedies.

The first thing to do is to figure out what kind of headache you have.

Tension headaches are the most common types of headaches that people seem to suffer from. These are the headaches that come up when the day gets hectic at the office, when your teen-age son plays his music too loud and refuses to turn it down, or when you have just run yourself into a frazzle without stopping or slowing down to rest or relax.

Tension headaches tend to affect the whole head rather than just one section of the skull. People often describe them as feeling like a weight on the top of their heads or a tight band around their heads. A tension headache may last for days at a time and happen several times each week or month.

Some people suffering from tension headaches will feel slightly queasy or nauseated, but vomiting is rare. People might describe a tension headache as "terrible," but the tension headache is usually not serious enough to keep you from your regular activities, including work.

The migraine headache is another common type of headache. These headaches usually hurt in the front of the head, with an occasional painful spot on the side of the head near the temples. Even when the whole head seems involved, many people complain of throbbing pain. A migraine almost never lasts for more than 48 hours, and most people have no problems or head pain in between attacks of migraines.

Most people who get migraine headaches complain of seeing an aura — a halo of light around objects. They also suffer from nausea and vomiting and extreme sensitivity to light. Some even complain of diarrhea.

Sinus headaches are those caused by a buildup of fluid and pressure in the sinuses in your head. These headaches feel more like pressure inside your head — like your head wants to explode or pop.

Many people with sinus headaches suffer from a feeling of pressure behind the eyes, across the forehead above the eyebrows, across the nose and just under the eyes, and even a feeling of "fullness" in their ears.

This kind of headache typically is worse in the morning but better by afternoon. It also is worse in cold, damp weather.

The hunger headache is another common kind of headache. This kind of headache occurs when you have waited too long to eat. The headache is your body's signal telling you to eat.

Heat headaches happen when you spend too much time in the direct sun. Getting overheated puts stress on you, and your head responds by hurting.

Drug headaches are the ones that are side effects of medications that you're taking.

Cluster headaches are unusual headaches. They come on very quickly and last for only an hour or so at a time. The pain is severe, sometimes incapacitating, and usually involves the head, eyes, neck, face and temples. And although the headaches go away quickly, they come back, often for several consecutive days.

A person, usually male, who suffers from cluster headaches will often feel fine for weeks or months and then suffer from an attack of cluster headaches in which the headaches happen several times a day for many days in a row. Then they'll go away again for a while.

Hypertension headache is the pain that results from your blood pressure getting too high. The increased blood pressure in your head causes the typical headache.

Now, depending on what kind of headache you have, there are different home remedies that can help bring you relief.

Tension headaches

❏ Try to avoid stressful situations that trigger the tension headaches. If that is impossible or impractical, try some stress-relief measures: taking 10 deep breaths; consciously relaxing your tensed shoulders, hands and jaw muscles; taking a brief walk to calm you down and clear your mind; listening to some quiet, calming music; doing simple stretch exercises to increase your blood flow and regulate your breathing; undertaking meditation and prayer.

❏ Massage your temples and forehead gently with your fingers. This increases the blood flow to these areas and can bring some relief from the pain.

❏ Avoid chewing gum. The constant motion and tightening of your jaw muscles can trigger a tension headache.

❏ Try putting a heating pad on your shoulders and neck to help relax those muscles. It might also help to put the heating pad on your head and use warm cloth compresses on your forehead.

❏ If heat doesn't seem to work, try using a cool cloth compress on your forehead and an ice pack on your head and neck. Sitting in front of a cool fan or air conditioner might also help relax you and ease your headache pain.

❏ If your headache is not too severe, try some mild exercises. The exercises will help relieve any tension and stress. Exercising also releases chemicals in your body known as endorphins — these are kind of like natural pain killers, and they might ease your headache pain. Exercise also improves the blood circulation to your head and scalp — the extra blood flow might bring you some relief.

❏ Try sleeping it off. Many times a quick nap will be all you need to settle down and get rid of that nagging headache. But don't stay in the bed too long — this can cause headaches in some people.

❏ Try some over-the-counter pain relievers like aspirin or acetaminophen. But never take more than the recommended dosage, no matter how bad your headache is.

❏ Get your eyes checked. Often people with bad vision strain and squint to help them see. The straining and squinting can cause headaches. Getting some reading glasses from your optometrist could be the only relief you need.

❑ During your next dental exam, tell your dentist about your headaches. Sometimes headaches can come from dental troubles, like an infected tooth, misaligned jaws, wisdom teeth coming in, or problems with the joints in your jaw. Fixing those dental problems may very well clear up your headache.

Migraine headaches

❑ Try to figure out what your triggers are — what foods, situations, etc., seem to trigger your migraine headaches. The best way to do this is to keep a careful diary. When you get a migraine headache, get your journal and write down all the foods you ate in the past two days, what you did during the two days before the headache started (worked, had a stressful doctor's appointment, etc.) and any other information that you think might play a part in your migraine headache trigger. Women should include dates of their menstrual periods because hormone changes can definitely trigger migraines. Then study the diary after you've recorded information about several headaches and try to determine what the common factor(s) is or are. When you think you have identified the triggers, try to avoid them and see if your headaches decrease in frequency or intensity. Some common foods that often trigger migraines are chocolate, caffeinated drinks, salty foods and alcoholic drinks.

❑ Try to sleep it off. Migraine headaches rarely last more than 48 to 72 hours. Often a good sleep will be enough to clear it up quickly.

❑ Avoid bright lights. Bright lights, especially direct sunlight, aggravates the pain of a migraine headache. Instead, try to stay in dimly lit rooms and avoid direct sun. If you must go outside, wear dark sunglasses and maybe even a wide-brimmed hat.

❑ Try to eat regular meals. Eating irregularly often triggers or worsens migraine headaches.

❑ Decide which works best for you: heat or cold. Some people get relief from ice packs on their heads and cool compresses on their foreheads. Others get more relief from warm compresses and heating pads. Try both and pick the one that seems to help you the most. Some people find that alternating heat and cold helps relieve their headache pain.

❑ Try an over-the-counter pain reliever like aspirin or acetaminophen. If your headaches are extremely severe, your doctor can prescribe a pain reliever with greater strength (Tylenol-3, etc.). Always take the pain reliever as soon as the headache starts. This will help prevent the headache from getting worse.

❑ Try drinking clear, carbonated beverages like ginger ale or Sprite to soothe your upset stomach.

❑ If your migraine headaches cause vomiting or diarrhea, drink plenty of liquids (clear liquids) to keep from getting dehydrated. You can buy over-the-counter medications to help relieve the diarrhea and vomiting.

Sinus headaches

❑ Take decongestants and antihistamines to help relieve the congestion in your sinuses that is causing your headache. When your sinuses clear up, your headache will go away.

❑ Place a washcloth soaked in warm water on your face — over your nose, cheeks and forehead where your sinuses are located. The moist heat should bring you some relief.

❑ Take a hot shower. The steam from the shower will help clear your sinuses and relieve your headache.

❑ Drink lots of liquids. The extra liquids will help drain and clear your sinuses and bring relief for your aching head.

Hunger headaches

❑ Stop what you are doing and eat. But avoid salty and fried foods. Eat some fresh fruit and vegetables or a high-carbohydrate meal (like pasta). A quick-energy drink is orange juice. Listen to your body — it knows when you need to slow down and nourish yourself.

Headaches from too much direct sun

❑ Get out of the sun and cool off. Drink some cool (not too cold) liquids and sit in front of a gentle fan until your body temperature goes back down to normal.

❑ When you go back out into the sun, wear a wide-brimmed hat to keep the sun off your head. Also wear lightweight, light-colored, loosely fitting clothes to help your body stay cool. If possible, take breaks and drink plenty of liquid to keep your body from getting overheated.

Drug-induced headaches

❑ Talk to your doctor or pharmacist about the medications you are taking. If one of the side effects is headaches, ask your doctor if he can prescribe a different drug or lower the dose. But never change medications or doses without talking to your doctor.

❑ Be sure to carefully read the label and package insert on any over-the-counter drugs that you use. Look for cautions and side effects that include headaches.

❏ Avoid drinking alcohol when you are taking medication. The combination can result in various side effects, including headaches.

❏ Do not take illegal, recreational drugs. They can cause headaches, coma and even death.

❏ Be careful about drug combinations — taking several different drugs at one time. Some drug combinations can cause headaches even though the individual drugs will not. Your local pharmacist can help you determine whether the drugs you take interact to cause your headaches.

❏ Carefully follow the instructions on the label of your medicines. Taking too much (or too little) of the drug or taking it at the wrong time can cause headaches.

Cluster headaches

❏ The majority of the people who suffer from cluster headaches are men who smoke and drink lots of alcohol. Scientists think the smoking and alcohol might trigger the headaches. To bring relief, stop smoking and cut way back on your alcoholic drinks.

❏ Cluster headaches come and go too quickly for any pain medicines to be effective against them. Instead, try placing cool compresses on your forehead or an ice pack on your head for some immediate relief.

❏ For those who do not get any relief from cool compresses or an ice pack, try a heating pad on your head and warm compresses on your face.

❏ People who suffer from chronic cluster headaches should see the doctor to get some kind of preventive medication to help reduce the number of headaches.

Hypertension headaches

❏ Keep your blood pressure under control.

❏ Avoid salty and fried foods that can raise your blood pressure.

❏ Avoid stressful situations that will cause your blood pressure to rise. If you have a stressful job or family situation, try to practice stress-relief tips, such as taking deep breaths, listening to calming music, going for a walk, taking up meditation and prayer.

❏ If you take blood-pressure medication, be sure to take it according to the directions on the label. Try not to skip doses, and avoid taking the medicine irregularly. Also, ask your doctor or pharmacist about any possible side effects of the medication (some might cause headaches).

❏ Watch your weight. Overweight people usually have a more difficult time controlling their blood pressure. If you are overweight, losing a few pounds might help lower your blood pressure and get rid of your headaches.

❏ Exercise regularly to help control your blood pressure.

MEDICAL SOURCES

The Practitioner (236,1513:449)
Headache (32,4:184 and 32,4:197)

Simple relief for migraine headaches

This kind of M&M won't melt in your mouth, but it might help melt away your headache.

The M&M stands for magnesium and migraine — don't have one without the other. Don't suffer from a migraine without trying some magnesium, that is.

Dr. Kenneth Weaver from Johnson City, Tennessee, recommends taking magnesium supplements to relieve the pain of migraine headaches.

Apparently, the magnesium helps the blood vessels relax, helps prevent the blood from thickening or clotting, and reduces the body's ability to make a substance known as thromboxane that might add to the headache pain.

MEDICAL SOURCE ————————————————————

Headache (30,3:168)

How to stop migraine headaches before they start

The gripping pain, nausea and fatigue seem too big for a baby to handle — but it depends on which baby you're talking about.

A baby aspirin each day could be able to handle the job of relieving your migraine headaches.

Researchers are suggesting that one aspirin taken every other day (or one baby aspirin every day) helps cut the risk of migraine headaches. The aspirin seems to work by keeping platelets from clotting in your blood.

Platelets are the components in your blood that help form scabs when you cut yourself.

They clot the blood and keep you from bleeding endlessly. Unfortunately, sometimes they clot when they don't need to, and they cause problems like migraine headaches.

Taking aspirin reduces the ability of the platelets to clot, and this lowers your chances of getting another migraine, according to this theory.

A team of researchers from Harvard Medical School and Brigham and Women's Hospital performed a study to test the effects of aspirin on migraine headaches.

They started with 22,000 male volunteers (ages 40 to 64) and studied them for five years. The men took an aspirin or a sugar pill every other day for the five years.

From the 22,000, they focused on 1,479 men who had suffered from migraines. The study showed that there was a 20-percent reduction in migraine risk among the men who took the aspirin.

The researchers suggest the results should encourage people who suffer from migraines to consider taking one baby aspirin a day to help cut down on their risk of migraines. But the researchers caution people about the possible stomach irritation that aspirin might produce.

MEDICAL SOURCES ————————————————————

Science News (137,7:103)
Journal of the American Medical Association (264,13:1711)

HEALING AFTER SURGERY

Go home! — Shorter hospital stays are better for many people

Save your health and your pocketbook — go home early!
From the hospital, that is.

Reducing the amount of time you stay in the hospital probably won't compromise your health and safety. In fact, going home early might even improve your health and recovery time.

Researchers from six hospitals in Boston and San Francisco studied 2,484 people who were in the hospital for the following situations: total hip replacement, coronary artery bypass graft surgery, heart attack, gallbladder removal and removal of the prostate gland through the urethra.

They studied the patients' medical records, and then checked on the patients for three to 12 months after the patients went home.

The researchers found that the patients' recovery times and progress didn't correspond to longer stays in the hospital.

In fact, for people who had coronary bypass and gallbladder removal, longer stays in the hospital seemed to lessen healing and to require longer recovery times.

It seems that many people are held in the hospital longer than is really necessary for optimal recovery. Going home early seems to help improve recovery times and certainly helps reduce skyrocketing health-care bills.

However, you should never check out of the hospital without your doctor's consent. That could put you in a life-threatening situation if you are still in need of hospital care.

If you are concerned about lengthy hospital stays for yourself or your family members, talk to your doctor. Your doctor might agree that a shorter hospital stay would be safe and healthy.

MEDICAL SOURCE ————————————————————

Medical Tribune (32,15:7)

HEARTBURN

Here's how you spell relief from heartburn and acid indigestion

It's that gnawing, burning feeling that starts soon after your meal — heartburn.

Some call it acid indigestion. Doctors call it gastroesophageal reflux. It's what happens during the digestion process when the acid from your stomach backs up into your esophagus, the tube that connects your mouth and stomach.

Your stomach is used to the acid. Your esophagus is not. That's why it burns.

The common symptoms of esophageal reflux include the following:

- Burning beneath the breastbone, typically moving upward.
- Pressure or discomfort above your stomach.
- Painful or difficult swallowing when you eat or drink.
- Unusual chest pain that doesn't seem to come from the heart.
- Regurgitation when you bend over, or for no apparent reason.
- A sudden filling of the mouth with salty fluid — this is known as "water brash."
- Sour taste in your mouth.

Almost half of the people in this country have heartburn at least once a month. More than 20 million Americans — 7 percent of the population — suffer from heartburn every day. Gastroesophageal reflux disease is common at all ages, but occurs most often between the ages of 60 and 70.

The main symptom of heartburn is usually a burning sensation in your chest that radiates upward.

When we eat, the food we swallow passes through the tube-like esophagus and into the pouch-like stomach on its way to the intestines. Muscles at the lower end of the esophagus contract to prevent contents of the stomach from going back up into the esophagus.

It's when the muscles relax excessively that you start to have problems. Contents of your stomach can back up into the esophagus or into your throat. Acid digestive juices from the stomach can irritate the lining of the esophagus and cause burning pain.

Antacids neutralize the acid in your stomach and usually can bring relief.

Certain substances that can cause the esophageal sphincter muscles to relax too much are alcohol, coffee, cigarettes, chocolate, peppermint and spearmint.

Some medicines that can increase reflux include theophylline, belladonna, calcium-channel blockers and progesterone.

Some foods that can irritate the lining of your esophagus and cause heartburn are citrus juices, tomato products, onions, cola soft drinks and beer.

Foods rich in fats cause delayed emptying of the stomach and can add to the reflux problem.

Being pregnant can put extra pressure on your stomach and can create or worsen gastroesophageal reflux.

It's a common problem with some simple solutions. Follow the tips below for some easy relief from heartburn:

❏ Stay away from foods that seem to aggravate your stomach: fried foods, spicy foods, chocolate, coffee and wine.

❏ Eat slowly, taking small bites and chewing your food thoroughly.

❏ Take time to eat. Don't eat while working, playing or driving.

❏ Don't stuff yourself. Here's the picture: Put a big rock in a bucket of water. See the water rise and slosh over the edge. That's the acid in your stomach backing up into your esophagus when you overeat.

❏ Eat four to six small meals a day, instead of two or three larger ones.

❏ Eat at least two to three hours before you go to bed.

❏ Put gravity to work for you. Avoid lying flat or leaning over if you experience heartburn. Lying down makes the problem worse. Standing or sitting helps to keep the acid from the stomach from backing up in the esophagus as badly as it does when you're lying down. Remain upright at least three hours after meals.

❏ Sleep with your head elevated at least six inches. Raise the head of your bed with wooden blocks under the bedposts. This helps to prevent the contents of your stomach from flowing back into your esophagus while you are asleep.

❏ Some medications cause esophageal reflux as a side effect. Ask your doctor about your drugs. Perhaps he can prescribe a different drug that doesn't cause heartburn.

❏ Wear loose clothing and avoid belts. Don't wear tight jeans or girdles. Some people say goodbye to heartburn when they say hello to suspenders.

❏ Avoid chewing gum. You swallow air when you chew gum, and this can cause reflux and heartburn.

❏ Watch your weight. If you are overweight, lose some, especially around the middle. Being overweight increases abdominal pressure and can cause reflux.

❏ Avoid straining and heavy lifting. Your abdominal muscles contract and squeeze the contents of your stomach up and out into your esophagus.

❏ Stop smoking. Don't use any tobacco products.

❏ Suck on sugarless candy-like lozenges during the day. Avoid peppermint-flavored ones, since they seem to aggravate heartburn.

Medical Sources

Heartburn Help, a news release published by the makers of Gaviscon
Modern Medicine (57,4:92)
Archives of Internal Medicine (151,3:448)
The Merck Manual, Sixteenth Edition, Merck Research Laboratories, Rahway, N.J., 1992
U.S. Pharmacist (17,10:21)

Is it indigestion, an ulcer or your heart?

Anyone who suffers from heartburn for more than a few days must begin to worry, "Is this an ulcer?" or even worse, "Is it a heart attack?"

Here are some general guidelines to help you.

First, is the pain caused by your heart? Probably not if the pain follows a large meal, gets worse when you lie down and is relieved quickly by taking over-the-counter antacids.

Pain from a heart attack often gets better when you lie down, gets worse if you stand or exercise, and isn't helped at all by taking antacids.

Ulcers might be the cause if the pain begins while your stomach is empty but gets better when you eat.

The two most common kinds of peptic ulcer get their names from their locations in the digestive tract. A duodenal ulcer is a sore on the lining of the first two or three inches of the duodenum. That's the lazy-S curve where the small intestine joins the stomach. A gastric ulcer is the same kind of sore on the lining of the lower curve of the stomach, just short of the duodenal junction.

One way to distinguish heartburn from duodenal ulcer is to note when the pain starts. If the discomfort comes soon after meals, it's not a duodenal ulcer.

If the pain comes two to three hours after a meal, or wakes you up in the middle of the night, it's much more likely to be an ulcer than to be ordinary heartburn. This kind of ulcer pain typically is relieved by eating, while heartburn pain seems to start soon after you eat.

These differences can help you rule out heartburn as the cause of your distress, but you can't do the opposite and rule out ulcer.

That's because, unfortunately, gastric ulcer has many of the same symptoms as heartburn, but is a much more serious situation. Gastric ulcer pain may be brought on by eating, or the pain may not show up for two to three hours after eating.

With an ulcer in the esophagus (known as esophagitis), you feel the pain when you swallow or lie down.

Chronic heartburn (two to three times a week for more than four weeks) should be a signal for you to see your doctor. If the pain hits in the middle of the night or hours after a meal, you need to get a medical checkup right away.

MEDICAL SOURCES————————————————————

The Merck Manual, Sixteenth Edition, Merck Research Laboratories, Rahway, N.J., 1992
U.S. Pharmacist (17,10:21)

Which antacid should you use?

For every 100 people with heartburn, 84 of them take antacids. These chemical combinations work by neutralizing the acid parts of gastric juices run together (primarily hydrochloric acid) that are attacking the sensitive lining of the esophagus.

❏ Most effective nonprescription antacids: liquid forms containing aluminum (Maalox), magnesium (milk of magnesia)or calcium (Tums). Hint: The antacids containing alginic acid seem to work best of all kinds in preventing heartburn.

❏ If you use tablets, chew them thoroughly before swallowing. Drink some water with them.

❏ Avoid taking calcium antacids for more than a few days for two reasons: might cause acid rebound, in which your stomach is stimulated to produce even more acids, or can lead to formation of kidney stones.

❏ Don't take sodium bicarbonate (baking soda). It releases carbon dioxide, which can cause bloating and can increase the amount of acid sloshing back into your esophagus. By the way, carbon dioxide is what causes the bubbles in the fizzy antacids.

❏ Take every four to six hours as directed to keep the acid buildup at bay.

❑ Start with the lowest dose suggested on the label and increase only as needed, per the directions.

❑ Watch out for interactions with other medicines: tetracyclines, quinolones, digitalis and iron-containing preparations. If you have to take both antacids and these other drugs, separate the doses by at least one hour, preferably two.

❑ Unless you have gas along with your heartburn, avoid antacids containing simethicone.

MEDICAL SOURCE ————————————————

U.S. Pharmacist (17,10:21)

HEART DISEASE

What you can do, and what you can't do for heart disease

Heart disease is a simple term for a complex of problems that affect the heart and its ability to pump blood efficiently. Generally speaking, heart disease implies that something is wrong with the heart muscle itself. Often, the problem involves the network of arteries and veins that provides the heart with its own blood supply.

Symptoms of blood supply problems to the heart include the pain and chest tightness felt with angina. When blood vessels become blocked, portions of the heart muscle literally starve for oxygen and fuel. When that happens, you suffer a heart attack, resulting in more or less permanent damage to the heart.

It's beyond the scope and intent of this book to try to tell you how to "treat yourself" for heart disease or an actual heart attack. You simply can't treat yourself for such a serious condition. Expert medical care is required, from diagnosis to treatment to rehabilitation.

However, there are a number of things that you can do to help prevent heart problems from arising, and we tell you about several of them in this section.

In addition, there are a few things that you can do to increase your chances of surviving a heart attack. The most important, of course, is to get medical help as soon as you feel the common symptoms of a heart attack.

The quicker you get to an emergency room, the better the chances doctors can save your life and minimize damage to your heart. People often "deny" the reality of severe heart problems, delaying treatment for hours when minutes count.

So, never treat lightly any signs of heart pain. Call for medical help quickly. Better a false alarm than a DOA.

How to tell if you're having a heart attack

❑ Severe chest pain. Usually the pain is a heavy or squeezing, deep, constant ache right behind the breastbone. Often the pain radiates to the back, left arm or jaw. Nitroglycerin — which usually banishes the pain of angina — has little or no effect on this pain. Antacids can't touch it. If the pain lasts for more than 10 minutes, you should get immediate medical help. However, about two out of every 10 heart attack victims have little or no pain. Some complain about uncomfortable pressure, fullness or squeezing in the center of the chest instead of pain. Again, if the sensations last more than 10 minutes, get medical help.

❑ Sweating, usually excessively, and cool, clammy skin. Occasionally, chills accompany the symptoms.

❏ Nausea, vomiting or feelings of severe indigestion.

❏ Shortness of breath, dizziness, lightheadedness or faintness.

❏ A sense of impending doom, severe nervousness or fear.

Many people get these warning signs but put off getting help. Initial denial of the seriousness of the situation is normal, but it's important to get past your denial quickly. Most people who die of heart attacks do so within two hours of the first signs of distress. Waiting simply reduces your chances of survival.

MEDICAL SOURCES ─────────────────────

The Merck Manual, Sixteenth Edition, Merck Research Laboratories, Rahway, N.J., 1992
Complete Guide to Symptoms, Illness & Surgery, 2nd Edition, The Body Press/Perigee Books, New York, 1989
1992 Heart and Stroke Facts, American Heart Association, Dallas, Texas, 1991

Simple changes in lifestyle — clean living and clean diet — can reverse heart disease

You know the old saying, "The more things change, the more they stay the same." Well, in the case of heart disease, the saying could go something like this: "The more things change, the more they go back to the way they were."

Making changes in your lifestyle can help your heart and blood vessels go back to how they were before your doctor told you that you have heart disease.

Following a low-fat vegetarian diet, clean living and stress management can reverse heart disease in many people in as little as a year, some scientists are saying.

In a one-year experiment, 41 volunteers (men and women ages 35 to 75) agreed to make some lifestyle changes to help reverse their existing heart disease.

An experimental group of 22 volunteers agreed to a substantial change in their habits: They ate a low-fat vegetarian diet, exercised regularly and went to a stress management class.

They also didn't smoke or drink caffeine, and the amount of alcohol that they drank was limited to two drinks a day.

The 19 volunteers in the control group stuck to a program that is usually recommended by doctors for heart patients: They didn't smoke, did moderate exercise and limited their dietary fat to 30 percent of total calories.

At the end of the study, 18 of the 22 volunteers who made substantial lifestyle changes showed reversal of their heart disease.

The arteries that had been clogged were clean. The blood vessels started looking as clean and clear as they had before they developed heart disease.

The people in this experimental group reduced their angina (chest pain) frequency by 91 percent, their angina duration, 42 percent, and their angina severity, 28 percent.

The study also indicated that the sickest people made the greatest improvements, and those improvements seemed to occur more readily in women.

Out of the group of 19 volunteers who followed the usual moderate medical advice, only eight showed any improvement. Ten others actually got worse. Their angina frequency, duration and severity all increased.

The changes and reversal of heart disease in the volunteers in the substantial-lifestyle-change group are similar to the changes doctors expect to see with cholesterol-lowering drugs.

But these people achieved their results with sensible changes in diet, stress management and exercise habits without having to depend on drugs.

Although eight of the people in the usual-care group got better, the study suggests that we should fight against heart disease more aggressively.

MEDICAL SOURCES ———————————————————

> *The Atlanta Journal and Constitution* (July 21, 1990, A8)
> *The Lancet* (336,8708:129)
> *Modern Medicine* (58,8:22)

How to counterattack against heart disease

The lifestyle changes that reversed heart disease damage included:

❑ Eating a vegetarian diet, which derived only 10 percent of its calories from fat.

❑ Managing stress by means of stretching exercises, breathing methods, meditation and progressive relaxation, at least one hour each day.

❑ Giving up the use of tobacco products.

❑ Exercising — usually walking — to 50 percent to 80 percent of individual target heart rates at least three hours a week.

❑ Gathering twice a week for group discussions to provide social support.

MEDICAL SOURCE ———————————————————

> *Geriatrics* (45,12:73)

Lower dietary fat to reduce heart disease, prevent heart attack

Can simple lifestyle changes prevent heart attack even though your arteries are clogged?

Lowering lipids (fats) in your diet can stabilize or reduce heart disease and can possibly prevent heart attack, some researchers believe. Even a modest improvement in an angiography (X-ray of blood vessels) is often associated with a significant decrease in heart attacks, coronary bypass surgery and angioplasty, some studies indicate.

When you decrease your fats even slightly, your angiography may not show you're making much progress in unclogging your arteries. But you are probably making huge improvements in unclogging the little coronary vessels that don't show up on the angiography.

Regression of atherosclerosis (hardening of the arteries) is mostly related to increases in high-density lipoprotein (HDL), the "good" cholesterol.

Stabilization of the clogged arteries seems to be associated with decreases in low-density lipoprotein (LDL), researchers say.

Dr. Jacques Rossouw, of the National Heart, Lung and Blood Institute, concludes that just as high LDL cholesterol levels call for treatment with diet or diet-drug combinations, so do mild elevations of LDL.

If coronary artery disease is present, Dr. Rossouw believes it is best to aim at an LDL level under 100.

He feels that dietary measures alone are very effective in slowing the progression of atherosclerosis, even when only modest reductions in LDL are achieved.

MEDICAL SOURCE ——————————————————

Medical World News (32,8:10)

Quick refresher on diet

Saturated Fats — "Bad"

- Obvious fat on or in meats
- Organ meats
- Dairy cream
- Butter
- Lard
- Coconut oil
- Palm oil

Polyunsaturated fats — "Good" if amounts are limited

- Corn oil
- Safflower oil
- Margarine

MEDICAL SOURCE ——————————————————

The Edell Health Letter (9,7:6)

An aspirin each day slashes heart attack risk in women 30%

A leading medical journal now recommends that women past menopause take an aspirin a day to prevent heart attacks and strokes.

Researchers suggest that taking an aspirin a day could reduce the risk of heart attack in women by 30 percent.

Aspirin keeps blood from getting too sticky and clumping together into clots. Many heart attacks and strokes are triggered by blood clots that form in arteries that are already narrowed by fatty deposits and cholesterol.

According to studies, women over age 50 who seem to be more

at "risk for coronary artery disease" get the most benefit from taking 325 milligrams (a full, regular tablet) of aspirin a day.

Doctors recommend aspirin for those who have a history of coronary artery disease, stroke or transient ischemic attacks (temporary interference of blood supply to the brain).

Avoid taking aspirin if you have a family history of strokes caused by hemorrhaging or other bleeding disorders, or if you already take anti-clotting medicine or have stomach ulcers.

Aspirin therapy tips

❑ Many doctors recommend taking an aspirin every other day to help prevent heart disease. Some studies recommend taking baby aspirin (81 milligrams per tablet) daily for anti-stroke therapy.

❑ Check with your doctor if you have questions about the proper dosage for anti-stroke therapy or heart disease prevention.

❑ Don't start taking aspirin on your own — talk with your doctor first.

MEDICAL SOURCE ─────────────────────────

Archives of Internal Medicine (151,6:1066)

All-natural way you can stop a racing heart

How to stop a racing heart?

Hold your breath and take an icy plunge in front of your doctor.

If you suffer from occasional heart palpitations or tachycardia, dunking your face in icy water can slow your racing heart, according to emergency room doctors.

Although tachycardia is not usually serious, it can be very uncomfortable and even scary for your heart rate to suddenly rise to 160 beats per minute. The normal heart rate for healthy adults is about 50 to 100 beats each minute.

Doctors usually treat tachycardia by massaging the arteries in the neck, or putting mild pressure on the eyes. But researchers looked to trained divers to find a totally natural and more effective technique.

When divers plunge into cold water, their body functions slow down automatically, in anticipation of receiving less oxygen. The same reflex takes over when you put your face into icy water, and the heart rate slows by more than 15 beats per minute.

To get the best results, a doctor might have you sit down in front of a container of very cold water — between 32 and 40 degrees Fahrenheit — hold your breath, and immerse your face in the water.

Then, the doctor would have you remove your face from the water when it becomes uncomfortably cold.

A word of warning: Don't try this cold-water technique on your own. Check with your doctor about the wisdom of using this technique. People who have chest pain or angina that becomes worse in cold weather should avoid this method of slowing the heart rate.

MEDICAL SOURCE ─────────────────────────

Emergency Medicine (23,21:95)

Listen ... your ears could warn you of heart disease

More news about earlobe creases.

If you have a crease in one or both of your earlobes that is a 45-degree downward angle toward your shoulder, it could be an early warning sign of heart attack.

According to a new report, Dr. William Elliot, assistant professor at the Pritzer School of Medicine, University of Chicago, studied 108 men and women for eight years. Some of them had coronary artery disease, and some had earlobe creases. After 8 years, those people with earlobe creases had a significantly higher rate of death from heart disease compared with those without an earlobe crease.

Dr. Elliot speculates that arteries that supply blood to the heart might be similar to those that supply blood to the earlobe. If this is true, then what happens to the heart arteries might also happen to the earlobe arteries at the same time.

Thus, a decrease in the blood supply to the earlobe could be a warning sign of possible heart problems. The earlobe crease seems to indicate such a decrease in blood supply to the earlobe tissue.

Although being overweight is a known risk factor for heart disease, researchers say that being fat does not influence whether people have ear creases. Both fat and thin people have them in equal numbers. Apparently, people don't usually get ear creases until they are about 50 years old.

Talk to your doctor if you have an earlobe crease or are concerned about heart disease.

MEDICAL SOURCES ─────────────────────────

British Heart Journal (611,4:361)
Science News (139,20:319)
Modern Medicine (57,10:126)

Smoking hides warning signals from the heart

Pains in the chest are usually early warning signals from the heart, telling you about possible problems.

However, you may not receive these signals if you smoke.

Smoking seems to block a smoker's perception of pain. This would be great news in some situations, but, in this case, some pain lets us know there's trouble ahead.

To demonstrate the effect smoking has on a person's pain perception, Dr. Paula Miller conducted a study by testing a group of male smokers. After each one smoked a cigarette, the researchers placed heat probes on their arms. The heat was turned up a few degrees after each cigarette, but none of the men could feel the difference.

The cigarettes seemed to act as a kind of "pain reliever."

Scientists are not really sure how smoking numbs the nerves, but this could be a reason why people who smoke don't notice the beginning of heart problems.

If you smoke and are concerned about how this may affect you, talk to your doctor immediately. Smoking a long time has been proven to be harmful to your health. This just may be another reason to think twice before lighting up.

MEDICAL SOURCE ———————————————————

American Family Physician (43,2:591)

Smoky places can cause sticky blood, raise heart attack risk for nonsmokers

You say you don't smoke, but are you sure about that?

What do you mean, Am I sure? you say. Of course I'm sure.

Well, you might not be an active smoker, but you could be a passive smoker. If you are exposed to smoke from other people's cigarettes (passive smoke) either at home or at work, you are considered a passive smoker. And, as a passive smoker, you have a greater risk of heart disease.

In fact, passive smokers are nearly two-and-a-half times more likely than other nonsmokers to suffer from a heart problem such as heart attack or death.

The problem is this: The smoke you inhale from other people's cigarettes causes your body to produce too much of a substance known as fibrinogen. Fibrinogen is a part of the blood that helps the blood form clots when needed, such as with a bleeding cut or wound.

However, too much fibrinogen in the blood causes clots to form too often and unnecessarily. Those unnecessary clots can block the flow of blood to the heart and cause heart attacks.

So, if you thought you were safe from health problems because you don't actively smoke, think again. The dangers of passive smoking are just as real, and just as deadly. Stay away from those smoky places for your heart's sake.

MEDICAL SOURCE ————————————————
    Medical Tribune (32,19:10)

'What's up, doc?' Not your risk of heart disease if you eat carrots

The fact that Bugs Bunny is always nibbling on a carrot when he asks the famous "What's up, Doc?" is more than just animated humor.

But perhaps the question should be "What's down, Doc?" Doc says your risk of heart disease and stroke goes down if you'll eat those carrots.

Women who consume more than 15 milligrams of beta carotene each day can reduce their risk of stroke by 40 percent and their risk of heart attack by 22 percent, reported Dr. JoAnn Manson to an annual meeting of the American Heart Association.

Dr. Manson reported the findings of a study that examined the relationship between dietary intake of foods rich in vitamin E and beta carotene and the risk of heart disease among a group of 87,245 nurses between the ages of 34 and 59.

The women who ate more foods rich in vitamin E and beta carotene had lower risks of coronary heart disease, researchers found during eight years of follow-up studies of the participants.

Apparently these vitamins help prevent plaque buildups that plug blood vessels. That lowers your risk of heart disease and stroke.

Dr. Manson also reported that women who took 100 milligram vitamin E supplements experienced a 36 percent lower risk of heart attacks. She stresses that the best way to lower your risk of coronary heart disease is to eat more foods that contain vitamin E and beta carotene, such as carrots, spinach, sweet potatoes and apricots.

"What's up" should be your daily intake of those fruits and vegetables. Then what's down will be your risk of heart disease and stroke.

MEDICAL SOURCE ———————————————

Medical Tribune (32,25:16)

Vitamin C plays role in keeping a heart healthy

Vitamin C does more than get you going in the morning. It keeps your blood going. And that is great news for your heart.

Researchers have now found a possible link between high intake of vitamin C and lower risk of atherosclerosis (hardening of the arteries).

Researchers studied 314 men and 142 women ages 20 to 95, separated into two groups of over age 58 and under age 58, because lipid levels had been found to peak in the late 50s.

Scientists studied their levels of vitamin C, triglycerides (a large portion of the fatty substances in the blood), LDL, HDL and HDL2 (which is the fraction of HDL that seems to be most protective against heart disease).

Vitamin C was associated with lower levels of LDL and higher levels of HDL and HDL2 (the "good" cholesterol) in older men and higher levels of HDL2 in older women.

You can get your vitamin C through natural sources like citrus fruits, cantaloupe, strawberries, tomatoes, green and red peppers, kale, collards, mustard greens, broccoli, cabbage and potatoes.

MEDICAL SOURCE ─────────────────────────

Medical World News (32,8:11)

Slash your risk of heart attack with this new weapon

Have scientists finally discovered a "new weapon" that will help prevent heart attacks?

Well, not exactly — but close.

The "new weapon" is a naturally occurring vitamin that is probably a part of your diet already. This surprising new weapon against heart disease is vitamin E, researchers report. Found in many common foods, vitamin E helps keep your heart healthy and helps prevent heart attacks.

In fact, low levels of vitamin E in your bloodstream might be more dangerous than either high blood pressure or high cholesterol alone, these researchers say.

That startling finding comes from a Swiss study sponsored by the World Health Organization (WHO).

But, the study cautions, beware of smearing on the vitamin E-rich mayonnaise, pouring on the salad oil and passing the nuts because those E-rich foods — vegetable oils, salad dressings and nuts — are also full of fat.

In other words, vitamin E is readily available in many natural food sources. But those food sources are also high in fat, so you shouldn't eat too much of them just to get more vitamin E in your diet.

Instead, researchers are suggesting that people start taking vitamin E supplements to help protect against heart attacks.

"Because of the well-known high variation of the vitamin E content in vegetable oils, vitamin E supplements may even be required to reach the present low RDA of 15 IU vitamin E," the study reports.

Death from blocked heart arteries can be predicted in more than six out of 10 cases just from low vitamin E levels in the blood. The predictability of fatal heart attack rises to eight out of 10 when low vitamin E and high cholesterol levels are taken together. And by the time researchers factored in the combinations of low levels of vitamins E and A, high cholesterol and high blood pressure, they were able to predict nine out of 10 fatal heart attacks, the report says.

So impressed were the researchers with the vitamin E findings that they rated low E levels as a higher risk factor than both high total cholesterol levels and high blood pressure.

Vitamins E and A, as well as some "previtamin-A" forms of carotene, are antioxidants. That means they absorb loose oxygen-carrying "free-radicals" in the blood before the oxidizing substances can damage artery walls. Damaged areas are prime targets for buildups of fatty plaque.

Plaque deposits cause arteries to harden and can even block the flow of life-giving blood to heart tissues. A heart attack results when an artery feeding part of the heart muscle becomes plugged.

Higher levels of vitamin E apparently neutralize more of the oxidizing radicals, minimizing artery damage, the study indicates.

But, one study of health-conscious elderly Californians raises a caution flag against megadoses of vitamin E. That study showed that the highest death rates occurred among people who took 66 times the RDA of vitamin E and among those who took no supplements at all.

For safety's sake, check with your doctor before taking vitamin E supplements or supplements of any kind.

MEDICAL SOURCES————————————————————

The American Journal of Clinical Nutrition (53,1:326S)
Medical Tribune (32,3:9)

Add this 'germ' to your diet to help lower your risk of coronary heart disease

Although the word "germ" is in its name, it is not associated with causing disease. In fact, it seems to be very helpful in fighting against disease.

The "it" is wheat germ. Wheat germ is the highly nutritious part of the wheat kernel used to enrich breads and cereals, and can also be found in most grocery stores. And recent research shows that it might help reduce your risk of coronary heart disease.

A low-fat, low-cholesterol diet might help reduce cholesterol levels in the blood and help reduce the risk of heart disease, many researchers currently believe. One way to lower your cholesterol intake is to replace animal proteins with vegetable proteins.

Wheat germ is a good vegetable replacement because it is rich in vegetable proteins (27 to 30 percent) as well as in dietary fiber (10 to 16 percent).

To test the effects of dietary wheat germ on cholesterol levels in the blood, researchers added raw wheat germ to the diets of about 20 volunteers (ages 37 to 69) for a period of about seven months. Researchers measured the blood-cholesterol levels of the test volunteers before beginning the study to provide a baseline measurement.

The volunteers were then instructed to eat 20 grams of wheat germ per day for four weeks, then 30 grams of wheat germ daily for an additional 14 weeks. Twenty grams is a little under two-thirds of an ounce, and 30 grams is approximately one ounce.

Researchers then continued to observe the volunteers for an additional 12 weeks without any wheat germ added to the diets. The test volunteers reported that the wheat germ did not produce any bad side effects such as intestinal discomfort or excess gas. Some even reported that the wheat germ produced positive effects on constipation.

Results showed that during the four-week, 20-gram-per-day period of the test, blood-cholesterol levels dropped by nearly 9 percent. These results demonstrate the short-term effects of dietary wheat germ. Researchers went on to report that the 14-week period of 30 grams of wheat germ per day resulted in a 7.5-percent, long-term decrease in blood-cholesterol levels.

The long-term effects of the wheat germ also included an 11.3-percent decrease in blood triglycerides and a 15.4-percent decrease in LDL cholesterol, the "bad" cholesterol.

These results from the 14-week period of the test demonstrate the long-term health benefits of adding wheat germ to the diet.

Talk to your doctor about adding raw wheat germ to your diet.

MEDICAL SOURCE —————————————————————

The Journal of Nutrition (122,2:317)

Lower heart disease risk the nutty way

Your friends might think you've gone nuts, but you could be lowering your risk of heart disease. If you start eating almonds, that is.

Too much fat and cholesterol in the diet are believed by many researchers to be risk factors for heart disease. However, eating the right kinds of fat can actually reduce the amount of "bad" cholesterol in your blood.

The "right" kinds of fats are the monounsaturated fats, and almonds contain this kind of "good" fat.

So scientists recently tested the cholesterol-lowering effects of adding almonds to the diet. Thirty men and women (ages 29 to 81) enrolled in a study at the YMCA Cardiac Rehabilitation Unit in Palo Alto, California.

The researchers measured the levels of cholesterol in the blood of each person in the study before they began a special diet.

There were four food categories based on the amount of "bad" saturated fats they contained: unlimited, limited, not allowed and unchanged.

The "unlimited" foods included grains and grain products, fruits, vegetables, nonfat dairy products, low-fat fish and legumes. These foods are low in saturated fats, and the people in the study could eat unlimited amounts of these foods on the diet.

The "limited" foods included lean beef, poultry, eggs, medium-fat cheeses and low-fat cookies or cakes. They could only eat two to three servings of these foods each week.

The "not allowed" foods included margarine, butter, vegetable oils, mayonnaise, most meats, shellfish, whole-fat dairy products, chips, ice cream, avocados and all nuts except the almonds given for the study. These foods are high in saturated fats.

The "unchanged" foods included tea, coffee and alcoholic drinks. The people in the study could drink as much of these liquids as they did before beginning the study.

The men and women in the study stayed on this low-in-saturated-fats diet for nine weeks. During that time, they ate 100 grams of almonds a day (50 grams as whole raw almonds, and 50 grams as ground almonds). That's the equivalent of almost four ounces per day of almonds. Each person kept a food diary, and the scientists took measurements of blood-cholesterol levels throughout the nine weeks.

At the end of the nine weeks, the investigators reported that the average total cholesterol level of 235 was reduced by about 20 points. The nearly 9-percent reduction in the total cholesterol level was due to a reduction in the level of LDL cholesterol in the blood (the "bad cholesterol"). Scientists explained that the almonds weren't fat-free. But, they contain monounsaturated fats (the good fat).

So, even though the people in the study actually ate more fat during the nine-week diet than normal, the fat they ate on the diet seemed to be good for them.

The increase in monounsaturated fats (almonds) and the decrease in saturated fats ("limited" and "not allowed" foods) helped lower blood-cholesterol levels.

Although almonds are a good source of monounsaturated fats, don't begin eating large amounts of almonds without checking with your doctor first. Any dramatic change in your diet could cause more harm than good.

MEDICAL SOURCE ————————————————

The Journal of the American College of Nutrition (11,2:126)

Doctors inject magnesium to cut heart attack fatalities

It's just a simple mineral, but it might double your chances of surviving a heart attack.

The mineral is magnesium, and doctors think that giving magnesium to heart attack victims could save thousands of lives each year.

The way that magnesium helps prevent death after a heart attack is by keeping the heart from beating irregularly. Many people live through the actual heart attack only to die from irregular heartbeat (arrhythmias) later.

Scientists hope that magnesium therapy at the hospital will help prevent deaths from arrhythmias after the heart attack.

To test the effects of magnesium therapy, investigators recently studied the cases of 1,301 people who had suffered from heart attacks. Some of the people in the study had received the standard heart attack medications alone. Others received the standard medications along with intravenous magnesium supplements.

The investigators found that 8.2 percent of the people who had received standard medication without magnesium died. However, only 3.8 percent of the people who had received the magnesium supplements with the standard medication died.

The study indicated that adding magnesium to standard heart attack treatment cuts the death rate by two-thirds.

The scientists state that magnesium therapy is inexpensive, and it has no bad side effects. This intravenous treatment is done only by doctors in hospitals.

MEDICAL SOURCE ————————————————————
Medical Tribune (33,1:10)

Low-intensity exercises help make a healthy heart

You know that frequent, high-intensity exercise is great for your heart, but running several miles three days a week just isn't your bag?

Well, you're not alone.

And you're not out of luck, either.

Research has long confirmed that frequent, high-level exercise is an important way to prevent heart disease. But if you can't manage to exercise vigorously for twenty minutes, four times a week, you might find this new research encouraging.

New studies indicate that you can get similar heart benefits from regular, low-intensity exercise. You can even profit from several short periods of exercise instead of one long interval.

For example, if you can't jog for 30 minutes a day, you can walk for 10 minutes three times a day and still get substantial health benefits.

Your main goal should be to use 1,200 to 2,000 calories per week in exercise regardless of the level of intensity.

Remember to check with your doctor before beginning a new exercise program. Together you can find a routine that works for you and your heart.

MEDICAL SOURCE ————————————————————
Medical Tribune (31,26:2)

Breaking out in sweat could reduce your heart attack risk

Exercise reduces the level of fibrinogen, a key protein present in the blood-clotting process. Vigorous exercise helps prevent clot formation in older men, which could significantly reduce the risk of heart attacks.

Scientists believe that fibrinogen is a risk factor for heart attacks and strokes and can be as damaging as smoking, high cholesterol and high blood pressure.

During a six-month study, 13 men between the ages of 60 and 82, and 10 men ages 24 to 30, took part in an intense exercise training program. The researchers defined "intense" as strenuous walking, jogging or cycling for 45 minutes, four to five times a week. The volunteers were all screened for coronary heart disease before the study, and monitored throughout the study. The researchers wanted to keep anybody from having a heart attack during exercise.

After six months, the exercise program seemed to make the older men's blood more "slippery." In other words, their blood was less likely to form dangerous clots.

In the process, fibrinogen levels in the older men's blood dropped 13 percent.

The level of naturally occurring tissue plasminogen activator (TPA), a clot-dissolving enzyme, increased by 39 percent. The level of a TPA blocker dropped 58 percent, says the report.

The younger men's blood showed no significant changes in the levels of these enzymes, probably because they were more active before the study, the report indicates.

Your blood's "slipperiness" varies during the day. It's usually low in the morning and high in the afternoon. This might explain why most heart attacks occur in the morning.

So, exercise might be most beneficial in the morning to give your blood an added boost when it needs it most. Always check with your doctor before starting any exercise program.

MEDICAL SOURCE ——————————————————————————

American Heart Association news release (May 9,1991)

Skipping breakfast might cause early morning heart attack?

People who miss their breakfast might spend their mornings at higher risk of heart problems and heart attacks. Hearty breakfast eaters have fewer heart attacks.

Doctors have noted that heart attacks are most likely to occur within a few hours after you wake in the morning. Although they are unsure exactly why that happens, researchers believe that early-morning changes in the body increase the risk.

Some believe that increases in blood pressure or heart rate in the morning raise the danger level. Other studies blame the problem on the increased tendency of blood platelets to clump or stick together when a person gets up in the morning. "Sticky" blood may reduce blood flow in arteries already narrowed by atherosclerotic plaque.

"**Skipping breakfast** may dramatically enhance the early-morning stickiness of the platelets," according to cardiologist Renata Cifkova of Memorial University of Newfoundland in Canada.

Cifkova did a study where she withdrew and analyzed blood from 20 healthy men and women. During each of the several visits, the healthy volunteers' blood levels of the protein beta-thromboglobulin (beta-TG) were normal, except in two participants. These two individuals showed more than seven times the normal amount of beta-TG on one morning.

The apparent reason — both skipped breakfast that morning.

According to the study, overnight fasting and skipping breakfast seems to increase platelet activation (stickiness of the platelets) and might contribute to the increased frequency of heart attacks during the morning hours of the day.

MEDICAL SOURCE ————————————————————

Science News (139,16:246)

'Silent danger' lurks in the night

Going to the bathroom might get to be a dangerous business for some people—if they are getting up at night to go. For some people with heart disease, the simple act of getting up in the middle of the night to use the bathroom or get a drink of water could lead to a dangerous condition known as "silent myocardial ischemia."

"Ischemia" means that some cells in the body are not getting enough blood. "Silent myocardial ischemia" means that the heart is not getting enough blood. It could lead to a heart attack.

Doctors call it "silent" because it doesn't hurt—you usually don't even realize when it happens. (Ischemia is not always "silent" — chest pain is sometimes a warning sign that your heart is not getting enough blood.)

In a controlled study, 30 volunteers wore ischemia-detecting devices for 24 or 48 hours straight and kept detailed diaries of their daily and nightly activities. The ischemia-detecting devices look much like Walkman tape players that you attach to your waistband, only you have patches that stick to your chest instead of ear phones.

The patches detect your heartbeat and any changes in rhythm, and the monitor on your waist records the information. So, doctors have the true story of what your heart is doing instead of the misleading story of what you might feel.

Of the 30 volunteers, 21 got up at some time during the night, some more than once, for a total of 36 times. On 24 of those 36 occasions, getting out of bed was accompanied by silent myocardial ischemia. That boils down to two out of every three times.

Apparently, the body has a "sleeping mode." During sleep, the heart and blood vessels seem to rest a little, too. But when you get up and start moving around, the heart and vessels have to "wake up" and adjust to your "awake mode." It is during this adjustment time that the heart has a greater risk of suffering from ischemia.

Research suggests that most heart attacks and other coronary events occur most often in the early morning hours, when most people are in that adjustment stage between sleeping and getting up and about.

Some scientists recommend that you lie awake in bed for a while when you first wake up in the morning (or in the middle of the night). Then slowly sit up. Finally, after sitting still for a while, put your feet on the floor and stand. Going through these motions slowly and deliberately might help your heart to adjust to being awake without causing a shortage of blood or ischemia.

MEDICAL SOURCE ────────────────────────────

American Heart Association news release (Nov. 13, 1989)

Stay warm in winter for your heart's sake

As the temperature drops, does your risk of heart attack rise? It could for some elderly people.

Levels of fibrinogen in older people seem to rise during the coldest months of the year, increasing the risk of heart attack and stroke. Researchers suggest that lower indoor temperatures appear to be an important factor in more deaths in the winter.

For a year, researchers studied 100 people aged 75 and over. The scientists monitored their body temperature, environmental temperature and risk factors for heart attack.

Levels of fibrinogen showed the biggest seasonal change. They were 23 percent higher in the coldest six months of the year than in the summer months. This seasonal change in fibrinogen levels is large enough to increase the risk of heart attack and stroke during the winter.

Fibrinogen is a protein in the blood that is essential for blood clotting, and the thickening of the blood is what seems to be related to heart attack and stroke.

Older people sometimes have a faulty "thermostat," meaning their body temperatures don't regulate well. Also, older people might be more prone to seasonal changes in their metabolism.

Some ways to help keep you warm and prevent hypothermia (lower than normal body temperature) include dressing warmly outside and inside, keeping a blanket or afghan handy, wearing socks to keep your feet warm, wearing a hat to keep your head warm, drinking warm fluids and keeping the thermostat set at a comfortable temperature.

Talk to your doctor if you are concerned about your health during the colder months of the year.

MEDICAL SOURCE ————————————————————
The Lancet (338,8758:9)

Up and down weight swings could lead you to an early grave

Get off the weight-loss yo-yo to improve your chances of a long life, researchers say. Fluctuating weight significantly increases the risk of premature death and heart disease.

The finding suggests that you might be better off staying at a constant weight instead of watching the scales bounce up and down in a continual lose-then-regain pattern.

Researchers studied 5,127 people between 32 and 62 years old. Their body weight was measured every two years.

Results showed that people whose weight fluctuated frequently had up to twice the risk of dying early from heart attacks or other causes as those who kept their weight relatively stable.

"The health risks posed by repeated weight gain and loss may even exceed those of being overweight," according to Kelly D. Brownwell, a professor of psychology at Yale.

According to Dr. Albert Stunkard, director of the Obesity Research Group at the University of Pennsylvania in Philadelphia, "The more weight a person loses, the more weight the person is apt to regain."

Dieters who can't keep the weight off and are constantly gaining and losing pounds are at high risk of dying from heart disease, according to researchers.

Researchers are not sure why fluctuating weight is a problem, but suggested that people who continuously lose and gain weight seem to have a high percentage of body fat. Body fat is a known risk factor for heart disease.

Researchers suggest that if you are dieting, and have lost weight, try to keep those pounds off.

Be sure to check with your doctor before you start a weight-loss program.

MEDICAL SOURCE ————————————————

The New England Journal of Medicine (324,26:1839)

Caution for men: What going bald may say about your heart!

A toupee or hairpiece may help cover a receding hairline or a bare crown that accompanies male pattern baldness, but it won't help cover heart disease.

Heart disease? you ask. What do heart disease and male pattern baldness have to do with each other?

Researchers think that they might be closely related, reports the American Heart Association.

Apparently, scientists at the State University of New York at Buffalo discovered that men with typical male pattern baldness often have greater levels of blood cholesterol.

They also have higher blood pressure levels than the men with full heads of hair or other types of baldness patterns.

These conditions might increase your risk of developing heart disease.

Based on their study of 872 Italian men, the researchers observed that the men with pattern baldness had cholesterol levels that were five to six points higher than men without the pattern baldness.

The higher cholesterol levels indicate a greater risk of heart disease.

However, researchers caution that this study is in the early, preliminary stages and cannot be extended to all men with pattern baldness.

More studies are currently in progress.

MEDICAL SOURCE ——————————————————

Heartstyle (1,1:6)

HEAT PROBLEMS

Stay cool and beat the heat!

The summer months can be some of the most enjoyable months of the year. But they can also be among the most dangerous. In addition to long, lazy days and glasses of lemonade, summer also brings hot weather and the risk of heatstroke.

Many think the only person in danger of heatstroke is someone stranded in the desert without water — but heatstroke can happen to anyone. So, in order to make the most of your summer, you need to know what heatstroke is and some simple tips on how you can help avoid it.

There are three kinds of heatstrokes that you need to look for.

The first kind is the most well-known: exertional heatstroke. This happens in healthy and not-so-healthy people during vigorous exercise (tennis, running, mowing the lawn) in hot weather.

The second kind of heatstroke is the nonexertional heatstroke. This happens when someone is exposed to extremely hot temperatures without being able to cool off.

The third kind, and the least well-known, is the drug heatstroke. This happens when a medication prevents the body from cooling properly during hot weather.

Now that you know what kinds of heatstroke there are, you need to know if you are at risk.

Doctors have shown that many people who suffer from any type of heatstroke (exertional, nonexertional or drug) usually have some underlying factors that probably contributed to the heatstroke. Some of these factors are:

- Being overweight
- Not drinking enough fluids (dehydration)
- Recent move from a cool or mild climate to a hot climate
- Recent illness that included fever or diarrhea
- Poor physical conditioning
- Recent problems with sleeping
- Use of excess protective clothing (by firemen or athletes)
- Use of medications that prevent heat loss from the body

Doctors warn that some diseases put people at higher risk for heatstroke.

If you suffer from diabetes, cardiovascular disease or other diseases of the heart, you might have an increased risk of heatstroke during the hot months of summer.

The body has natural ways of cooling itself. Sweating is one such way the body regulates its temperature. Anyone who has an inability to sweat also has an increased risk of heatstroke.

People who have suffered from burns or extensive skin diseases might have problems with sweating.

Elderly people have an especially high risk of heatstroke during the heat waves of summer. Elderly people often don't sweat as much as they used to, and they don't seem to feel as thirsty as they used to, so they don't drink as much as they should. These two factors greatly increase their risk of getting overheated and suffering from heatstroke.

Drug heatstroke usually occurs because the drug changes the way the blood vessels carry blood around the body. This can change the body's natural ability to cool off.

Some of the drugs that might increase your risk of heatstroke are beta blockers, calcium channel blockers, diuretics, antihistamines, antiparkinsonian agents, phenothiazines, tricyclic antidepressants and alpha-agonists.

If you take any medications and are not sure whether they fit these categories, ask your pharmacist or doctor. They can tell you if your medicine will increase your risk of heatstroke.

If you get outside during the summer, here's how to enjoy the season without falling victim to it:

❑ Drink lots of water. Whether you are weeding your garden, walking around the block, watching a baseball game or playing a competitive game of tennis, make sure you drink plenty of water — before, during and after the time you are out in the heat.

❑ Avoid drinking alcoholic beverages. Alcohol flushes water out of your body, dehydrating you.

❑ Stay out of the sun as much as possible. Sit under an umbrella at the pool, wear a broad-brimmed hat in the garden, and sit under the overhang at the ball game. Getting out of the sun may not keep you from getting warm, but it will help keep you from getting heat-blasted.

❑ If possible, go indoors and cool off every now and then instead of staying outside in the heat for several hours without a break.

❑ Try to gradually build up the amount of time you spend outdoors each day. Spend 30 minutes outside the first day. Then 45 minutes the next day, and so on. This helps your body get used to the heat.

❑ If you are taking drugs that might increase your risk of heatstroke, talk to your doctor about lowering the dosage or changing the medication during the hot months. But never change your medication without talking to your doctor first.

❑ Avoid strenuous exercise during the hottest part of the day.

Try to do your yard work or exercises in the cooler morning or evening hours and stay indoors in the cool air during the middle of the day when the temperature is highest.

❑ If you start feeling dizzy, queasy or faint while you are out in the heat, go inside immediately and cool off. If you don't feel better after a while, call your doctor.

If you know someone who you think is suffering a heatstroke, call for medical help immediately. While waiting for an ambulance to arrive, try to cool the person. You can do this by getting the person out of the heat and direct sun — move indoors if possible.

Cool, wet rags and fans will help lower the person's temperature. Also, removing any excess or heavy clothing will help cool the person.

How will I know if someone has had a heatstroke? you ask. Doctors say that a person has had a heatstroke if that person has a body temperature of 106 degrees or higher, no sweating and altered mental status (unconscious, delirious or very confused and disoriented).

If you have questions about heatstroke, call your doctor. She can help you make sure the summer months are safe and risk-free.

MEDICAL SOURCE ─────────────────────

Postgraduate Medicine (91,4:379)

Hypothermia presents chilling winter problem for elderly people

Jack Frost and Old Man Winter bring beautiful snowflakes and icicles each winter. But they may bring more than just snow-covered sidewalks.

Winter months and chilly winds also may bring older people a special problem known as hypothermia.

Hypothermia is a condition in which the body loses more heat than it can produce. The body no longer produces enough heat to maintain body functions. This condition is extremely dangerous, and it can be deadly if it's not treated right away.

Perhaps the most dangerous aspect of hypothermia is that it may occur before you are even aware that you are too cold.

You can develop hypothermia from exposure to cool water, a cold wind or from being underdressed in cold weather. It's even possible to get hypothermia indoors.

It doesn't even have to be especially cold for hypothermia to occur.

You can develop this condition on a sunny day on the lake with a breeze blowing through your damp clothes, and the air temperature in the 70s. Older people are especially vulnerable to hypothermia for several reasons.

They usually have decreased muscle and body mass, and this makes it hard for their bodies to conserve heat. Also, the body's ability to respond to cold temperatures diminishes with age.

Usually, the body's circulatory system responds to cold temperatures with increased metabolism and muscular shivering. These automatic responses help produce enough heat within the body to fight the cold.

However, older people lose some of that ability to respond to the cold. Fatigue and iron deficiency anemia can also contribute to hypothermia.

You can recognize the early stages of hypothermia by these signs: the person may be pale, sleepy or confused.

Body temperature will register more than four degrees below normal (98.6 degrees Fahrenheit). A person suffering from hypothermia may also seem lethargic and may lose voluntary muscle control. And a person in the later stages of hypothermia may be unconscious.

Take these simple precautions to help prevent hypothermia:

❏ Keep your home adequately heated.

❏ Eat well and drink lots of fluids.

❏ Layer your clothing to provide more protection from cold weather, whether you're indoors or outdoors.

❏ Wear a hat. You can lose a great deal of your body's heat through an uncovered head.

If you suspect that a person is developing hypothermia, get medical help right away. If you must wait more than a few minutes for medical help to arrive, here's what to do:

❏ Remove the person from the cold environment, if possible.

❏ Provide shelter and heat.

❏ Remove any wet garments and replace with warm, dry clothes.

❏ Warm the body trunk, not the limbs, of the person.

❏ Layer the clothes and blankets. Heating blankets or rewarming blankets (used in hospitals) help to rewarm the trunk of the body. Rewarming the limbs of a person suffering from hypothermia may cause an additional drop in core body temperature, so concentrate on warming the trunk, which contains the vital organs.

❏ Give the victim a warm, sweet drink (nonalcoholic) if the

person is conscious.

MEDICAL SOURCE ────────────────

Postgraduate Medicine (88,8:55)

Check your pantry for some ironclad protection against hypothermia

If you're low on iron, you may have an increased risk of developing hypothermia.

According to the latest research, iron deficiency anemia reduces the body's ability to produce heat in response to cold conditions.

To make sure that you're getting enough iron, include these foods in your diet:

> * Beef or calves' liver
> * Meat
> * Whole-grain breads and cereals

Before taking any iron supplements, make sure you check with your doctor.

MEDICAL SOURCE ────────────────

The American Journal of Clinical Nutrition (52,5:813)

Hemorrhoids

Hemorrhoids — almost everyone gets them at some time

It's a painful, aggravating problem that no one seems to want to talk about. And the reason no one wants to talk about it is clear enough — it's embarrassing.

Hemorrhoids are just not the kind of thing people like to discuss.

And all the secrecy is probably the reason most people don't know what to do for them — they're embarrassed to ask. That's surprising because hemorrhoids "occur universally in adults and children," says one standard medical treatment volume.

In fact, half of all people over the age of 50 live with this painful nuisance.

Hemorrhoids are very similar to varicose veins in the legs — they are swollen, tender veins either inside the rectum or outside around the anal area. The veins get swollen and tender from too much pressure.

The pressure comes from the strain of constipation, diarrhea or pregnancy, or it comes from disorders such as obesity and liver disease. When the veins swell, they become tender and often painful.

You can have two kinds of hemorrhoids — internal ones and external ones. The internal hemorrhoids usually are painless, and the only reason you know you have them is the occasional bright red blood on your stools or on the toilet paper.

Occasionally, you might notice a feeling of incomplete evacuation, a sense that the bowel movement isn't finished. That sensation comes from the pressure of an internal hemorrhoid.

External hemorrhoids are the ones that cause most people trouble. The veins around the outside of the rectum get swollen, and these swollen veins bleed easily from straining or rubbing. They also tend to itch and be painful.

Hemorrhoids are more of a nuisance than anything. If left untreated, they won't turn into cancer or some other horrible disease. They'll just continue to aggravate you, unless you take some simple steps to avoid them.

The treatment of hemorrhoids begins with simple advice: "No strain, no pain." Ways to prevent hemorrhoids include the following:

❏ Stop straining when you go to the bathroom. Let your bowel movement come naturally. Resist the urge to "help" it to completion.

❏ Eat more fiber to avoid constipation and hard stools. The best way to stop straining is to control your constipation with a diet that is high in fiber. If you get plenty of bran, grains, fruits and vegetables in your diet, your stools will be soft and bulky and easy to eliminate. You won't have to strain anymore. You can also use bran supplements to add fiber to your diet. Some of the common over-the-counter sources of fiber include Metamucil, FiberCon and Citrucel. You can buy these products at most supermarkets or pharmacies. Just follow the instructions on the label. Be sure to increase the amount of fiber in your diet gradually — adding too much at one time will result in some constipation at first before you get the stool-softening benefits.

❏ Drink more liquids. Drinking lots of liquids also helps to soften your stools. And you don't have to drink just water. Fruit juices and vegetable juices are good liquid sources. But stay away from caffeine and alcoholic beverages — these tend to pull water out of your system and can lead to dehydration. Avoid using laxatives that contain ingredients other than simple stool softeners. Stronger laxatives can cause diarrhea, and that is just as bad on your hemorrhoids as constipation is.

For active hemorrhoids that are irritating you now, try these remedies:

❏ Sit in a warm sitz bath. Sometimes a warm bath is all you need to cure what ails you. And what is a sitz bath? It simply means taking a bath sitting down in a tub with water soaking the anal area. There are no special chemicals or medicines that you need to add to the bath water. Just run warm to hot water in a stoppered tub to a depth above and covering the hips — more if you prefer — and lean back and enjoy a good soak. If you can, raise your legs above your hips to fully expose the anal area to the soothing water. If the pain continues, sit in hot water for up to 20 minutes several times a day.

❏ Compress the hurting area. Many people find relief with cool compresses — soft cotton cloths soaked in cool or cold water and applied to the hemorrhoids.

❏ Try using some witch hazel, available without a prescription at any pharmacy. Dab a little on a cotton ball and apply it to the swollen veins. Sometimes chilling the witch hazel gives you even more relief. Or, try a witch hazel compress — cotton cloths soaked in witch hazel and applied to the anal area.

❏ Consider using softer toilet paper, or even medicated tissue, to cut down on harsh rubbing. You can buy specially medicated wipes made for hemorrhoid sufferers. Otherwise, use only nonperfumed, white (uncolored) tissue. Soften it up a bit by running water gently on the tissue before wiping. But be sure not to neglect your personal hygiene just because it is a little uncomfortable. Uncleanliness can lead to infection of the damaged skin and more serious problems.

❏ If sitting is painful or uncomfortable, try using a pillow or a doughnut-shaped cushion (or pool float) to sit on. This will sometimes relieve the pressure on those veins and help the healing process.

❏ Don't hesitate to use some of the over-the-counter hemorrhoid remedies like Preparation H. But choose a cream instead of a suppository. The suppositories often dissolve too far up into the rectum to do your hemorrhoids any good, even the internal hemorrhoids. Creams can relieve the symptoms of both internal and external hemorrhoids. Just follow the instructions on the label.

❏ Avoid heavy lifting or vigorous exercise. Such activities can irritate tender hemorrhoid tissue.

❏ Make any bathroom visit a quick trip. Reading on the porcelain "throne" might improve your mind, but it plays havoc with your hemorrhoids. Every minute you sit on the toilet is a minute of extra pressure on those veins in the rectum.

You may suffer severe pain if a blood clot forms in an external hemorrhoid, a condition known as a thrombosed hemorrhoid. But Dr. Lee E. Smith of the George Washington University Medical Center says that these blood clots are like a black eye and usually disappear after a few days.

For those of you who are afraid of surgery, don't worry. Hemorrhoid surgery is almost never absolutely necessary. Most hemorrhoid problems will clear up on their own over time if you take the proper steps.

People who have surgery usually just want some quick relief from a particularly painful case of hemorrhoids instead of waiting for it to go away on its own.

There's "rubber-band" surgery. That's where the doctor pulls the internal hemorrhoid out like a rope loop and puts a tight constricting band around it. The loop loses its blood supply, dies and drops away virtually without pain.

If you want to get rid of an external hemorrhoid, the doctor might choose to freeze it, applying super-cold instruments to the tissue.

For severe, prolonged pain from "an acute attack of the piles," doctors usually inject painkillers into the hemorrhoid.

A word of warning: Remember that the blood from hemorrhoids is bright red. If you have stools that are dark colored from blood, you should see your doctor.

That blood came from somewhere in your intestines (not in the rectum), and you should have it checked out right away. If you have dark, tarry stools or bleeding that lasts for more than a minute from the rectum, you should see your doctor. Hemorrhoids don't cause cancer, but bleeding from the rectum might also be a sign of colon or rectal cancer.

MEDICAL SOURCES ———————————————————————

FDA Consumer (26,2:31)
The Merck Manual, Sixteenth Edition, Merck Research Laboratories, Rahway, N.J., 1992
Complete Guide to Symptoms, Illness & Surgery, 2nd Edition, The Body Press/Perigee Books, New York, 1989

Foods for hemorrhoid sufferers

A couple of natural ways to keep hemorrhoids from developing are to drink several glasses of water daily and eat a fiber-rich diet. Here are some excellent natural sources of fiber:

> - Bran cereals
> - Fruits
> - Potatoes
> - Beans (kidney, navy, lima and pinto)
> - Vegetables — especially asparagus, brussels sprouts, cabbage, carrots, cauliflower, corn, peas, kale and parsnips

Limit low-fiber foods like ice cream, soft drinks, cheese, white bread and meat.

When your hemorrhoids are acting up and causing pain, avoid cola drinks, coffee, beer and strong spices. Residues in these foods can irritate inflamed anal tissues during a bowel movement and increase your pain.

MEDICAL SOURCE ——————————————

FDA Consumer (26,2:32)

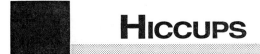

HICCUPS

Tips to get rid of the hiccups

It never fails — just when you are about to meet a new business colleague, make an important presentation, or engage in a serious conversation, you start hiccuping. It's distracting and embarrassing. And you have got to get rid of them pronto. So, what do you do?

Well, try massaging your earlobes. Yes, your earlobes. Sounds crazy, but many people claim that it works. No known connection, but the hiccup control center is close by in the upper part of the spinal column in the back of your neck.

If an ear massage doesn't do the trick and you happen to be close to the coffee machine at the office, try swallowing a spoonful of granulated sugar.

The sugar seems to trigger some kind of nerve impulse in your mouth that somehow helps to calm down your spastic diaphragm (the muscle just under your lungs that is causing this problem). Other people report relief just from holding the sugar in their mouths until it dissolves.

If that doesn't work either, here are some age-old tricks that many people will swear by:

❑ Hold your breath for as long as you can, and swallow each time you feel the urge to hiccup. Try this a few times, and the hiccups should go away.

❑ Try the old paper-bag remedy. Breathe for about a minute into a paper bag gathered tightly to your lips. The buildup of carbon dioxide might shut down the hiccups. Don't try this for more than a minute at most.

❑ Get a small cup of water, bend over, hold your breath and drink the water upside-down. The hiccups should be gone by the time you swallow the last gulp, stand up and let out your breath.

❑ Chug-a-lug a glass of water quickly.

❑ Eat some dry bread.

❑ Swallow some crushed ice.

❑ Sit on the floor and pull your knees up to your chest. Wrap your arms around your knees and squeeze — this compresses your chest and forces all the air out of your lungs. Hold it for a moment, then relax. It should clear up those pesky hiccups.

❏ Yank on your tongue. Others recommend a gentle pulling.

❏ Tickle the top of your mouth with a cotton swab.

❏ Gently massage your eyes through closed eyelids. Another source suggests simply putting mild pressure on your closed eyes.

❏ Put your thumb inside your mouth between your teeth and upper lip. Pinch inward with your index finger, pressing just below the right nostril.

❏ Gargle with some mouthwash. It helps clear up the hiccups and leaves you with fresher breath.

MEDICAL SOURCES ————————————————

The Lancet (338,8765:520)
Your Good Health, Harvard University Press, Cambridge, Mass., 1987
Complete Guide to Symptoms, Illness & Surgery, 2nd Edition, The Body Press/Perigee Books, New York, 1989

HIVES

Take the heat out of hives

Hives are the eruption of itchy whelps anywhere on the body. They are caused by contact with or ingestion of an allergic substance, food, food additive or drug.

Sudden sharp changes in climate may produce hives in people who are allergic to heat or cold. Some get hives from stress or tension, while others break out when the skin is scratched or exposed to heat. Others break out for no apparent reason. You can be certain it's hives if the itchy whelps "move around," disappearing on one patch of skin only to show up somewhere else shortly after.

Usually the condition, which is annoying but harmless, will clear up by itself. If the hives are caused by a food allergy, they will appear within minutes of eating the offending food. If the cause of your hives is not that obvious, you might want to check with your doctor or allergist; the culprit could be a dye or additive in your food.

There is another form of hives called angioneurotic edema, which occurs when the tissue under the hives swells, particularly in the face area. Should your lips or the skin around your eyes swell, get medical help immediately.

The best defense for hives is to identify what you are allergic to and stay away from it. Here is a checklist for treating hives:

❑ Watch for other signs that might signal life-threatening anaphy-laxis, a severe allergic reaction. If the itchy whelps on your skin are followed by wheezing, runny nose, paleness, cold sweats or dizziness, call an ambulance immediately.

❑ Stop exercising until several days after hives have disappeared.

❏ Don't get hot, sweaty or excited. This aggravates hives.

❏ Don't take hot baths or hot showers.

❏ Stop taking any drugs, including over-the-counter ones, unless they are specifically prescribed for you. Call your doctor if you're taking a prescription drug.

❏ If your doctor agrees, you might try a nonprescription antihistamine containing either diphenhydramine or chlorpheniramine. These drugs fight the whelping, itchy process.

❏ Don't eat or drink any more of what you ate or drank during the last three to four hours before the itching began. Eliminate those foods to see if the hives go away. Keep a food diary to determine what triggers the attack.

❏ Lay off alcoholic beverages, coffee and other caffeine-containing foods or drinks. These make hives worse.

❏ Wear only loose, nonconstricting underwear. Protect your skin from irritations to avoid another flare-up.

❏ Take a bath in cool or lukewarm water. Soak for up to half an hour several times a day for relief.

❏ Apply cool, moistened cotton cloths as compresses to the itchy areas several times a day. Experiment with rubbing an ice cube on an especially itchy whelp. If it helps, try some more ice cubes.

Medical Sources

The American Medical Association Family Medical Guide, Random House, New York, 1987
Complete Guide to Symptoms, Illness & Surgery, 2nd Edition, The Body Press/Perigee Books, New York, 1989
The Merck Manual, Sixteenth Edition, Merck Research Laboratories, Rahway, N.J., 1992

Hyperventilation

Recognize the symptoms of hyperventilation

Your heart is racing, your mouth is dry, your fingers feel tingly, you feel light-headed and you can't catch your breath — what is happening to you?

You're probably hyperventilating.

Hyperventilation is a situation in which you begin taking abnormally long, rapid and deep breaths. When this happens, too much air gets into the lungs, and the balance in your lungs between oxygen and carbon dioxide gets thrown off.

In order for your body to function correctly, your lungs maintain a certain balance between the amount of oxygen you breathe in and the amount of carbon dioxide you breathe out. When that balance gets messed up, you start having funny feelings — the symptoms of hyperventilation.

In many cases, hyperventilation is caused by a sudden fright, overwhelming anxiety or panic (as in "panic attacks"). In these cases, the hyperventilation is not serious and will probably go away when the person settles down.

However, hyperventilation can be caused by more serious medical problems, such as epilepsy. And even if an episode of hyperventilation is triggered by anxiety or fright, hyperventilation in people with heart disease could be a life-threatening situation.

Doctors in the past recommended that people who are hyperventilating should breathe into a paper bag until they calmed down and their breathing returned to normal. Now, the doctors caution against the use of a paper bag.

Apparently, in people with heart disease, breathing into a bag can prevent their hearts from getting enough oxygen. This could result in collapse or even death.

So, doctors are now recommending that people who are hyperventilating should breathe into their cupped hands, try to calm down and call a doctor. Sometimes the hyperventilation episode can be triggered by a small heart attack or a case of myocardial ischemia — a situation in which the heart doesn't get enough blood.

If the hyperventilation was triggered by something (heart attack or ischemia) other than fright, anxiety or panic, the doctor will need to make sure the heart is not damaged or in danger.

Here are the symptoms of hyperventilation:

- Chest pains
- Shortness of breath or difficulty breathing
- Fluttering or irregularly beating heart
- Abdominal discomfort or pain
- Dry mouth
- Difficulty swallowing
- Abdominal bloating
- Numbness or tingling in your arms, legs or skin
- Muscle spasms
- Feelings of fear or apprehension
- Giddiness
- Irritability
- Light-headedness
- Seizures
- Altered consciousness (confusion, delirium or unconsciousness)
- Fainting

MEDICAL SOURCES

Postgraduate Medicine (88,1:191)
Modern Medicine (57,12:80)

HYPOGLYCEMIA

Blood sugar disorder: Nuisance for some, serious problem for others

The dizzy, shaky feelings of hypoglycemia—not enough sugar in the blood—can develop for a variety of reasons.

Some causes are serious, and some are of minor importance. But hypoglycemia can be uncomfortable and, at times, dangerous.

Hypoglycemia occurs when the level of sugar (glucose) in the blood falls too low. It's the opposite of hyperglycemia. Hypo is too low, while hyper is too much.

Since the brain's only fuel source is glucose, severe hypoglycemia can be serious. And, if it continues unattended long enough, it can be fatal.

Fortunately, most people can learn to control hypoglycemia naturally, just by making simple changes in diet and routine.

Who gets hypoglycemia?

❑ Insulin-dependent diabetics. After a person eats, the body normally releases insulin to help absorb glucose into the muscles and tissues of the body. Sometimes a diabetic who must take insulin gets too much at one time. When that happens, the diabetic's blood sugar level falls too low, and he begins to experience the warning signs of hypoglycemia.

Insulin-dependent diabetics may also trigger hypoglycemia by eating too little food or by exercising so much that the delicate balance between glucose and insulin levels is upset. Diabetics who are dependent on insulin should work with a health care team to learn how to avoid hypoglycemia. Such a team could include your doctor, nurse, nutritionist, pharmacist and family.

It may help you to know that some drugs, including alcohol, can encourage hypoglycemia or alter the ability to recognize the signs of hypoglycemia. Other factors can also affect how the body uses insulin.

For example, the longer you have been dependent on insulin, the more likely you are to become hypoglycemic. Your health team can help you evaluate all the factors that affect how your body uses insulin.

❑ Children with hereditary disorders. A physician should evaluate and treat a child who becomes hypoglycemic because of an inherited condition.

❑ People with postprandial (after-eating) hypoglycemia. Some people suffer from a form of hypoglycemia called reactive hypoglycemia.

These people may produce too much insulin after a large meal. Blood glucose then falls below normal levels, causing hypoglycemia. This problem can be solved by eating frequent, smaller meals. Another kind of after-meal hypoglycemia sometimes develops in people who have had part or all of the stomach removed by surgery.

Because the whole stomach isn't there to slow the passage of food to the small intestine, the bloodstream absorbs the food too quickly.

This causes a speedy rise in blood sugar. A quick rise in insulin follows and triggers an abrupt fall in blood glucose. Again smaller meals at frequent intervals may prevent this type of hypoglycemia.

❑ People with fasting hypoglycemia. For these people, eating habits are not the problem.

Instead, they may become hypoglycemic for other, more serious reasons.

Following is a list of the causes of fasting hypoglycemia:

> • Problems with adrenal gland
> • Alcoholism
> • Severe liver damage
> • Tumors
> • Prolonged fasting

If hypoglycemia is a problem for you, your doctor can help you pinpoint the cause and learn the right solution for you.

MEDICAL SOURCES ————————————————

> *U.S. Pharmacist* (15,11:6 Supplement)
> *Postgraduate Medicine* (88,1:175)

Warning signs

Watch for these warning signs of hypoglycemia:

> • You feel shaky, hungry or anxious.
> • You tremble and break out in a cold sweat.
> • Your heart races or flutters.
> • You become faint or light-headed.
> • You feel irritable and unable to concentrate.
> • You develop an unexplained headache.
> • Your hands, feet or head develop an uncontrollable shaking.
> • You suddenly can't see well.
> • You become confused or start doing things that are unlike you.
> • If hypoglycemia happens during the night you may have nightmares, feel restless, sweat heavily and wake up with a headache.
> • In the advanced stages of hypoglycemia, you may become unconscious.

Without treatment, severe hypoglycemia may result in seizures, coma and death.

MEDICAL SOURCE ————————————————————

> *The Merck Manual, Sixteenth Edition*, Merck Research Laboratories,
> Rahway, N.J., 1992

First aid for low blood sugar

For relief of mild hypoglycemia, try these quick sources of energizing blood sugar:

- Glucose tablets or dextrose solution
- Nondiet carbonated soft drink
- Skim milk
- Honey, corn syrup or sugar
- Fruit juices such as orange juice, pineapple juice, cranapple juice and apple juice
- A hard candy like Lifesavers
- Sugar cubes
- Saltine crackers
- Graham crackers

Ask your doctor about the right amount of carbohydrates to relieve hypoglycemia. More severe hypoglycemia may require a shot of glucagon and hospitalization to stabilize your blood levels.

MEDICAL SOURCE ————————————————————

> *U.S. Pharmacist* (15,11:14 Supplement)

Cornstarch might be the missing ingredient for hypoglycemia

The cornstarch in your kitchen could be the missing ingredient in the diets of those who suffer from certain types of hypoglycemia.

Researchers report that cornstarch heads off trouble for people who develop hypoglycemia several hours after eating and for children who have specific types of hereditary disorders.

The cornstarch helps you to maintain normal levels of glucose in the blood because it is a form of starch that's digested and absorbed slowly.

Researchers had the best success with the cornstarch when they mixed it with a sugar-free soda. Cooked cornstarch or starch mixed with lemon juice doesn't work.

Naturally, you should check with your doctor before treating yourself with cornstarch for hypoglycemia.

MEDICAL SOURCE ─────────────────────────────

The American Journal of Clinical Nutrition (52,4:667)

HYPOTHYROIDISM

Hypothyroidism may be the culprit behind fatigue, weight gain, constipation and depression

Are you shivering while everyone else is toasty? Don't blame your thermal underwear. You might be suffering from hypothyroidism.

The thyroid gland straddles the windpipe below the voice box in your neck, and it affects practically every cell in your body. So, when it fails to produce enough hormones (hypothyroidism), you can suffer a wide variety of complaints.

Women in particular are prone to hypothyroidism. And your chances of getting the disease increase with age. In fact, studies indicate that one out of every 10 women over 40 suffer from an underactive thyroid. The most common symptoms include fatigue, depression, intolerance to cold, weight gain and constipation.

However, you don't need to panic if you've gained a few extra pounds lately. Not everyone who gains weight or suffers from depression or constipation is suffering from hypothyroidism. These symptoms can obviously result from other medical problems or changes in lifestyle.

But, if you experience one or more of these symptoms over a period of months, without a change in lifestyle, ask your doctor about getting your thyroid checked.

In other words, if you keep gaining weight, but you haven't been eating any more than usual, you should check with your doctor.

However, occasionally doctors have a hard time reading the results of thyroid tests, and an accurate diagnosis can be tricky. Sometimes even a lab report that shows your thyroid hormone levels in the "normal" range can be misleading. You might suffer a "sub-clinical" form of underactive thyroid. Insist on thyroid tests that are very sensitive.

Avoid medicating yourself with over-the-counter "thyroid" supplements. They can cause serious problems, including hyperthyroidism or excessive thyroid hormone output.

For more information, contact the American Thyroid Association at 1-800-542-6687.

MEDICAL SOURCE ————————————————

Pharmacy Times (57,1:43)

Common symptoms of hypothyroidism

- Dry skin
- Stiff muscles, cramps
- Hair loss
- Elevated cholesterol
- Abnormal menstrual periods
- Infertility
- Headache, dizziness
- Slowed heart rate
- Hoarse voice

MEDICAL SOURCE ————————————————————————

Pharmacy Times (57,1:43)

IMPOTENCE

Weight loss might be the key to improving problems with impotence

Impotence is a problem experienced by men everywhere, and no matter who you ask, the problem is unpleasant and embarrassing. For some men, it's even psychologically damaging.

In many cases, impotence is caused as a side effect of medication. Men who take diuretics, or "water pills," to help control their high blood pressure often experience this unpleasant side effect.

But recent studies suggest that losing weight can help reverse the impotence caused by the blood pressure medicine. Scientists placed 35 male volunteers on a weight-loss program. All of the men were taking medication to control their high blood pressure.

After about six months on the weight-loss program, the group lost an average of 11 pounds each, and the men reported a pleasant benefit of the weight loss: Only three of the men in the group suffered from impotence.

Without weight-loss programs, about 30 percent of men taking high blood pressure medicine experience some problems with impotence. But only 10 percent of the men in the study experienced impotence after losing weight. That means 90 percent of the men who lost weight didn't suffer the unpleasant side effect of impotence.

Researchers advise men who are suffering from drug-induced impotence to talk to their doctors about a safe and effective weight-loss program. Losing weight could mean an end to a distressing problem.

MEDICAL SOURCE ─────────────────────────

Science News (138,12:189)

Infections

Selenium helps fight infections

Yeast enriched with selenium appears to strengthen the immune systems of elderly adults.

As people age, their immune systems tend to weaken, so susceptibility to infections increases.

Researchers report that a dietary supplement of selenium-enriched yeast boosts the immune system in elderly adults.

MEDICAL SOURCE ————————————————————————

The American Journal of Clinical Nutrition (53,5:1323)

Contaminated makeup can cause skin irritations, even blindness

It's an essential part of a morning ritual for millions of American women. And, most women wouldn't think of beginning the day without it. You can find it in almost every bathroom and purse in America — makeup.

Women use it to enhance their beauty and hide any blemishes, but do they ever stop to question the safety of using cosmetics? It's a question all makeup-users should ask. The makeup itself is usually not the problem. It's what is found in the makeup.

Contaminated makeup can cause serious health problems, including anything from minor skin irritations to permanent blindness.

The Food and Drug Administration (FDA) reports that cosmetics are not necessarily free from contamination when first opened, nor will they remain free from contamination during consumer use.

In fact, a survey revealed that over 5 percent of new samples of cosmetics were seriously contaminated with dangerous microorganisms, bacteria, molds or fungi.

According to the FDA report, most of the contamination in the new packages of makeup is caused by manufacturers using inadequate preservatives in the makeup to help keep it fresh and contamination-free.

Aside from faulty manufacturing, however, your daily use of the cosmetics also allows microorganisms to get in and contaminate your makeup.

Most forms of cosmetics contain preservatives that should kill any foreign microorganisms that might get into the makeup, but those preservatives are not foolproof.

Contaminants occasionally escape the action of the preservatives found in the makeup. When this happens, you run the risk of infection from the contaminating agents.

Reactions to contaminated cosmetics can be as simple as an irritating itch to something as serious as blindness resulting from an eye infection caused by contaminated mascara.

If you develop any problems from the use of your makeup, stop using the makeup right away, and see your doctor.

Also, call your local FDA office and report the type and brand of makeup that you are having trouble with. Consumer feedback is one of the few ways the FDA will know if the makeup on the market is really as safe as it should be.

MEDICAL SOURCE ———————————————————

FDA Consumer (25,9:19)

Tips on how to protect yourself from makeup contamination

❑ Throw makeup away immediately if you notice that the color changes or an odor develops. The preservatives in the makeup can degrade over a period of time and allow contamination.

❑ Keep makeup containers closed tightly at all times except when using them.

❑ Never share your makeup with anyone. Sharing spreads germs.

❑ Keep your makeup out of direct sunlight. The strong sunlight can damage the preservatives.

❑ Never add any liquid (water, etc.) to the cosmetic product to soften it. If the product is too old and stiff, buy some new.

❑ Never use cosmetics near the eyes or on the skin if you are suffering from some type of allergic reaction.

❑ Be careful about using makeup when you have active cold sores around your lips. The Herpes simplex type I virus in the cold sores can spread to your eyes, a very serious situation. Wash your hands after touching the infected areas and before you apply makeup around the eyes. By the way, it's a slightly different virus — type II — that causes genital sores.

❑ Read the label and follow the instructions correctly. Use the makeup only in the places specified on the package.

❑ If you want to know how long you can safely use your cosmetics before buying new, call the manufacturer and ask. The customer service department is there to help answer questions.

MEDICAL SOURCE ─────────────────────────

FDA Consumer (25,9:19)

Ferocious felines — what to do for cat scratches

Your kids loved playing with the neighbor's cat, until one accidentally stepped on the cat's tail and got scratched.

Should you just wash and bandage the wound, or take your child to see a doctor?

The answer depends on the wound. The type of wound and the depth of the wound are the important factors you should consider. Although any cut, abrasion or laceration from an animal (cats, especially) can get infected, puncture wounds and deep, full-thickness wounds have the greatest chance of getting infected.

Why? Because they are harder to clean well, and the bacteria gets trapped in the tissue and starts the infection process.

No matter what the cut, abrasion or puncture looks like, the first thing to do is clean it well. Wash the wound with a mixture of water and povidone-iodine solution. If the cut or puncture is deep, try using a Water Pik (that you use to clean your teeth) and spray the water into the wound. That will help flush out any deep dirt and bacteria. Wash the wound for at least five minutes.

If the wound is bleeding, apply a clean cloth or gauze pad with pressure, and stop the bleeding. Then bandage the wound to prevent it from getting dirty and infected.

If the wound looks very deep, or if it starts turning red, swollen and tender, see the doctor right away. He can prescribe antibiotics that will prevent bacterial infection of the wound.

If the cat scratch doesn't look infected (swollen, red, tender or pus-filled) after 24 hours, then it probably isn't going to get infected. The first 24 hours after an animal bite usually determine whether or not the wound will get infected.

Animal bites or scratches have greater chances of getting infected than other wounds because of the extra bacteria the animal carries. Up to about 90 percent of all cats carry the bacteria Pasteurella multocida. If you become infected with this bacteria after a cat scratch or bite, your wound will begin to show infection right away, including pus drainage and occasional fevers and swollen glands.

Any signs of infection should alert you to see your doctor.

You can also get the illness tetanus — once known as lockjaw — from animal bites. So if it has been five or more years since your (or your children's) last tetanus shot, get one right away.

Over-the-counter pain relievers like aspirin or acetaminophen will help soothe any pain and discomfort that the wound might cause. See your doctor if the wound doesn't improve or gets worse.

MEDICAL SOURCE —————————————
  Emergency Medicine (24,4:195)

This is no fish tale — catfish wounds can be serious

You've been catching fish all day, but they were all bream that were no bigger than butter beans. So when you catch that whopping catfish, you are determined to put it on your empty stringer. And that's when it happens — one of the fins from the fish punctures your hand.

You might consider it an honorable battle scar, but it might turn out to be a high price to pay for a measly fish story. You see, catfish usually swim in slow-moving, muddy waters. The only problem is that bacteria can survive and flourish in this slow-moving water. So, the catfish's skin, including the fin that just speared you, is probably covered with bacteria.

If that bacteria gets into your wound and bloodstream, it can cause an infection that could be serious enough to require amputation of a finger or portion of your hand.

When bacteria invades a wound, it begins infecting the surrounding tissues, and occasionally, it infects the closest bones. The bone infection is known as osteomyelitis, and it is a very difficult infection to manage. People suffering from osteomyelitis often have limbs amputated to prevent the bacteria from spreading to the rest of the body.

Now, obviously, not everyone who gets finned by a catfish will develop a dangerous bone infection. However, the risk is always there.

To lower your risk of becoming infected:

- Use thick gloves when handling catfish.
- Let the catfish go. Cut the line without trying to retrieve your hook. Being on the safe side of avoiding infection is worth the price of losing a single hook.
- Take some anti-bacterial soap and some anti-bacterial, first-aid spray with you in your tackle box. If you get finned, clean the wound immediately with the soap, then spray on some of the first-aid spray to help reduce your chances of a bacterial infection.
- If your wound becomes tender, red or swollen, go see your doctor right away. Early treatment could prevent the wound from becoming seriously infected.

MEDICAL SOURCE ————————————————
Emergency Medicine (24,3:6)

Oysters could be a raw deal for some

If you are elderly, suffer from diabetes or liver disease, or have had some kind of stomach surgery, you probably should avoid eating them raw — raw oysters, that is.

Oysters are commonly infected with a bacteria known as Vibrio. This kind of bacteria can cause illnesses such as cholera, intestinal disorders, blood infections or tissue infections.

People with diabetes or liver disease and those who are elderly or who have had stomach surgery are more likely to become infected with an illness if they eat an oyster that carries the bacteria.

Cooking oysters usually kills any bacteria present in the popular seafood choice. It's eating them raw that presents a danger.

To avoid coming down with a serious illness, order your's steamed or fried instead of raw.

MEDICAL SOURCE ——————————————————————

Medical Tribune (32,19:18)

Microwave your food to reduce your risk of contracting hepatitis

You may be getting a little more than you ordered from your local fast-food restaurant.

Scientists conducted a recent investigation to determine the cause of an outbreak of the infection hepatitis A. Hepatitis A is a serious illness marked by an infected liver.

The infection was traced back to a cook at a local, fast-food restaurant who had been an intravenous drug user. He had not been wearing gloves while handling the food and transferred the virus to the food.

A group of factory workers nearby routinely ordered food from this restaurant. One particular worker would go and pick up the food for himself and twelve other people.

As it turned out, he was the only one who got the hepatitis-A infection, because he ate his food on the way back to work while the others heated their food up before they actually ate it. Those who heated their food in the microwave before eating it never became ill.

Microwaving the food seemed to raise the temperature of the food high enough to kill the infectious germs from the hepatitis A infection.

"Microwaving food appears to protect against hepatitis A infection and clinical disease," says the report.

MEDICAL SOURCE ——————————————————

Modern Medicine (59,2:127)

INFERTILITY

Conquering or coping with infertility

Infertility is the inability to become pregnant after one year of regular sexual intercourse without contraceptives. Infertility is also defined as the inability to carry a pregnancy to live birth.

There are many theories about the causes of infertility. The following are among the most common:

❏ Sexually transmitted diseases, which result in pelvic inflammatory disease and infertility.

❏ Working women are exposed to hazards that affect reproductive activity.

❏ Environmental toxins.

❏ Women delay childbearing until they are in their 30s when their fertility begins to decrease.

❏ There aren't more infertile women, just more infertile women seeking help.

Couples who seek help at a fertility clinic or center should be aware that the process is often lengthy, expensive and frustrating. According to *The Columbia University Complete Home Medical Guide*, "Determining whether pregnancy is probable and what must be done to make it possible requires far more cooperation on the part of patients than in almost any other medical specialty."

The first order of business at a fertility center will be to have you give a thorough family history to detect possible genetic disorders. Following that, the doctor will ask you about your own personal health history with particular attention to any medical condition that might affect fertility. For example, if the husband had mumps as an adult, that could be a factor. The health history will also include listing medications that might kill sperm, as well as the use of alcohol, so-called "recreation" drugs, tea or coffee, all of which can affect sperm count.

You and your spouse will be asked detailed questions about your sexual history. The history will include the date of the onset of menses and the type and frequency of monthly periods, any therapeutic abortions, miscarriages or sexually transmitted diseases.

You'll also be asked if you use certain lubricants during intercourse. That's because a lubricant like petroleum jelly slows sperm down and decreases the number of live sperm getting into the uterus.

The woman will learn how to measure and record her basal body temperature and then to chart it, so that in a few months she will know when she is ovulating.

The man will be asked the date of his circumcision and if he had any problems with the descent of his testicles.

Both will be asked about their sexual behavior and activity.

After all the data are gathered, you both will undergo extensive physicals. First, the doctors will check the sperm for both quality and quantity. If the sperm is defective, the doctors will ask about extensive use of hot tubs; saunas; long, hot showers; chronic illnesses; alcoholism; or hormone imbalance. In some cases, the woman is allergic to the man's sperm, in which case one or both will be given medications.

If there seems to be no problems with the man's sperm, the doctors will scrutinize the woman's background to see if there is a history or episodes of dieting so severe that her periods stopped, chronic illness, drug abuse or alcoholism.

As each possibility is eliminated, the doctors will move to another until the problem is uncovered and, in many cases, treated. But, doctors caution, in one out of every 10 infertility cases, no cause is ever found.

MEDICAL SOURCES

The Columbia University Complete Home Medical Guide, Crown Publishers, Inc., New York, 1985
Your Good Health, Harvard University Press, Cambridge, Mass., 1987

Shocking news — electric blankets do more than warm the bed

They are warm and cozy on a cold winter evening, but their effects could be silently devastating. The danger comes from the electromagnetic field that is produced when the electric blanket is on.

Many household appliances and even power lines above your house create electromagnetic fields. The problem with the electromagnetic field produced by electric blankets is that many people spend up to eight hours or more directly under that field when they sleep.

Strong electromagnetic fields might be linked to cancer and fertility problems, some researchers believe. And although the fields produced by electric blankets are relatively weak, spending so much time that close to the blanket might cause problems.

Many scientists suggest that women who regularly use electric blankets have difficulty getting pregnant. And those that do get pregnant are more likely to have miscarriages or to have babies of low -birth weight.

Some researchers suspect that those babies have a greater chance of developing leukemia or brain cancer.

To avoid the potential side effects of the electromagnetic field produced by an electric blanket, follow these safety steps:

- Turn on your electric blanket 20 to 30 minutes before you go to bed.
- Turn the blanket off before getting into bed.
- Unplug the blanket, even though you switched it off, to avoid any magnetic fields in the blanket's wiring.
- Enjoy your freshly warmed sheets, and remember to leave the blanket unplugged all night.

MEDICAL SOURCE ─────────────────────────────

Health Gazette (14,3:1)

INSECT BITES

This tiny tick can cause tall troubles

It's only the size of a pinhead, but it can cause a truckload of problems. It's the Ixodes dammini tick — often known as the deer tick — and it's responsible for the spread of the dreaded Lyme disease.

The ticks are usually found in tall grass and brush, in or near wooded areas. The ticks are parasites — that is, they live on a variety of animals, including deer, field mice, dogs and people.

It's not the tick itself that causes the Lyme disease illness. The tick is a carrier of a germ-like organism known as a spirochete. When the tick bites you and begins feeding, the spirochetes carried inside the tick enter your blood and cause the infection.

Not all deer ticks are infected with the spirochete that causes Lyme disease. However, you can't tell which are and which are not carriers of the disease, so you always need to take the proper safety steps when you find a tick on yourself.

Tick bites can happen any time throughout the year, but the summer months are the time when the ticks are the most numerous.

There are three stages to Lyme disease (if you do not get treatment for the disease).

Stage I, a rash, occurs about three to 14 days after the tick bites you. It starts as a round or oval rash at the site of the tick bite. About 85 percent of all people with Lyme disease develop this rash. The rash can be two to several inches wide.

Many times the rash looks like a bull's-eye, with a lighter

colored area in the middle of the rash. The area of skin that contains the rash is sometimes raised or elevated compared to the surrounding skin. And some people develop other skin lesions that are similar to the rash, but smaller in size.

The rash will probably go away on its own in about a month. However, doctors know of cases in which the rashes lasted up to a year.

During the first month, you will probably have some flu-like symptoms along with the rash. You might experience fever, headaches, muscle and joint pains, fatigue and a stiff neck.

Stage II comes if you don't receive antibiotic treatment. The main symptom of Stage II Lyme disease is joint pain. This happens in about six out of 10 people who don't get antibiotic treatment. The joint pain and stiffness are similar to that in arthritis, and the knee is almost always involved, although any joint could be affected.

About 15 percent of untreated people also develop nerve problems that can cause headaches and the loss of function of the muscles in the face. Some people even develop heart problems.

Stage III of Lyme disease is really just a worsening of Stage II. The joint pain becomes a progressive arthritis, and the nerve problems can cause mental problems and disorders.

Most people notice the rash right away and get antibiotics from their doctors. The antibiotics usually clear up the infection with no further problems.

The best way to deal with Lyme disease is to avoid getting bitten by a tick. Follow the steps below to reduce your chances of getting bitten:

❏ Avoid wooded or grassy areas that have large populations of deer.

❏ When you go into wooded or grassy areas, never go barefoot or in sandals. Always wear shoes.

❑ When you go into wooded or grassy areas, always wear long pants and long sleeves. And tuck your pants legs into your socks to keep the ticks from getting to your skin. Also, tuck your shirt into your pants.

❑ Wear light-colored and tightly woven clothes on your outings. The light color will make it easier to see any ticks that try to grab onto your clothing. The tight weave will help prevent the ticks from grabbing on and staying on.

❑ Check your clothes and your body for ticks as soon as you get home. Then shower and check again.

❑ Put insect repellent on your pants, socks and shoes. Use an insect repellent that contains the ingredient DEET. DEET is an effective tick repellent. Be sure to read the instructions on the repellent container. You can put some insect repellents directly on the skin. Other types of repellent have warnings or cautions about putting the repellent directly on the skin. Follow the instructions on your repellent package.

❑ If you apply insect repellent to your skin, remember that it washes off if you sweat or get in the water. Reapply the repellent as needed.

❑ Stay near the center of trails and roads and avoid heavy brush and grass as often as possible.

❑ Check your pets regularly for ticks. Pets can get Lyme disease, but they can't transmit it to you. But, pets can carry the ticks inside your home. So, protect your pets with tick collars and regular baths.

Even when you follow all the proper safety tips for avoiding tick bites, it is possible that you could still get bitten. If you discover a tick on yourself or any member of your family, take the following steps:

❑ First, remove the tick. Use fine-tipped tweezers to grasp the tick's mouthparts as close to the skin as you can. Pull out steadily and firmly, making sure that you remove the whole tick. If you do not have tweezers, you can pull the tick out with your fingers. Cover your fingers with rubber gloves or tissue, and pull the tick out just like you would with tweezers, grasping the tick at its mouthparts.

❑ Wash your hands and the area around the bite and apply antiseptic cream or spray to cut down on the chance of infection.

❑ Tape the tick onto an index card with clear plastic tape. On the card, write down the date of the bite, the part of your body bitten, and where you were when the tick might have gotten on you (your neighbor's cow pasture, etc.).

❑ Pay close attention to any symptoms that you might develop. Make a note of what they are and when they started.

❑ Call your doctor if you have symptoms of Lyme disease.

For more information about Lyme disease, write the Lyme Disease Foundation, P.O. Box 462, Tolland, Conn., 06084. You also can call the foundation at 203-871-2900. This is not a toll-free number, and will be charged to your telephone bill.

MEDICAL SOURCES ───────────────────────────

Drug Therapy (19,8:25)
American Family Physician (45,5:2151)
The Physician and Sportsmedicine (20,4:140)

Get 'tick'ed off early to prevent Lyme disease

Now you see it, now you don't.
That's part of the difficulty in detecting Lyme disease.

It has a variety of symptoms that can appear and then subside, and sometimes you can't tell whether a symptom points to Lyme disease or some other problem.

Even doctors sometimes have trouble identifying Lyme disease, according to Dr. Saul Rosen.

Dr. Rosen uses the example of a young woman with a typical case of Lyme disease to show how this confusing illness can cause weeks and months of discomfort.

In this case, a 29-year-old woman finally went to the doctor in September because her knees and elbows were hurting as if she had arthritis.

But her trouble really started in mid-June when she was working as a camp counselor on the Chesapeake Bay in Maryland. While at camp she was probably bitten by a deer tick carrying a spirochete called Borrelia burgdorferi.

The first symptom she remembered, according to Dr. Rosen, was an itchy spot on her thigh in early July. It developed into a circular rash that looked something like the bull's-eye on a target. The rash grew and then gradually disappeared.

In late July, a new set of symptoms appeared. She felt unusually hot and tired, and had headaches and nausea for five days. She also had trouble concentrating and sleeping. One eye hurt and she had trouble with peripheral vision in that eye. These symptoms all went away within a week.

By the end of August, one of her knees began to swell and ache. As soon as the knee began to feel better, an elbow started to swell and hurt.

She then saw a doctor who put all the facts together and concluded that Lyme disease was causing all of these problems.

Others who have Lyme disease have reported additional symptoms:

- fever
- flu-like chills
- stiff neck
- sore throat
- anorexia
- headache
- back or muscle ache

MEDICAL SOURCES

Journal of the American Medical Association (267,10:1381)
Drug Therapy (20,7:86)

Can tick bites cause strokes?

Sounds crazy, but it could be true! Doctors recently reported that a healthy 20-year-old soldier suffered from a stroke after returning home from a visit to Germany. Apparently, he had complained of headache, double vision, light-headedness and other symptoms before his stroke.

A few weeks later, he suffered another stroke that left his face mildly paralyzed. Doctors were baffled over the case until they tested the soldier's blood and found Borrelia burgdorferi, the culprit that causes Lyme disease. After more research, they found other cases of strokes associated with Lyme disease.

Strokes usually are caused by blood vessel disorders, but they apparently can also be caused by tick bites. Those who have suffered strokes might have their doctors test them for Lyme disease.

MEDICAL SOURCE

Medical Tribune (31,18:3)

Unexplained loss of vision might be related to tick-bite disease

Suffering from unexplained vision loss? Maybe it's reversible, according to a new report.

Do you recall experiencing disturbances in your color perception and loss of vision in the central part of your eye? If so, you could have Lyme disease, the infectious disease transmitted by the deer tick.

Lyme disease occasionally causes a kind of vision problem known as optic neuritis, an inflammation of the optic nerve that causes vision loss.

Doctors in the Marshfield Clinic in Wisconsin recently discovered that out of 20 people suffering from optic neuritis, four had Lyme disease.

They remembered being bitten by deer ticks. But, none had suffered any of the characteristic symptoms of Lyme disease such as the "bull's-eye" rash, headache, chills, fatigue and muscle or joint pain.

The four patients were treated for Lyme disease with antibiotics, and each recovered their vision.

Doctors caution against testing for Lyme disease in all people with unexplained vision problems.

Lyme disease only causes optic neuritis, not other types of vision problems. So, doctors should test for Lyme disease only in people who have been diagnosed with optic neuritis.

If you are having trouble with your vision and you suspect you might have optic neuritis, talk with your doctor about the possibility of Lyme disease.

A simple antibiotic could clear up your problems right away.

MEDICAL SOURCE ————————————————————

Medical Tribune (32,12:2)

What's bugging you? Tips for dealing with bee stings

Afternoon rain showers, tender new leaves and fresh flowers are all hallmarks of spring and summer. And, unfortunately, the flowers can't come without the bees.

If you and your family spend any time in the great outdoors, you're bound to have at least one run-in with one of these stinging creatures.

Although the wasp and hornet can cause their fair share of pain, the stings from the honeybee and the yellow jacket usually cause the most exaggerated problems. The sting is ordinarily followed by intense pain or stinging for a few minutes. The area around the sting then begins to turn red and starts to swell. If you are not allergic to bee stings, the sting will usually go away in a few days with no additional trouble except some occasional itching.

The honeybee is the only bee that leaves its stinger and sack of poison in your skin. When you get stung by a honeybee, you need to get the stinger out as soon as you can.

Don't try to pull the stinger out with your fingers or tweezers, and try not to squeeze the area around the stinger — this will force more poison (venom) out of the venom sac and cause more trouble.

To remove the stinger, gently scrape it with a knife blade or your clean fingernail until the stinger comes out of your skin. Then clean your hands and the sting with soap and water.

After removing the stinger, put some ice or a cold compress on the sting for about 20 to 30 minutes. This will help take away some of the stinging and will also help reduce swelling.

Mix together some baking soda, meat tenderizer and a few drops of water to make a paste to put on the sting. The meat tenderizer contains an ingredient called papain that can make the bee venom ineffective and relieve some of the symptoms.

If you got stung on your leg or foot, keep it elevated and still for a little while.

Aspirin will help relieve any pain and inflammation, and some over-the-counter anti-itch medications (Benadryl tablets and cream or cortisone creams) can help with any itching.

People who are allergic to bee stings might start to experience wheezing, dizziness and cramps, or in serious cases, choking, unconsciousness and even death. These people should be rushed to the doctor as quickly as possible. If they have an emergency bee sting kit, use the proper medications on the way to the doctor's office or hospital.

If you have ever experienced mild symptoms like dizziness, shortness of breath, difficulty breathing or cramps after a bee sting, but you didn't go to the doctor because the symptoms went away after a while, you need to see your doctor and tell him about your experience.

In many (or most) cases, a person who experiences a mild allergic reaction to a bee sting on one occasion will most likely experience a serious allergic reaction the next time he comes into contact with the allergen (the thing that causes the reaction — the bee sting, in this case). Next time, your symptoms might be much worse — even deadly. Your doctor can give you a bee sting kit to keep with you (in your car or purse) to use if you ever get stung again. If you are allergic to bees, these kits can save your life.

To avoid all the symptoms of a bee sting, try to avoid getting stung in the first place. Here are some simple precautions to take to avoid being stung:

❑ Stay away from insect nests. If you need to remove one from an area close to your house, use the kinds of bug sprays that have six-foot or nine-foot sprayers. If you are allergic to bees, call an exterminator to get rid of any bee nests or hives near your home.

❏ Don't wear bright-colored flowery clothes — the bee could mistake you for a flower and be attracted to you. Also avoid wearing dark, rough clothes. Light-colored, smooth fabrics are the best things to wear to avoid being stung.

❏ Don't wear brightly colored jewelry or hair ribbons or other shiny metal objects that might attract the bees.

❏ Wear insect repellent when you go outside. Put the repellent on your clothes and on any exposed skin.

❏ Keep your garbage cans covered to avoid attracting the bees, and stay away from other garbage cans where bees are looking for food.

❏ Keep screens on your open windows and doors to keep the bees from entering your house.

❏ Always wear shoes outside. Many people are accidentally stung because they stepped on a bee that was minding its own business. Many bees gather food from clover and other flowers that are close to the ground, and some bees even live in the ground. Going barefoot makes your feet a prime target.

❏ Use caution when cutting or smelling fresh flowers. And carry some bug spray out to the garden in case you run into some angry bees that don't want to leave you alone.

MEDICAL SOURCES

Emergency Medicine (24,7:171)
Healthprint (7,4:1)

INSECT REPELLENTS

Safety tips for using insect repellents

You and your family are ready for your weekend camping trip. You've got the tents, sleeping bags, marshmallows and the insect repellent.

You know how to use the tents and sleeping bags, and you know what to do with the marshmallows. But are you sure you know how to use the insect repellent? And use it safely?

It sounds like a ridiculous question. But, unfortunately, people have been hurt and have gotten sick because they used the repellent improperly.

Accidentally swallowing bug repellents or getting any repellent in the eyes can be extremely hazardous to your health and your children's health. Many people have complained that insect repellents cause them to break out in rashes and hives, and there have even been cases of serious nervous system illness from the use of insect repellents.

Spraying the repellent into your eyes, or touching your eyes with your repellent-covered hands can lead to problems that range from minor eye irritations to serious corneal abrasions and ulcers.

To guarantee the safest and most effective use of your insect repellent, follow these few safety tips:

❏ Always read the repellent label and package insert carefully and completely before using the product. Notice any cautions or warnings. And follow the directions as carefully as possible concerning where to use the spray (just on clothing, or on bare skin), when to use it (how often you need to reapply the repellent) and other important instructions.

❏ Use just enough of the insect repellent to cover exposed skin and clothing.

❏ Try applying a little bit of the repellent to a small patch of skin before covering all exposed skin. If the small patch of skin becomes red or irritated, don't use the repellent.

❏ Apply the repellent to yourself in open spaces — don't spray it on in your tiny bathroom. Go out onto your front porch to spray it.

❏ Avoid spraying the repellent directly onto your face.

❏ Don't spray or apply the repellent to the hands of children. They can put their hands in their mouths or eyes and cause possible problems.

❏ When you come in from your outdoor excursion, wash all exposed skin with soap and water, and immediately wash all treated clothes.

❏ If you accidentally get repellent in your eyes, flush your eyes with water. Forcefully hold your eyelids open, and let the water rinse your eyes. The longer you let the water cleanse your eyes, the better. The water might be uncomfortable, but it could save you from some serious problems that can result from the repellent. See your local eye doctor if your eyes seem damaged or irritated.

❏ If you accidentally swallow some insect repellent, rinse your mouth out with water several times. If you have any liquid antihistamine medication, rinse your mouth out with that, too. This helps avoid any possible allergic skin reactions in your mouth.

❏ If your skin breaks out after using insect repellent, stop using the product immediately. If the skin reaction looks like a rash, use an over-the-counter cortisone cream to relieve the irritation. If the reaction looks like hives, you could be suffering from the first stages of a serious allergic reaction, and you should see a doctor as soon as you can.

MEDICAL SOURCE —————————————————————

The Physician and Sportsmedicine (20,4:57)

Natural insect repellent from dried grass

You can dry the grass, steam the dried grass leaves, and you've got your own natural insect repellent.

Citronella oil is the name of the oil that comes from the Java citronella grass. Use it in oils for insect repellents, but do not swallow the oil — it can be poisonous.

You can purchase citronella candles, oils and extracts at most local pharmacies.

MEDICAL SOURCE —————————————————————

The Lawrence Review of Natural Products (October 1991)

JELLYFISH STINGS

Underwater dangers — what to do for jellyfish stings

The waves and warm ocean water were glorious, until you had the sudden feeling that your leg was on fire.

You swim to shore as quickly as you can and inspect your leg. You see a red, painful and swollen sore or swelling right where that jellyfish got you.

Most jellyfish stings are not dangerous — they're kind of like large bee stings, and you can usually treat them as you would a bee sting.

After cleaning the area where you were stung, put an ice pack or some cold compresses on the sting to relieve some of the burning and to reduce any swelling and inflammation.

Then you can use some soothing lotion, aloe vera or anesthetic spray (spray that mildly numbs the skin) to relieve any pain. Aspirin is also helpful. Some people even recommend rubbing aspirin on your damp skin or crushing an aspirin and rubbing it onto your skin with some cream to help relieve some of the pain and inflammation.

If the sting begins itching, try some cortisone cream or some over-the-counter antihistamine (Benadryl pills or cream).

Although many jellyfish stings are not serious and require little more than some ice to relieve the stinging, some species of jellyfish are more dangerous.

For example, the Portuguese man-of-war jellyfish is an extremely poisonous jellyfish, and people have even died from these stings.

If you begin experiencing dizziness, shortness of breath, cramping or difficulty in breathing, get to a doctor as soon as possible. You could be having an allergic reaction to the sting, or you could have been stung by a more poisonous jellyfish.

It's really hard to avoid getting stung by jellyfish if you swim in the ocean because you usually don't see the jellyfish before it stings you. However, you can talk to some local oceanographers or wildlife rangers that might know which times of the year the jellyfish are most numerous in that area.

MEDICAL SOURCES ──────────────────────────────

The Physician and Sportsmedicine (18,8:93)
Healthprint (7,4:1)

How to treat jellyfish stings

Take the following steps, in order, as first aid for stings:

1) Pour ocean or salty water over the injured area.

2) Remove the visible tentacles or stingers with gloves, tweezers or forceps.

3) Saturate the painful area with a soupy solution of baking soda (sodium bicarbonate) and water for 10 minutes. As an alternative, soak the injury in vinegar for 30 minutes. (Don't mix the two solutions.)

4) Pour flour or baking powder (not baking soda) all over the wound area, and then scrape off the powder with a knife.

5) Rinse the area with water (fresh water will do).

6) Apply a nonprescription skin cream or lotion containing corticosteroid, antihistamine and pain-killer. SeaBalm is one brand that works well.

Other remedies reported to ease the pain include the following:

- Soak the area in ammonia. Note: Don't mix this with vinegar or try using both at the same time. An unpleasant chemical reaction will occur.
- Apply a meat tenderizer like papain to the wound.
- Soak the area in a boric acid solution.
- Splash on lemon juice or the juice of figs.
- Soak the painful area in rubbing alcohol.

If you feel faint, if you become short of breath, or if your heart flutters or races, get immediate medical help.

MEDICAL SOURCES

The Physician and Sportsmedicine (18,8:93)
The Merck Manual, Sixteenth Edition, Merck Research Laboratories, Rahway, N.J., 1992

JET LAG

Jettison jet lag

Jet lag is the state of feeling unwell and excessively fatigued after crossing several time zones in a hurry. The condition — known medically as circadian dysrhythmia — is caused by the disruption in the body's normal habits or rhythms. The symptoms include tiredness and hunger at unexpected times, as well as irregular bowel and bladder movement.

Since time zone lines run north and south, jet lag is produced when traveling east and west.

To cut the effects of jet lag:

❑ Gradually shift your eating and sleeping patterns before the flight to match your destination time zone.

❑ Try to eat and drink only low-calorie, high-protein foods for about a day before the flight.

❑ Drink little or no alcohol during your flight because alcohol slows the body's ability to adjust.

❑ Drink lots of nonalcoholic beverages.

❑ Often the legs or feet swell from sitting for long periods of time, so avoid tight shoes or boots.

❑ Wear loose, comfortable, nonrestricting clothing.

❑ Plan on at least a 24-hour rest or adjustment period after you arrive.

❑ If you take a long-lasting type of insulin, you might need to switch to regular insulin until you adjust to the new location. Check with your doctor.

❑ Adjust your schedule for taking medicines based on actual elapsed time, not the local clock time.

❑ Avoid making any major decisions within the first day of arrival. You're just not at your peak mental condition during this transition period, which may inconvenience you for up to 48 hours after you arrive.

MEDICAL SOURCES ────────────────────────

The Marshall Cavendish Illustrated Encyclopaedia of Family Health, Marshall Cavendish House, London, 1986
The Merck Manual, Sixteenth Edition, Merck Research Laboratories, Rahway, N.J., 1992

KIDNEY STONES

Breaking up is hard to do: all about kidney stones

Kidney stones begin with a tiny speck of solid material in the middle of the kidney that, like a snowball, picks up other tiny specks until it becomes a solid piece or stone.

About one out of a thousand people has to be hospitalized for stones. Most stones — called calculi — are calcium compounds, usually calcium oxalate.

The larger the stone, the greater the discomfort because pain occurs when the stones enter the ureter — the tube that carries urine from the kidney to the bladder. The stones stretch the tube and block the normal flow of urine.

In addition to pain, the blockage of urine can lead to an elevated fever and infection, causing an emergency situation where you need to seek medical attention immediately. Usually, the pain associated with kidney stones comes in waves.

For the most part, however, kidney stones pass through the ureter into the bladder and are eliminated through the urine. Once the stone moves to the bladder, the pain stops, and as long as there is no infection, there is rarely any reason for surgery or ultrasound, which is used to break up the stones.

Kidney stones tend:

- To run in families.
- To be more prevalent among men.
- To be more common in hot climates.

Typically, the person with kidney stones sweats a great deal and loses a lot of water, but produces little urine. The urine that is produced tends to be high in calcium.

To help prevent the problem, see your doctor at least twice a year to make sure there is no permanent damage to the kidneys. Also, you should drink eight or more glasses of water a day and take aspirin for the pain.

MEDICAL SOURCES ───────────────────────────────

The Columbia University Complete Home Medical Guide, Crown Publishers, Inc., New York, 1985
The Merck Manual, Sixteenth Edition, Merck Research Laboratories, Rahway, N.J., 1992

 # KNEE PAIN

Exercise is 'oil' for the knees

When you look at your knee, think of a door hinge because that's how the human knee is constructed. Just as it's important to oil your door hinge regularly so that it doesn't become stiff and squeaky, so it's important to exercise your knees regularly for the same reason.

The more you exercise and condition your knees before activities, the better your "door hinges" will serve you.

Often when people age, their knee joints stiffen, most often in the mornings, though that stiffness usually improves as the day progresses.

Should you twist or sprain your knees, apply ice immediately. For minor twists, wrap the knee in an Ace bandage (trade name for an elastic bandage made of woven material) for support, and apply ice packs.

If, however, your knee pain is accompanied by swelling or fever, you should contact your doctor immediately.

Medical Source ─────────────────

The Marshall Cavendish Illustrated Encyclopaedia of Family Health, Marshall Cavendish House, London, 1986

LACTOSE INTOLERANCE

Lactose intolerance? Yogurt with live cultures aids digestion

Could this be you?

The simple delights found in eating an ice cream cone or drinking a smooth milkshake are unknown pleasures for you. Just looking at dairy products makes you feel sick. You avoid dairy products in any form because the nausea and cramping are too intolerable to bear.

You and many others suffer from lactose intolerance.

Lactose intolerance is a common condition in which the stomach does not contain the necessary enzymes to properly digest the lactose sugar found in dairy products.

This condition is not hazardous to your health — you just avoid dairy products.

Unfortunately, avoiding dairy products can sometimes lead to a deficiency in calcium, especially in women.

However, scientists report that lactose in certain types of yogurt that contain live bacteria is better tolerated than lactose in other dairy products,.

Apparently, the live bacteria found in some types of yogurt manufacture an enzyme known as beta-galactosidase that digests lactose.

Since the bacteria manufacture the enzyme, the human stomach doesn't have to do it. In other words, the bacteria contained in the yogurt digest the lactose in the yogurt.

Therefore, people who can't digest the lactose themselves won't suffer from lactose intolerance symptoms because the lactose will be digested by the bacteria. (The bacteria contained in the yogurt is "good" bacteria, not harmful to you.)

As well as being a healthy and tasty snack, yogurt is an excellent natural source of calcium.

So those who suffer from lactose intolerance won't need to suffer from a calcium deficiency as well.

Scientists report that not all brands of yogurt contain the live bacteria that manufacture the important enzyme. Be sure to check yogurt labels for contents. If the label does not give enough information, consider calling the yogurt manufacturers or the Food and Drug Administration.

MEDICAL SOURCE ─────────────────────────────

The American Journal of Clinical Nutrition (54,6:1041)

Who gets this condition, and what you can do about it

Surprisingly, it seems linked to race. Except for white people with origins in northwest Europe, lactose intolerance is a common condition. Nearly eight out of 10 nonwhite people lose the ability to digest lactose by age 20. It happens to nine out of 10 Orientals. Whites who suffer from lactose intolerance number less than two out of 10 people.

A simple nonprescription remedy is to buy lactase enzyme and add it to dairy products before you eat. Another is Lactaid, tablets that you eat with lactose-containing foods. Follow directions on the packages to find the best results for you.

MEDICAL SOURCE ─────────────────────

The Merck Manual, Sixteenth Edition, Merck Research Laboratories, Rahway, N.J., 1992

LARYNGITIS

Talk back to laryngitis

Laryngitis is usually caused by bacterial or viral infections of the larynx or voice box; or, it can be caused by an irritation or inflammation without infection. In rare instances laryngitis is a symptom of tuberculosis. It can also be the result of a tumor in the larynx, though that is unusual.

When laryngitis is caused by a bacterial or viral infection, the mucous membranes of the larynx swell and become inflamed. When the condition is caused by an irritation or inflammation without infection, it typically follows a bout of smoking or drinking or excessive talking, singing or shouting.

In either case, the main symptom is hoarseness, which may lead to a loss of the voice.

Speaking is often painful, and there may be fever or other flu-like symptoms.

If you have a bout of laryngitis and otherwise are in good health, you should:

- Stay at home.
- Rest your voice.
- Don't smoke.
- Don't drink alcoholic beverages.

Steam inhalation sometimes helps, as does a cough suppressant. If your laryngitis persists for more than a week, you may have chronic laryngitis, in which case you should seek medical attention.

MEDICAL SOURCE ————————————————

The American Medical Association Family Medical Guide, Random House, New York, 1987

LEG PAINS

Recognizing intermittent claudication

Intermittent claudication is often one of the early symptoms of arteriosclerosis obliterans when the major arteries that carry blood to the legs and feet become narrowed by fatty deposits on the walls of the arteries. Sometimes collateral blood vessels that branch off the major arteries take over, but they are often inadequate to meet such demands as walking more than a short distance.

You can suspect intermittent claudication if you experience cramp-like pains, aching or muscle fatigue in the calves of the legs during even moderate exercise. Intermittent claudication can make it difficult for minor foot injuries to heal. A small cut that won't heal can get infected and, at the worst, can lead to amputation.

The treatment will depend on the severity of the condition. The following measures are often helpful:

- Stop smoking.
- Exercise, particularly walking.
- Lose weight.
- Learn methods to control diabetes or to lower high blood pressure, if you have either of those conditions.
- Wear comfortable, well-fitted shoes and socks that will adequately protect your feet from injury or infection.
- Inspect your feet daily, and seek prompt medical care for such problems as corns, calluses, injuries or infections.

MEDICAL SOURCE

The Columbia University Complete Home Medical Guide, Crown Publishers, Inc., New York, 1985

LICE

Home remedy for getting rid of lice

Your child came home from school with a note from the school nurse: Billy has head lice. Do not let him return to school until the lice are removed.

You're horrified and angry at the same time. But your real concern is how to get rid of the lice.

There are many prescription-strength "pesticides" that you can get from your doctor to get rid of lice. However, many people don't want to use such strong chemicals on their children's skin. And many people have very sensitive skin that would react to the prescription-strength chemicals.

So, if you are looking for a safe and sure-fire home remedy for removing the lice, look under your bathroom sink — for the mineral oil.

Pour the nonprescription mineral oil over the entire scalp and leave it on for about 10 minutes. You might want to warm the mineral oil a little to make it a bit more comfortable on the head. After 10 minutes, wash out the mineral oil with shampoo.

After shampooing, use a fine-toothed lice comb to gather the suffocated lice.

Repeat this procedure every two days for ten days. At the end of ten days, the lice and all their eggs should be gone.

Be sure to thoroughly wash all clothing and bed linens that might have come into contact with your child's head to guard against reinfestation.

You can also use mineral oil to suffocate lice found on other areas of the body, including eyelashes.

Petroleum jelly is a good alternative for body areas other than the scalp.

MEDICAL SOURCES ─────────────────────────

Emergency Medicine (24,3:164)
The Merck Manual, Sixteenth Edition, Merck Research Laboratories, Rahway, N.J., 1992

LONGEVITY

Live longer and regain strength with exercise

If you think that retirement means resting on your laurels and taking things easy, think again. More and more people are beginning to realize that an active lifestyle improves not only the quality of life, but also how long you live.

Many people have a tendency to become less active as they age. However, experts agree that a lot of the aging process is psychological—we think that as we get older we have to slow down. That's not the case.

Studies show that you can regain a great deal of strength, agility and independence if you exercise regularly, no matter what age you begin.

Researchers recently completed a study focusing on 10 people between the ages of 86 and 96.

After using standard muscle-resistance training over an eight-week period, all 10 showed signs of increased muscle strength.

Unfortunately, many people don't begin to worry about fitness until they are a little older and notice that they can't do as much as they used to.

Usually by age 50, a lot of damage has already been done, because of poor nutrition, bone loss and the general aging process. And, it's harder to undo the damage than prevent or delay it.

However, don't despair if you are over 50 and don't exercise. Starting an exercise program now will still give you many health benefits.

No one can put off the effects of aging permanently, and you may still suffer from disease. But, you can avoid or delay diseases associated with aging by staying active. Exercise can even help people who suffer from diabetes, hypertension and heart disease.

An active lifestyle and exercise improves your heart and blood-vessel functions, and it can help you live longer. A study of 16,936 people showed that active people lived from one to over two years longer than people who didn't exercise.

When thinking about an exercise program, keep these things in mind. The exercises should be within your capabilities, and should allow you to gradually improve your capabilities. They should be kept to a reasonable time and level of intensity. And they should be fun.

Always consult your doctor before starting any exercise program, because there are a lot of "dos" and "don'ts" that you may not think of.

For instance, do you know that eating can lower your blood pressure, so you shouldn't eat for one hour before or after exercising?

And did you realize that warm-up and cool-down periods are essential to move the blood flow from the large leg muscles and prevent dizziness?

Some people occasionally "go off the deep end" and end up

doing more harm than good. So, be sure to check with your doctor before beginning your exercise program. She can help you design a program that's best for you.

MEDICAL SOURCE ——————————————————————

The Physician and Sportsmedicine (18,11:83)

Go hungry and live longer?

Counting calories could add up to a longer life.

Yes, restricting your intake of calories might actually lengthen your life.

Cutting calorie intake helped slow down age-related diseases. Studies show that mice with restricted diets live 29 percent longer than those with normal diets, and also have fewer cancerous tumors.

Even after two years, mice with unrestricted calorie intake had about four times as many tumors as those with restricted diets.

Dietary restriction appears to protect DNA from damage, increases enzymes' ability to help repair DNA and significantly reduces the effects of proto-oncogenes (genes that can cause cancer when altered).

Scientists conclude that chronically hungry mice seem to live 15 to 50 percent longer and remain livelier than the mice with full bellies.

Some scientists believe that the results of these studies might be applicable to humans. But, remember, cutting calories is different from cutting nutrition. Your body still requires a minimum amount of vital nutrients — vitamins, minerals, proteins, etc. — each day to stay healthy.

MEDICAL SOURCE ——————————————————————

Science News (140,14:215)

MEMORY

Sweeten your memory with sugar

A spoonful of sugar might do more than make the medicine go down when it comes to memory. Sugar might actually help improve long-term memory.

In a recent study scientists recruited 17 healthy volunteers (ages 62 to 84) to test the effects of sugar on memory. The volunteers fasted at night, then went to the lab in the morning and drank an eight-ounce glass of lemonade. Half the glasses of lemonade were sweetened with sugar. The other half were sweetened with saccharin, a sugar substitute.

The scientists carefully monitored the blood-sugar levels of the volunteers for the next two hours while the volunteers took memory tests. One of the tests involved listening to a tape-recorded message, then telling about it five minutes later and 40 minutes later. Another test involved trying to repeat a list of 12 words.

The researchers found that the volunteers who drank the lemonade sweetened with sugar performed better on the two tests than the volunteers who drank lemonade sweetened with a sugar substitute.

The sugar seemed to help improve long-term memory. The scientists think that the sugar helps the body to transmit chemicals in the brain (known as neurotransmitters) that might influence memory.

Although the sugar seems to help memory, researchers caution that too much sugar in the diet is not healthy and can increase the risk of diseases such as diabetes.

MEDICAL SOURCE ————————————————————

Science News (138,12:189)

Menopause

New treatment for women's 'old' heart disease problems

Here's a simple therapy that could radically change the lives of each one of you 50 million American women approaching menopause.

It's known as estrogen-replacement therapy, and it could help reduce a woman's risk of heart disease by as much as 44 percent and her risk of death from heart disease by 39 percent.

When a woman goes through menopause, her body undergoes a series of changes.

One of the more dramatic changes is the large drop in estrogen production in the body. Along with other things, this reduced level of estrogen in the blood results in an increased risk of heart disease.

In fact, white women past age 50 have about a 30 percent chance of dying from heart disease, and black women past age 50 have a surprising 38 percent chance of dying from heart disease.

However, replacing the estrogen in the body through simple estrogen-replacement therapy can substantially reduce that risk of heart disease.

Estrogen replacement usually is prescribed to do two things: to reduce the rate of bone loss that occurs after the female body stops making its own estrogen, and to ease the hot flashes, insomnia, fatigue and other distressing symptoms of menopause. The heart-helping action is purely incidental.

Scientists think that estrogen helps reduce the risk of heart problems by affecting cholesterol levels in the blood. The estrogen somehow helps to lower the amount of harmful LDL cholesterol in the blood and raise the amount of healthy HDL cholesterol. The increased ratio of HDL to LDL cholesterol in the blood reduces the risk of heart problems.

Despite the great cardiovascular effects of estrogen-replacement therapy, it's not for everyone.

High levels of estrogen in the blood have been linked to breast cancer and endometrial cancer.

Some researchers estimate that estrogen-replacement therapy increases the risk of breast cancer by about 30 percent and doubles the risk of endometrial cancer.

So, women who have family histories of breast cancer or endometrial cancer should use estrogen-replacement therapy with extreme caution, if at all.

However, for women past the age of menopause with at least one other risk factor for heart disease, estrogen-replacement therapy seems to be worth the risk, because the benefits of reducing heart-disease risk far outweigh the risk of cancer.

Estrogen-replacement therapy is also beneficial because it lowers the risk of dying from a hip fracture by about six-fold.

Talk to your doctor about the potential risks and benefits of estrogen-replacement therapy.

MEDICAL SOURCES ———————————————————
> *Medical Tribune* (32,20:1)
> *The New England Journal of Medicine* (325,11:756)

'Trim and slim' through mid-life for your heart's sake

For smooth sailing through menopause, don't take extra pounds along.

Extra pounds during mid-life could put you at a higher risk for heart problems. Excess weight is often followed by blood pressure and heart problems.

Researchers conducted a study in which they focused on problems associated with weight gain in the years just before and after menopause.

In the three-year study, the 485 healthy women ages 42 to 50 experienced significant gains in weight and body mass, whether premenopausal or postmenopausal.

Average weight gain was about five pounds, but 20 percent of the women added closer to 10 pounds. Low-exercise levels seemed to be a factor in weight gain.

There were strong associations between weight gain and increases in blood pressure readings, total blood cholesterol and triglycerides (a large portion of the fatty substances in the blood). These are all risk factors for coronary heart disease.

Keeping those extra pounds off helps to avoid changes that can trigger increased risk for heart disease.

MEDICAL SOURCE ————————————————

Archives of Internal Medicine (151,1:97)

Menopause for left-handers comes early?

If you're a left-handed woman, you might want to prepare for an early menopause.

The women taking part in two national surveys were between 35 and 74 years old and had experienced menopause at least one year previously.

Researchers found that the average age for left-handed women to reach menopause is 42.3 years.

The average menopausal age for right-handed women is 47.3 years.

That means that left-handed women go through menopause an average of five years earlier than do right-handed women, according to these figures.

MEDICAL SOURCE —————————————————————————

American Family Physician (43,3:962)

MENSTRUAL CRAMPS

Conquering the cramps

There are many reasons for a woman to experience cramping during her menstrual periods.

Commonly, when painful cramps are accompanied by nausea and diarrhea, the cause is an excess of a certain type of prostaglandin in the uterus that is "leaking" into the intestines. (Prostaglandins are substances found in the body, one of which causes the uterus and intestinal muscles to contract.)

When there is too much prostaglandin in the body, the normally painless, rhythmic contractions of the uterus during menstruation become longer at the tightening phase, keeping oxygen from the muscles.

The lack of oxygen is what causes the pain. Since the uterus is a muscle, relaxation exercises help, as does massage. Anticipating the pain, however, makes it worse.

Many women find that dietary changes help to relieve the symptoms.

Such changes include these:

- Add more whole grains, whole flours, beans, vegetables, fresh fruits and brewer's yeast.
- Eliminate or at least radically cut down consumption of sugar, salt, alcohol and caffeine.
- Eat small, frequent meals, rather than three large ones.

Other tips include the following:

- Allow time for extra sleep if needed.
- Do some stretching exercises.
- Try some herbal teas.
- Use heat pads on the stomach or lower back.
- Take some aspirin or acetaminophen.
- Try taking extra doses of calcium or magnesium.

For the depression, bloated feeling and tension that often accompany the cramps, try extra doses of vitamin B6 and decrease your intake of sodium. Whole grains, yeast and fresh fish are loaded with vitamin B6.

If you feel exceedingly tired or "dragged out," have your blood checked for iron. You may be slightly anemic.

MEDICAL SOURCE ————————————————

The New Our Bodies, Ourselves, Simon and Schuster, Inc., New York, 1988

MENTAL PROBLEMS

Researchers suspect Alzheimer's disease has three different 'links'

Researchers are looking at two broad types of Alzheimer's disease.

One kind seems to be family-linked, passed on from parent to child. This kind of "early-onset" Alzheimer's senility affects mostly members of the same family in their forties and fifties. It may involve a mutated gene, a damaged chemical messenger inherited by the child.

The other kind usually hits people over age 70. Scientists believe this kind of senility is not inherited. As many as half of the people over age 85 come down with this kind of Alzheimer's disease, some statistics indicate.

Strong links to the disease include the following:

❑ Aluminum — Although we get a lot of aluminum in our diet, scientists know of no dietary need for the light mineral. In other words, aluminum is nutritionally unnecessary.

The mineral has been found in abnormally high amounts in the brains of Alzheimer's victims. In such amounts, aluminum acts like a brain poison.

The controversy is whether the aluminum deposits cause the disease or whether the disease causes the deposits.

❑ Genetic problems — A lot of research is concentrating on a body substance known as amyloid precursor protein. Some research suggests that a damaged gene for that protein might cause the hereditary form of Alzheimer's that afflicts some families.

❏ Previous head injury — People who have received head injuries are nearly three times more likely to develop Alzheimer's than those with no history of head trauma.

❏ Tobacco smoke — At least one research study in recent years suggested that smokers are four times as likely as nonsmokers to develop Alzheimer's disease.

❏ Zinc — This nutrient is needed to repair brain and nerve cells. Some researchers think that low levels of zinc in the body might contribute to senility.

While scientists argue about causes, there is no disagreement about the outcome: Alzheimer's disease is incurable and always fatal, usually within five years of its first symptoms. An estimated 100,000 Americans die each year of Alzheimer's disease, making it the fourth leading cause of death among adults.

On the other side of the equation, researchers have identified at least two apparently protective factors against Alzheimer's.

❏ Aspirin and other anti-inflammatory drugs like ibuprofen; also cortisone-like drugs and medicines for malaria. Alzheimer's and other dementias are rare among people with rheumatoid arthritis, most of whom take these painkillers daily.

❏ Fluoride in water, especially sodium fluoride. A Canadian report says that aluminum and fluoride compete in the digestive system. "The more fluoride in the diet, the less aluminum is absorbed," the report says.

However, take note of the reports later in this chapter about the "leaching" effect associated with cooking with fluoridated water in aluminum pots.

MEDICAL SOURCES ───────────────────────────

Postgraduate Medicine (89,4:231)
Science (251,4996:876)
Journal of the American Medical Association (262,18:2551)
The Lancet (1,8632:267 and 335,8696:1037)
U.S. Pharmacist (15,5:62)
Men's Health Newsletter (6,4:1)
Canadian Journal of Public Health (83,2:97)

Simple tips on how to limit your exposure to aluminum

❏ Water — Get your home water tested. Public water systems normally put more aluminum compounds in your water during the summer than during the rest of the year. If the aluminum content is higher than 50 parts per billion, then you might want to consider a filtration system that acts on aluminum. Activated carbon filters don't work well on aluminum. Your best bet might be reverse osmosis-type filter systems.

❏ Foods — Watch out for processed cheese, especially grated, canned Parmesan cheese. White self-rising flour and baking soda also might contain aluminum compounds to help the products "flow" better.
Soft drinks in aluminum cans might contain raised aluminum levels, but it might be because of the water used rather than because of the can itself. Other sources include prepared cake mixes, frozen dough, pancake mixes and pickled vegetables.

❏ Table salt—Same thing here. Your table salt probably contains sodium aluminum silicate to keep the salt pouring during wet weather.

❏ Medicines — The majority of antacids contain aluminum. Other over-the-counter products with aluminum include buffered aspirin, antidiarrheal products, douches and hemorrhoidal preparations.

❏ Antiperspirants and cosmetics—Aluminum is the active ingredient in underarm deodorants.
The aluminum compounds rubbed on the skin "knock out" the sweat glands for a time. To do that, the compounds must be absorbed. Some facial creams also contain aluminum that may be absorbed.

❏ Aluminum cooking pots and pans — Foods with high-acid content, like tomatoes, might "leach" aluminum and absorb the compound into the food itself.
One test from Sri Lanka indicated that cooking with fluoridated water in aluminum cookware increased by up to 1,000 times the aluminum levels found in unfluoridated cooking water. Also, avoid storing high-acid foods in aluminum foil.

MEDICAL SOURCES ————————————————————

British Medical Journal (301,6746:286)
U.S. Pharmacist (14,12:57)
The Lancet (1,8629:59)

Aluminum acts like a 'deadly poison'?

Aluminum in food, water and medicines seems to act like a deadly poison in some people with kidney problems, new research indicates.

This follows British and French studies linking higher aluminum levels in drinking water to higher rates of Alzheimer's disease and to unusual levels of aluminum deposits in bones.

The latest warning flag has been raised about people undergoing dialysis for kidney failure. It turns out that people on dialysis face poisoning from even small amounts of aluminum.

Dialysis helps weakened kidneys by "washing" a person's blood and cleaning out impurities. Medicines commonly used in treating kidney failure contain aluminum.

These researchers recommend a change in treatment for dialysis patients because of the aluminum problem. Chief researcher I.B.

Salusky recommends changing from aluminum hydroxide to calcium carbonate to lower abnormally high blood levels of the nutrient phosphorous.

"One must wonder ... whether there is any safe dose of aluminum" for people with serious kidney problems, writes Dr. Donald J. Sherrard about the study.

The editorial tells about a dialysis patient who died unexpectedly because he was taking a nonprescription pain reliever containing citrate.

Citrate is a common compound that seems to increase absorption of aluminum in people with kidney failure, the editorial says.

In addition, Dr. Sherrard, for the first time in a major American medical journal, raises the question "about the potential for problems in the general population" caused by aluminum in the everyday diet.

Most American doctors are reluctant to point accusing fingers at aluminum.

After all, aluminum is the third most common element on earth, and it's nearly everywhere — naturally present in vegetables, a standard water treatment chemical, and a common ingredient in everything from over-the-counter antacids to underarm deodorants.

British and European researchers for several years have suspected aluminum might not be as harmless as most medical people have assumed.

A U.S. government study in 1987 estimated that you probably get between 9 and 14 milligrams of aluminum every day naturally from your food and drinks.

Another study says that you may get an additional 20 to 50 milligrams per day from food additives.

Leaching from aluminum cookware may add an additional 3 to 4 milligrams a day, according to a news release from the Aluminum Association, Inc.

Wichita State (Kansas) University researchers tested water from a new electric heating pot and found it contained 30 times the recommended limit of aluminum in the water. The heating pot apparently added about 74 times more aluminum than was contained in plain tap water.

If you take antacids for heartburn, you might add more than 1,000 milligrams of aluminum a day. One antacid tablet contains about 50 milligrams of aluminum, and a buffered aspirin up to 20 milligrams.

Your baby gets about 100 times more aluminum in soy-based formula than from mother's milk.

The body begins to accumulate more aluminum than it can get rid of when your daily intake is somewhere between 125 and 1,000 milligrams a day, says the aluminum trade association. And that's when it can become a health hazard.

However, the Food and Drug Administration continues to consider aluminum nontoxic to humans, says the Aluminum Association news release.

MEDICAL SOURCES ——————————————————

The New England Journal of Medicine (324,8:558)
The Journal of the American College of Nutrition (11,3:340)
Archives of Internal Medicine (149,11:2541)
The Lancet (1,8641:781 and 1,8636:490)

Phosphate deficiency can have you 'seeing pink elephants'

This simple truth became a nightmare for one 59-year-old woman who suffered from frightening visual hallucinations for almost two full days.

According to the report, this lady was admitted to the hospital for treatment for complications of diabetes. On admission to the hospital, she was alert and mentally aware.

However, after 24 hours, she began suffering from frightening hallucinations. She had no history of mental problems or of alcohol or drug abuse.

When her hallucinations worsened, the medical staff tested her blood and found that she was suffering from a deficiency of phosphorus.

They immediately started her on phosphorus replacement treatment, and the hallucinations disappeared within four hours.

She had been suffering from a phosphorus deficiency known as "hypophosphatemia," a condition which can occur among diabetics and alcoholics.

Researchers suggest regular phosphorus measurements for people who have diabetes or alcoholism.

If you experience visual or auditory (hearing) hallucinations, see your doctor immediately and ask him to test your blood phosphorus level.

Some natural dietary sources of phosphorus are meats, poultry, fish, eggs, grains, nuts, dry beans and peas.

MEDICAL SOURCE ————————————————————

The Lancet (338,8774:1083)

Mental confusion, shakiness linked to swollen bladder

Older folks may become confused for many reasons. But new research suggests an unexpected link between confusion and urine retention in studies of three men over the age of 70.

Because of urinary problems, these men retained too much urine in their bladders.

As a result, the men rapidly became confused, shaky and unable to communicate.

But as soon as doctors treated the three to relieve urine retention, the men's confusion disappeared, and they returned to normal within minutes.

This news encourages doctors to consider urine retention as a possible cause for unexplained mental confusion.

A simple visit to the doctor may relieve the problem of mental confusion in men over 70.

MEDICAL SOURCE ————————————————————

Archives of Internal Medicine (150,12:2577)

MOTION SICKNESS

Say 'bon voyage' to seasickness — tips on how to deal with motion distress

Are you one who loves to go deep-sea fishing, sailing or even on ferry rides, but the wave of nausea that always covers you prevents you from enjoying these pleasurable pastimes?

If so, you're certainly not alone. Research shows that one out of three adults experiences seasickness on boats. In fact, as many as 30 percent of all experienced navy crewmen suffer from seasickness during routine ship duty — and that's without rough waters. Up to 90 percent of the people in the navy experience seasickness during storms and rough waves.

Most people who experience seasickness complain of nausea, dizziness, heaving, sweating and vomiting. Some people suffer from heart flutters and shortness of breath.

It's an aggravating sickness, because it keeps you from enjoying your water activities. And, to make things worse, if you're on a boat, you can't just get away from what is making you sick. You have to just deal with the seasickness until the boat docks.

For some, it is such a miserable experience that they never want to see a boat again.

Fortunately, seasickness does not have to ruin your boating plans. Following a few simple tips will help you sail away from seasickness and on to a pleasurable activity.

❏ Avoid boating activities on stormy days when the waves are high and the waters rough.

❏ Go out in larger boats. The smaller the boat, the more it will bob and bounce in the water. Larger boats are more stable, and less bouncing results in less seasickness.

❏ **Stay in the center of the boat and avoid the ends of the vessel.** The ends of the boat bob up and down more than the center. Staying near the boat's center of gravity will reduce the rocking sensation from the boat and decrease the severity of the seasickness you experience.

❏ **Avoid boating activities if you have ear problems.** The fluid in the inner ear helps you maintain your balance and sense of equilibrium.

When the fluid is disturbed, you feel dizzy and queasy. In fact, the feeling of seasickness results from disturbances in the fluid in your inner ear.

So, getting on a boat when you already have problems with your ears (infections, hearing problems, etc.) is just asking for trouble. Ask your doctor if your ear problems will increase your risk of seasickness (or any other kind of motion sickness).

❏ **Try using anti-seasickness medicines.** These are now available in patch forms — you just stick the patch to your skin like you would a Band-Aid, and the medicine is absorbed through your skin. The best place to stick these patches is on the skin just behind your earlobe — this location provides the best relief from seasickness symptoms.

Anti-seasickness medicines are also available as pills or injections, but doctors recommend the patches because the patches cause fewer side effects and the benefits last longer. Pills and injections start wearing out after about two hours.

Anti-seasickness benefits from the patches usually last up to eight hours. However, the peak performance of the patches occurs about four to six hours after you put it on. So be sure to put on your patch a good four hours before your excursion to get the best results while you are out on the water.

Possible side effects of anti-seasickness medicines include dry mouth, blurred vision, headache and decreased attentiveness. Always follow the instructions on the label to make sure you are taking the drug correctly and getting the best results.

❑ Taking antihistamines might also help reduce your symptoms of seasickness.

❑ Stay on the deck of the boat, instead of going into the cabins below. Your symptoms will not be as severe on the deck.

❑ Try to stay warm — either with warm clothes, blankets or a hot water bottle.

❑ Try to eat, but stay away from large, heavy meals. Eat snacks that will help soothe your stomach — crackers, bread or toast. As you begin to feel better, add more foods.

❑ Drink clear liquids, such as ginger ale, to help calm your stomach.

❑ When riding on the deck, focus on the horizon instead of looking at the tossing waves.

❑ Try some ginger. This common spice will help relieve nausea. You can take ground ginger root capsules to help soothe your tossing stomach. Eating ginger snaps or drinking ginger ale might also help settle your stomach.

❑ Try massaging the skin in between your thumb and index finger. Many people claim that it helps relieve nausea.

MEDICAL SOURCES ——————————————————

The Physician and Sportsmedicine (20,7:35)
Complete Guide to Symptoms, Illness & Surgery, 2nd Edition, The Body Press/Perigee Books, New York, 1989

Ginger root vs. Dramamine

Ginger root capsules might be a better way to stave off motion sickness than Dramamine, according to a controlled clinical study.

People taking 940-milligram capsules of powdered ginger root had fewer episodes of vomiting during spins in a tilting chair than those who took dimenhydrinate (Dramamine).

The dose is equivalent to less than one-tenth of an ounce of store-bought ginger powder, or about a pinch between your fingers.

MEDICAL SOURCE ──────────────────────

Popular Nutritional Practices, Sense and Nonsense, Dell Publishing, New York, 1988

NIGHT BLINDNESS

Seeing through night blindness

You can suspect night blindness if your vision is normal in good light, but not so good in dim light. The ability of the eye to adapt to light and dark depends on photoreceptors in the retina. One particular type of photoreceptor regulates vision in dim light.

Night blindness can be a symptom of severe vitamin A deficiency. It can also signal retinitis pigmentosa, an inherited degenerative disorder of the retina.

If the problem is a vitamin A deficiency, it can be treated with vitamin A supplements. But if the problem is retinitis pigmentosa, there is no treatment.

Vitamin A is abundant in fish liver oil, liver, whole milk, fortified margarine, butter, whole-milk cheeses, egg yolks and dark green, yellow and orange vegetables.

Fatigue seems to make night blindness worse, as does smoking.

Don't overdose on vitamin A. The Recommended Dietary Allowance (RDA) for men is 1,000 micrograms (which is one milligram) and 800 micrograms for women. People taking 100 times that daily dose have suffered brain swelling and severe vomiting. People taking daily doses of about 15 times the RDA have developed chronic vitamin-A poisoning after several weeks. People who eat large amounts of animal liver risk getting too much of this vitamin.

MEDICAL SOURCES ────────────────────────────

The New Good Housekeeping Family Health and Medical Guide, Hearst Books, New York, 1989
The Merck Manual, Sixteenth Edition, Merck Research Laboratories, Rahway, N.J., 1992
Recommended Dietary Allowances, 10th Edition, National Academy Press, Washington, D.C., 1989

NOSE PROBLEMS

Removing foreign objects from your child's nose

It has happened to every parent. Your child walks in crying, holding his nose. You think he has probably fallen.

Then you discover that he accidentally (or purposefully) put a small button, eraser or toy up his nose and can't manage to get it back out.

Should you laugh or cry?

The answer is, you should get some nose spray.

Spraying some nasal decongestant (not antihistamine) into your child's nose will help reduce some of the swelling and mucous accumulation. This will allow your child to blow the object out of his nose with a strong blow.

If this doesn't work, or if there is the likelihood of internal injury, get medical help.

MEDICAL SOURCE —————————————————————

Emergency Medicine (24,4:191)

NOSEBLEEDS

What to do for nosebleeds — leave the cotton in the field

Nosebleeds are messy and aggravating, but usually pretty easy to deal with. Whether your nosebleed is from an overdry nasal mucosa, nose picking or a run-in with the door frame or your neighbor's fist, a few home remedies should have you fixed up and ready to go.

The first thing to do is to remember to leave the cotton in the field.

Never, no, never use cotton to plug up a bleeding nose. Yes, it is true that the cotton fits into the nostril well and absorbs lots of blood real well.

The trouble with cotton is that the fibers stick to the wound. And when the blood finally clots, the cotton fibers do, too. Pulling out the cotton fibers usually reopens the wound and starts the bleeding again.

And even if the nose doesn't start bleeding again, many of the cotton fibers stick to the lining of the nostrils and continue to irritate the sensitive skin long after the bleeding stops.

Instead of cotton, use a rectangular piece of petroleum-jelly-coated gauze to pack the nose and stop the bleeding.

While the gauze packing is in place, pinch the fleshy part of your nose right between your eyes with your thumb and index finger. But don't lean your head way back while you are doing this. Sit upright, with just a little upward tilt on your head

Pinch just below the bony bridge of your nose for about five to 10 minutes, and the bleeding should stop. If it hasn't stopped, try pinching for another 10 minutes or so.

Think of the inside of your nose as two pliable plates that you want to press closely together tightly enough to restrict breathing through your nose.

Also try placing an ice pack on your nose to help reduce the bleeding and relieve any stinging you might feel.

About ten minutes after the bleeding stops, put some water in your hands and splash your face to wet the gauze, then gently remove it from the nostril.

After your nose stops bleeding, try to avoid any trauma (hitting or picking your nose) for about a week to make sure the bleeding site heals properly.

If you have problems with frequent nosebleeds or a nosebleed that just won't stop bleeding, see your doctor. That could signal underlying problems, such as vitamin deficiencies, nasal tumors or bleeding disorders.

MEDICAL SOURCE ———————————————————————

Emergency Medicine (24,6:26)

NUTRITION

Plain speaking about healthy ways of eating

"Follow these rules for healthy eating" — only problem is, the rules are hard to understand.

The "rules" are just good eating advice from the American Heart Association and the National Cholesterol Education Program.

They recommend dietary guidelines for adults to prevent heart and blood vessel diseases by lowering cholesterol in the blood. Once translated, the guidelines are really quite simple.

There are two things you need to know about: The first thing is fat.

The human body stores fat as a form of fuel for muscles and organs — it's the gas for the body's engine, in other words. And, just like different kinds of gasoline, there are different kinds of fats that you can eat, and the body uses some fats more efficiently than others.

The most efficient fuel for the body is unsaturated fats. The least efficient fuel is saturated fats. The difference between saturated and unsaturated fats has to do with the way the molecules are put together.

An easy way to remember the difference: Saturated fats are solid at room temperature.

This usually includes animal lard, solid cooking shortening and most butters and margarines. These are the ones to cut way back on.

Unsaturated fats are usually liquid at room temperature. This includes most liquid shortenings and liquid forms of margarine.

These are the better ones to use.

Sometimes manufacturers use the terms "hydrogenated," "partially hydrogenated" or "nonhydrogenated" instead of saturated or unsaturated. Don't be confused.

Hydrogenated is the same thing as saturated — stay away from these. Unsaturated is the same as nonhydrogenated — these are the good fuels. Partially hydrogenated is somewhere in the middle — not as good as unsaturated, but definitely better than saturated.

The second thing is cholesterol.

Cholesterol is a substance that is made by all cells in animal bodies. Your body requires a minimum amount of cholesterol, but it usually makes all it needs internally.

Plants cannot make cholesterol in their cells. So, the sources of dietary cholesterol obviously come from animal sources, such as eggs, meats and some dairy products.

Although you might want to lower the amount of cholesterol in your diet, you might not want to eliminate all foods from animal sources.

These foods contain valuable nutrients. Instead, eat smaller amounts of these foods.

You can also be aware of the kinds of meat products you are eating.

Meats with the most fat have the most cholesterol — so eat meats with less fat.

Most cuts of beef and pork have the greatest amount of fat; poultry with the skin removed is in the middle; and fish has the least amount of fat and cholesterol.

MEDICAL SOURCE ─────────────────

Journal of the American College of Nutrition (10,5:443)

Simple tips for decreasing the amount of fat and cholesterol in your diet

❑ Avoid fried foods. Instead of frying your meats, bake or broil meats in a broiler pan so the fats in the meat drip into the pan rather than stay in the meat.

❑ Eat only lean, well-trimmed meats. Fish, chicken and turkey have the least amount of fat.
However, if you need some more variety, avoid "well-marbled" cuts of beef, and trim as much fat off the meat as you can before you cook it.

❑ Eat more fish and seafood. Seafood has very low fat content. (Remember to avoid fried foods — try broiled shrimp instead of fried shrimp.)

❑ Eat only five to six ounces of meat each day, no matter what kind of meat.

❑ Use low-fat dairy products. Buy low-fat milk and cheese — you usually can't even taste the difference.

❑ Only use margarines that contain one gram of saturated fat or less per spoonful. Most tub margarines fit into this group. Liquid margarines might even be better. Be sure to check the label.

❑ Choose "lite" condiments, when possible. For example, "lite" mayonnaise and salad dressings usually have half the fat of normal brands.

❑ Use substitutes. Frozen egg substitutes and butter-, cheese- and cream-flavored powders make good low-fat alternatives.

MEDICAL SOURCE ——————————————————

Journal of the American College of Nutrition (10,5:443)

How to prevent dietary deficiencies on a vegetarian diet

For some, it's a fad or a passing whim. For others, a religious tradition.

And still others are doing it for their health. But no matter what the reason, maintaining a vegetarian diet can be risky if you're not careful.

The more you restrict your diet, the harder it is for you to get all the nutrients that your body needs to function at its best. So, being a vegetarian is just not as simple as leaving out the beef in your lasagna.

There are really six different kinds of vegetarians, based on what foods they will or won't eat:

❑ Semi-vegetarians eat dairy foods, eggs, chicken and fish, but no other meat.

❑ Pesco-vegetarians eat dairy foods, eggs and fish, but they do not eat meat.

❑ Lacto-ovo-vegetarians enjoy dairy foods and eggs, but no other animal products.

❑ Lacto-vegetarians will eat dairy products, but no other animal products.

❑ Ovo-vegetarians will eat eggs, but no other meat or animal products.

❑ Vegans, the most extreme type of vegetarian, will not eat any meat or other animal products.

Vegans have with the greatest risk of nutritional deficiencies, because many animal products contain vital nutrients that the vegetarians in the other groups can get from the animal products they eat (eggs, milk, etc.).

Vegans have the greatest risk of suffering from a vitamin-B12 deficiency. This can result in serious mental problems and even irreversible nerve damage.

The need for vitamin B12 goes up during pregnancy, breast-feeding and growth spurts, so the risk of deficiency increases during those life stages.

Vegetarians also have an increased chance of suffering from a vitamin-D deficiency.

Almost all milk products in the U.S. are fortified with vitamin D, so the people who eat dairy products probably get enough of this important vitamin. Too little vitamin D prevents the bones from forming properly — this can result in rickets in children and osteoporosis in adults.

Iron deficiency is also a concern for vegetarians. Although many vegetarians get a normal amount of iron in their diets, the other foods they eat so much of (bran, fiber and soy products) often prevent the iron from being absorbed well into the bloodstream from the intestines.

And all vegetarians are at risk of inadequate caloric intake. They might not be getting enough food calories to keep their bodies healthy. This can be especially harmful in children and pregnant women.

To help avoid or to remedy these nutrient deficiencies and to assure the healthiest vegetarian diet possible, follow these simple dietary guidelines:

❑ Take daily vitamin supplements that contain calcium, riboflavin, iron, vitamin D and vitamin B12, because these nutrients are hard to get from plant sources. Infants, children and pregnant women need to be extra careful about getting the proper amounts of these nutrients each day.

❏ For vitamin B12, try using vitamin-B12-fortified soy milk and cereals in addition to vitamin supplements.

❏ To help avoid vitamin-D deficiency, try adding vitamin-D-fortified margarines to your diet. Sunlight is also a good source of vitamin D, so spend some time out in the sunlight each day. Vitamin supplements can also help boost your vitamin D.

❏ Be sure to get enough calcium by eating some calcium-rich foods: tofu, broccoli, seeds, nuts, bok choy, legumes and calcium-enriched grain products.

❏ Make sure your body's immune system is up to par by getting enough zinc in your diet (especially in children's diets). Some foods that contain zinc are legumes, nuts, tofu and whole-wheat bread.

❏ If you feel fatigued or a little run down, you could be suffering from anemia — not enough iron is getting into your bloodstream. Try some of the following iron-rich foods: legumes; tofu; green, leafy vegetables; dried fruits; and iron-fortified cereals and breads.

The amount of iron that your intestines will absorb will be greater if you eat it with some vitamin C. Foods that contain vitamin C that will improve your iron absorption include citrus fruits and juices, tomatoes, strawberries, broccoli and potatoes with skins.

❏ Look for "substitute meats" to spice up your diet. These "meats" are usually made from soy products, and you can get them as hot dogs, ground beef and even bacon. An extra bonus: Many of the substitute meats are fortified with vitamin B12.

❑ To make sure you are getting enough protein, combine legumes with grains in your meals. Examples of legumes are soy beans, lima beans, kidney beans, lentils, black-eyed peas, chickpeas, peas and navy beans. Examples of grains to combine with your legumes include rice, wheat, corn, rye, oats, millet, barley and buckwheat.

❑ To get the greatest benefits from your vegetarian diet, stay away from less-nutritious foods, such as sweets and fatty or fried foods.

❑ If you eat dairy products, choose the low-fat varieties.

❑ Choose whole and unrefined grain products instead of refined or heavily-processed grain products.

❑ Check with your doctor or a nutritionist to make sure your infants, children or teen-agers are getting enough calories and vitamins in their diets to assure their proper growth.

❑ If you are pregnant or nursing, take special care to make sure you are meeting all the recommended daily allowances of vitamins and minerals. Vitamin deficiencies during pregnancy can result in miscarriages, low-birth-weight babies, and even birth defects. Consult a registered dietition or other nutrition professional, especially during periods of pregnancy, breast-feeding and illness.

❑ If you are switching from a regular diet to a vegetarian diet, do it slowly. For starters, replace the fattiest meats with fruits, vegetables and cereals.
Then after your body adjusts to the increased fiber intake, start replacing other foods (lean meats, eggs, chicken, etc.). Switching to the new diet slowly is good for your health, but it also helps you from getting discouraged and bored with your new,

meat-free diet right away.

As you learn to cook more with fruits, vegetables and grains, you can begin substituting some of your new favorite dishes for some of the old ones.

MEDICAL SOURCE ————————————————————

FDA Consumer (26,4:21)

Fish for this fat: the omega story

The American Heart Association and the National Cholesterol Education Program recommend a diet that contains less than 30 percent fat calories each day.

They say that the amount of saturated fats in the diet should make up no more than 10 percent of your daily fat intake and should be less than 300 milligrams of the total amount of cholesterol.

Seafood is a great addition to your diet because it is a good substitute for many foods that are high in fat and cholesterol. One of the reasons seafood is such a healthy addition to your diet is because it contains the unsaturated fats known as omega-3 fatty acids.

The omega-3 fatty acids help prevent blood clots from forming in your blood vessels and help prevent the buildup of plaque on the walls of the blood vessels. This helps cut your risk of heart disease and stroke.

Seafood also provides one of the leanest sources of protein you can get in your diet, and it contains many valuable vitamins and minerals.

Most fish is low in total and saturated fats, but even the fish that has higher amounts of fat or cholesterol is good for you because of its omega-3 fatty acids.

The problem most people have when they try to add more fish to their diets is that they don't know what kind of fish to buy.

The following chart gives you an idea of which kinds of fish are low in fat and high in omega-3 fatty acids.

Fish*	Fat grams	Omega-3 grams
Albacore tuna	4.9	1.5
Atlantic mackerel	13.9	2.6
Atlantic salmon	5.4	1.4
Bluefin tuna	6.6	1.6
Bluefish	6.5	1.2
Catfish	3.1	0.3
Clams	1.5	0.1
Cod	0.7	0.2
Flounder	1.4	0.2
Halibut	1.2	0.4
Lake trout	9.7	2.0
Mullet	4.4	1.1
Mussels	1.6	0.5
Ocean perch	1.5	0.2
Orange roughy	0.3	0.1
Oysters	1.2	0.6
Rockfish (snapper)	1.8	0.5
Scallops	0.2	0.2
Shrimp	0.8	0.3
Sockeye salmon	8.6	1.3

*Based on an uncooked serving size of 100 grams (3.5 ounces)

MEDICAL SOURCE —————————————

U.S. Department of Agriculture, Human Nutrition Information Service

How to buy good fish

Now that you've decided what kind of fish you want to buy, you need to know how to buy it.

How to buy it? you ask. What's so hard about buying fish?

The federal government does not inspect fish the way it does beef or poultry, so you need to take extra care when selecting your fish. To make the best selection, keep the following tips in mind:

❑ Be careful and choosy about where you buy the fish. Go to a reputable store or market where the managers will tell you where the fish came from and how fresh it is. (Avoid buying fish off the back of someone's truck like vegetables.)

❑ Smell the fish. Yes — smell it. If it smells too "fishy," it's probably not as fresh as it should be. Fresh fish does not smell fishy. It should have an ocean-like smell, a seaweedy smell or even a cucumber-like smell. If it smells like ammonia, sour or too fishy, you probably should look somewhere else. Fresh fish does not smell offensive.

❑ Quickly refrigerate the fresh fish or any leftovers from your fish dinner to prevent bacteria from contaminating it. (Some people freeze their fish in Zip-lock bags with a little water around the fish to help preserve the fresh flavor when they thaw and cook it.)

❑ If you catch your own fish instead of buying it at a fish market, be sure to find out from the local fishing and game authorities which bodies of water are free of pollution or contaminants. Never eat fish caught in polluted waters.

MEDICAL SOURCES ─────────────────────────────

The Physician and Sportsmedicine (18,4:19)
Tufts University Diet and Nutrition Letter (7,4:3)

Get omega-3 oils from plants, too

The following are plant sources high in omega-3 fatty acids. The comparisons are based on a serving size of 100 grams (approximately three and one-half ounces).

Food	Total Fat in grams	Omega-3 in grams	Omega-3 % of fat
Rapeseed oil	100.0	11.1	11.1
Walnut oil	100.0	10.4	10.4
Wheat germ oil	100.0	6.9	6.9
Soybean oil	100.0	6.8	6.8
English walnuts	61.9	6.8	10.9
Black walnuts	56.6	3.3	5.8
Tomato seed oil	100.0	2.3	2.3
Soybeans, sprouted, cooked	4.5	2.1	46.6
Dry soybeans	21.3	1.6	7.5
Oat germ	30.7	1.4	4.5
Leeks, raw	2.1	0.7	33.7
Radish seeds, sprouted	2.5	0.7	28.0
Wheat germ	10.9	0.7	6.4
Common dry beans	1.5	0.6	40.0
Navy beans	0.8	0.3	37.5
Pinto beans	0.9	0.3	33.3
Kale, raw	0.7	0.2	28.5
Spinach, raw	0.4	0.1	25.0

MEDICAL SOURCE —————————————————————

U.S. Department of Agriculture, Human Nutrition Information Service

Should there be RDA for fatty acids?

In what may be the first such official argument, Norwegian researchers are suggesting that a minimum level should be established for "essential fatty acids," just as there are standards currently for vitamins, minerals and other basic nutrients.

The Norwegian researchers, led by Kristian Bjerve, discovered that omega-3 fatty acids are essential for the normal metabolic processing of omega-6 fatty acids.

Omega-6 oils, close relatives of omega-3 oils, are found in things like safflower oil and other cooking oils.

The Norwegians found a direct relationship between daily doses of omega-3 oils and healthy levels of certain blood substances. In their study, they found that 350 to 400 mg of omega-3 acids in the form of purified fish oil are needed daily to maintain normal plasma and lipid levels.

"Omega-3 fatty acids possibly also have some specific function in the retina (in the eye) and in the central nervous system," Bjerve says.

MEDICAL SOURCE ———————————————————

The American Journal of Clinical Nutrition (49,2:290)

Lean, red meat supplies vital nutrients

Wait! Don't hurry by the meat counter just yet.

Red meat is an excellent supplier of protein, iron and zinc, which are vital to the body's smooth performance and good health. Whatever your dietary requirements, you still need the nutrients that meat ordinarily supplies.

Why? you ask. Because one of those nutrients, protein, is essential for healthy muscles.

In fact, small servings of lean meat should be a part of the diet of anyone who needs protein, iron and zinc. A four-ounce serving of beef contains between 70 and 80 milligrams of cholesterol. The American Heart Association recommends capping cholesterol at 300 milligrams daily.

Many people shy away from beef or pork, thinking its cholesterol content is too high. But the 70 to 80 milligrams found in four ounces of lean meat is comparable to that found in four ounces of fish or chicken.

Also, the National Academy of Sciences says that there is no link between meat antibiotics and human health problems. Those who are concerned about hormones in meat might be comforted by reports from the Food and Drug Administration declaring that hormones found in meat are inactive after cooking.

MEDICAL SOURCE ─────────────────────

The Physician and Sportsmedicine (19,1:31)

Boost your performance with a healthy breakfast

Remember the old Cheerios commercial jingle, "This boy is running out of energy because he didn't fuel up with a good breakfast"? Well, it's more than a jingle—it's the truth. Eating a healthy breakfast helps to fuel your body's energy supply, and it increases your tendencies to eat healthier throughout the rest of the day.

If you exercise or train early in the morning, before work or school, and skip breakfast, you aren't doing yourself any favors. In fact, you're actually hurting your performance. Your blood sugar levels are low, and the exercises will feel more strained and tiring.

Instead of skipping breakfast, you should eat a small, pre-exercise snack like a slice of toast or a small banana. That small snack will boost your blood sugar levels and enhance your performance.

Then after the workout, you should eat the rest of your healthy breakfast. Many people have lost their appetites after exercising, but they need to eat anyway to help restore the energy reserves used during the exercises.

The breakfast can be a liquid breakfast, so try a glass or two of a fruit juice followed by a glass of low-fat milk. Then on your way out the door, grab a bran muffin, bagel or some other carbohydrate-rich food. This kind of breakfast gives you the fluids, carbohydrates, proteins and vitamins you need.

If you are not a morning person, and you prefer to exercise later in the day, you still need to eat a healthy breakfast. And that breakfast (or your breakfast plus a mid-morning snack) should provide at least one-third of your daily calories.

That means active women need about 600 to 700 calories for breakfast (1,800 to 2,100 total calories each day) and active men need about 800 to 900 calories for breakfast (2,400 to 2,700 average calories per day). And you can get your necessary calories from a bowl of cereal, a banana, a muffin and a glass of juice.

If you're thinking that you would never eat that much for breakfast, take the banana or muffin to work or school with you for a mid-morning snack.

If you prefer cooked breakfasts instead of cold cereal, try boiled eggs with toast and jam, oatmeal or other hot cereals, or waffles. These will also give you the necessary vitamins, minerals and calories.

If you skip breakfast because you think you can lose weight by skipping those extra calories, think again.

Eating a healthy breakfast seems to cut down on the amount that most people eat throughout the rest of the day. On the other hand, people who skip a healthy breakfast are more likely to be starving by lunchtime and grab the quickest junk-food snacks they can find.

If you are dieting, just eat a smaller, healthy breakfast — 400 to 600 calories instead of the full amount. You are still providing your body with necessary fuels and energy, but you will be able to lose weight because of the reduced calories.

Eating breakfast is just as important to your exercise and sports activity as your sporting equipment is. You wouldn't jog in cowboy boots — you need running shoes. Breakfast is just as important. Leaving without it is just like leaving your running shoes at home before a race.

MEDICAL SOURCE ————————————————

The Physician and Sportsmedicine (20,7:29)

Poor diet, lack of appetite can cause health problems in elderly

Since your retirement, have you noticed that you don't cook as much or as often as you used to? In fact, the only times you really cook much of anything are when the family visits on holidays and special occasions.

If that is true for you, you are one of a growing number of retired people who are at risk for illness and early death.

Illness and early death? you ask unbelievably.

Yes — illness and early death caused by a poor diet and the resulting malnutrition. Old age doesn't have to include illness and poor health, but for many people it does simply because they're not eating enough food or the right kinds of food.

People who are otherwise perfectly healthy are getting sick and even dying just because they don't get enough to eat.

They get weak from lack of proper nutrition, and their bodies are no longer able to fight off disease. The problem is that most people who are not getting a proper diet don't realize it because their eating habits changed gradually over a long period of time. The "risk factors" that have damaged their diets evolved slowly over time.

What risk factors? you ask. There are several. One of the most frequently seen risk factors is living alone. As far back as history records, eating has been a social event as well as a bodily need.

Eating with other people makes mealtimes more enjoyable, and preparing food for a family or for friends is often more enjoyable than preparing food for just yourself.

As a result, many people who live alone simply don't prepare meals. Instead, they snack on foods that do not provide all the nutrients they really need. Or, if they do prepare the meals, many people don't eat what they've cooked because eating alone causes depression and loneliness. So they end up just picking at their food without consuming a nutritious meal.

Physical limitations are another risk factor that keep many people from getting proper meals. For example, many people with arthritis have difficulty opening cans and packages. Since most foods are packaged in cans or other packages, those people are immediately limited in what they can prepare without assistance from someone else.

Others who have vision problems may have difficulty reading cooking directions or adjusting the settings on the stove or microwave.

The frustration that results from these limitations often discourages people so much that they stop trying to prepare meals, and they end up eating nonnutritious snacks instead.

Other people who are unable to drive or get to public transportation are severely limited in their ability to get food from the grocery store.

Another risk factor involves those people who have cultural, ethnic or religious preferences that differ from the majority of the population.

Cooking ingredients for special meals may be difficult to find, so they eat fewer kinds of food and get less nutrition.

Other risk factors include the use of canes, walkers or wheelchairs. People who need assistance with walking have greater difficulty standing in the kitchen to prepare meals. They also have trouble carrying pots and pans or cooking ingredients, so they tend to avoid cooking meals.

A frequent risk factor for poor nutrition among older adults is oral health problems. People who have poorly fitting dentures, tooth loss, dry mouth or gum problems usually suffer from decreased nutrition. Eating becomes a painful chore, so people eat less.

Other people suffer from decreased senses of taste and smell. These sensory losses cause foods to taste bland and boring, and the enjoyment of eating good food is greatly diminished. The use of drugs, medications or alcohol also can significantly affect a person's eating habits. Side effects from medicines can cause loss of appetite, nausea and vomiting, bad taste in the mouth and fatigue.

Drinking too much alcohol can lead to decreased ability to taste foods and can cause the body to lose valuable nutrients. The result is malnutrition.

If you recognize one or more of these risk factors in yourself or in someone you know, take extra care to make sure you or your acquaintance maintains a proper diet. The malnutrition that comes from a poor diet puts you at greater risk for illness, disease and death.

If you have questions about your diet or risk factors for poor nutrition, talk to your doctor. He can help you set up a diet that will meet your nutritional needs.

MEDICAL SOURCE ————————————————————

American Family Physician (44,6:2087)

Recommended Daily Food Consumption for Older Adults

Food group	Servings per day	Equivalent serving sizes
Milk	2 or more	1 cup milk, yogurt, custard, pudding, soft-serve ice cream or frozen yogurt 1.5 oz. cheese 1 1/2 cups cream soup made with milk 2 cups cottage cheese, ice milk/ice cream
Meat/Substitute	2 or 3	2 - 3 oz. lean meat, fish (a piece the size of a deck of cards) or 2 eggs, 1 chicken breast or leg and thigh 2 - 3 oz. cheese 1/2 - 3/4 cups cottage cheese, tuna or other flaked meat or fish 1 - 1 1/2 cups dried beans or peas 4 - 6 teaspoons peanut butter 2 - 3 slices low-fat cold cuts
Fruit	2 or more	1 serving of fruit or fruit juice with vitamin C
Vegetables	3 or more	1/2 - 1 cup dark green/deep yellow vegetable
Bread/Cereal	6 or more	1 slice whole grain or enriched bread 1/2 bun, bagel or English muffin 1/2 cup rice, pasta, cooked cereal 1 oz. (1 cup) cold cereal 3 - 6 crackers

MEDICAL SOURCE ―――――――――――

American Family Physician (44,6:2087)

Designer foods can help prevent cancer and heart disease

Move over, Ralph Lauren and London Fog. Here's the latest in designer fashions: designer foods. Designer foods? you ask.

Believe it, says the National Cancer Institute, because the designer foods might soon be on their way to the market. The new foods are vogue and stylish, and they're being designed to fight cancer.

The National Cancer Institute, along with several research institutions, private companies and the Food and Drug Administration, has begun a "designer food" program aimed at creating food products fortified with various cancer-fighting compounds.

Among the cancer-fighting compounds that researchers hope to add to these foods are phytochemicals. These "chemicals" are found naturally in fruits, vegetables and other plants; and they are known to interfere with the processes that lead to cancer.

By adding these phytochemicals to other foods, researchers hope to spread the cancer-prevention effects of fruits and vegetables into many other families of food to reach a larger number of people.

Right now, scientists are studying the cancer-fighting effects of extracts from citrus fruits, garlic, flax, soybeans and other vegetables, such as carrots, parsley, celery and parsnips.

The cancer-fighting effects of garlic are under special scrutiny. In fact, researchers at the University of Nebraska Medical Center are studying the way that garlic affects the body's response to acetaminophen, the active ingredient found in many popular over-the-counter painkillers.

The reason scientists are studying garlic's effects on acetaminophen in the body is because the body processes some cancer-causing agents in the same way it processes acetaminophen. By understanding how garlic affects that process with acetaminophen, researchers hope to understand how garlic interferes with environmental cancer-causing agents.

So far, studies suggest that garlic helps protect against cancer. Garlic helps block the development of colon, esophageal and skin cancers in lab animal tests. An additional benefit of eating garlic: Garlic helps lower cholesterol levels. Recent studies suggest that garlic can help reduce cholesterol levels as much as 12 percent.

Flax is another food that is under study for its cancer-fighting effects in the "designer food" program. Flax is the plant from which linen and linseed oil are formed. Flaxseed, the part of the plant being studied for anticancer effects, contains omega-3 polyunsaturated fatty acids. These fatty acids seem to be helpful in reducing risk of heart disease.

Natural Oven bakeries in Manitowoc, Wis., have been baking bread with flax for the past several years because of the positive health benefits associated with flax. Researchers are working with Natural Oven bakeries in their attempt to create healthy designer foods.

Upcoming studies will focus on two major groups of vegetables: the cruciferous vegetables, such as broccoli, cabbage and cauliflower; and some solanaceous vegetables, such as tomatoes, peppers and eggplant.

Scientists hope to come up with the most powerful cancer-fighting agents available. They also hope to fortify a wide range of foods including beverages, bologna and other processed meats, sauces, soups and spreads.

MEDICAL SOURCES ——————————————————————

Journal of the National Cancer Institute (83,15:1050)
Harvard Health Letter (16,10:1)
Medical Tribune (32,10:4)

Cool foods for hot days

Summertime brings long days and lemonade and other enjoyable pleasures.

It also brings heat and humidity. And many people fail to get nutritious meals because they don't want to spend a hot day cooking in a hot kitchen.

The answer is not your local fast food joint. Instead, pick out some cool foods for those hot days. Having cool meals available for you and your family during the summer months will involve a little bit of pre-planning on your behalf.

First, think of your family's favorite meals that you eat cold — fruit salad, cold chicken, raw vegetables and dip, yogurt and fruit, etc.

Now, think of ways to combine those favorites to ensure that you always have a healthy meal waiting that won't require too much time in the kitchen.

For example, pasta salads are great meals that will provide important carbohydrates and other vital nutrients. Make your pasta, then add vegetables, low-fat cheese, and some tuna, chicken or light seafood (shrimp or imitation crab), and top with some low-fat dressing or oil.

The cheese gives you calcium and protein; the vegetables provide vitamins and fiber; and the meats provide protein, minerals and healthy omega-3 oils (fish products, only). It's quick, easy and delicious.

Other tasty summer meals are fresh, green salads, filled with fresh vegetables, low-fat cheese and meat strips, like chicken, turkey or ham. Whole-wheat rolls on the side finish off a great meal.

Fruit salads with different fruits and nuts provide yummy, fun meals that are sure to be a hit every time. And potato salads are summertime favorites that provide important starches in the diet. Chicken, tuna and turkey salads are great ways to use your leftover meats — add a wedge of cantaloupe or a pineapple slice and you've got a deli delight in minutes.

Jell-O salads with fruit, cottage cheese and nuts are great examples of light desserts that you can keep on hand with minimal time spent in preparation. And fruit-flavored yogurts drizzled over freshly cut fruit is a special summertime dessert your family is sure to love.

Some other quick, easy and tasty summer favorites include the following:

- Cantaloupe or other melon stuffed with cottage cheese or Jell-O.
- Apple or banana with low-fat cream cheese or peanut butter.
- Cold cereals and low-fat milk.
- Sliced raw vegetables (carrots, cauliflower, celery, squash, broccoli, etc.) with low-fat salad dressing dip.
- Sliced fruit with low-fat Cool Whip dip.
- Bran muffins, blueberry muffins or English muffins.
- Low-fat yogurt mixed with fruit or granola.
- Low-fat cheese slices wrapped around low-salt pretzels or apple slices.
- Homemade Popsicles made from orange juice, apple juice or other fruit juices.

Staying away from the hot stove doesn't have to mean that you skimp on nutrition. Use a little creativity and fun, and keep your family cool and healthy during the summer months.

MEDICAL SOURCE ―――――――――――――――――

The Physician and Sportsmedicine (20,6:19)

Boiling coffee without a filter is a no-no

Does coffee raise cholesterol? Can it affect blood pressure? Will your method of brewing make a difference to your health? Which is better for you, regular or decaffeinated?

These are just a few of the questions you want answered.

The results of recent studies are varied.

An important Dutch study focused on the effects of caffeine on blood pressure and cholesterol. All of the people in this study drank filtered, decaffeinated coffee.

Half the group also took caffeine pills. Neither blood pressure nor cholesterol changed for either group. The caffeine didn't seem to make a difference.

Researchers say the secret to healthy coffee is in the brewing. This study suggests that when you brew your coffee by mixing it with hot or boiling water, you run the risk of raising your cholesterol levels.

Filtering, on the other hand, seems to remove the danger.

What's a coffee-lover to do? you ask. If you're concerned that the coffee you drink is affecting your cholesterol or blood pressure, you may want to experiment with giving up coffee for several weeks.

Or change your method of making coffee. Switch from brewing your coffee to filtering it. Then have your blood pressure or cholesterol checked.

Your doctor can tell you if these lifestyle changes are helping to improve your health.

MEDICAL SOURCES —————————————————

The American Journal of Clinical Nutrition (53,4:971)
British Medical Journal (302,6780:804)

Don't get your sweet-tooth fix from licorice

If you suffer from a chronic sweet tooth, reach for something other than licorice to satisfy it. The licorice might help satisfy your sugar craving, but it could also cause serious metabolic disorders.

Eating too much licorice can cause problems ranging from sodium and water retention to high blood pressure to hypokalemia, a disorder caused by dangerously low levels of potassium in the body.

How can a simple piece of candy do all that? you ask.

Well, the body works like a finely tuned Swiss watch — every little action depends on another action somewhere else. If there is a problem with one mechanism somewhere in the "machine," it almost always causes problems in many other areas.

Licorice interferes with one mechanism in the body by blocking a pathway inside the body — but that one problem area causes a variety of other problems.

It prevents the body from converting a substance known as cortisol into cortisone, a natural hormone in the body. (Don't be confused: Cortisone is also the name of a drug. Licorice interferes with natural cortisone the body manufactures.)

The block in this pathway causes a lack of cortisone and a buildup of cortisol. This can produce serious deficiencies in your body's electrolyte balance.

The good news is that the problem doesn't have to be permanent. If you stop eating so much licorice, your body can resume normal functions, and the problems should disappear within a week.

MEDICAL SOURCE ——————————————————————
The New England Journal of Medicine (325,17:1242)

Alter your lifestyle just for 3 or 4 extra months?

Living this present life forever is out of the question. But how about living longer?

But, here's a harder question: Would you trade a big change in your lifestyle and diet to add an extra three or four months, tops, at the end of your life? That's the dilemma that has been raised by a controversial study .

Current wisdom is this: Change your eating habits by consuming less than 30 percent of your daily calories in the form of fats.

That's the standard advice now being given by most national health organizations and many doctors.

Most Americans eat an average of 37 percent of their daily calories as fat.

Looking just at statistics, based on the report, this low-fat diet would defer deaths from coronary heart disease by 5 percent in the elderly and up to 20 percent in younger people.

The effect of the reduced-fat diet is larger on cancer death rates. According to the report, cutting fat to below 30 percent of daily calories would lead to a 21 to 33 percent deferral in deaths from prostate cancer, the statistical report says. A reduced-fat diet would give similar results among death rates from breast cancer and colon cancer as well.

Scientists suggest that restricting fat to less than 30 percent of daily calorie intake could eventually result in about 42,000 "deferred" deaths each year among adults.

But, that's where the statistics mislead. The same study says that making these stiff reductions in fat intake would add, on average, only about three to four months of life to these 42,000 people.

Again, those are "statistical" months. Some individuals would add many months, possibly even years; others would add few or none. And most of the reductions would occur in men over the age of 60 and in women past the age of 70. These age groups have the greatest number of deaths from fat-related diseases, so they would have the most to gain.

Is the trade-off worth it to you? That's a question only you can answer.

MEDICAL SOURCE ───────────────────────────

Journal of the American Medical Association (265,24:3285)

Controversy coming about cholesterol-lowering benefits

Keep your eyes on this battle that swirls around a startling statistical finding in the prestigious *British Medical Journal.* The finding is this: Lowering your cholesterol doesn't help your arteries and won't prevent heart attacks or death.

Current medical wisdom about the benefits of lowering cholesterol is based more on wishful thinking than on solid science, asserts a Swedish medical reviewer in the *BMJ.*

How could this be? you ask. Because researcher after researcher chose to use only those studies that supported their preconceptions and tended to ignore an almost equal number of studies that showed no effect or proved the opposite, says the reviewer, Uffe Ravnskov.

Most new cholesterol studies cite only those earlier studies that say what the researchers want them to say, the article asserts. The *BMJ* article says flatly that studies that conflict with current medical wisdom are ignored, even though there are an equal number of them.

Ravnskov conducted a "meta-analysis" of 22 major cholesterol studies done in the past 30 years. He grouped all the studies together and checked "to see if the claim that lowering cholesterol values prevents coronary heart disease is true or if it is based on citation of supportive trials only." He looked for two outcomes: heart disease or death.

His conclusion is a bombshell: "Lowering serum cholesterol concentrations does not reduce mortality (death) and is unlikely to prevent coronary heart disease."

Ravnskov might be the modern medical equivalent of the little boy in the children's tale who shouted, "The emperor has no clothes."

Here's what he found: "The preventive effect of [cholesterol-lowering] treatment has been exaggerated by a tendency in trial reports, reviews and other papers to cite supportive trials only."

Even in the studies that supposedly showed some connection between lowering average group cholesterol levels and death rates, the actual deaths of the people in the study occurred whether the victims had high, low or normal cholesterol. Whether they lowered their cholesterol or kept it the same, they still died, the *BMJ* article says.

The one positive note he found was a 32-percent reduction in nonfatal heart disease among all the trials. But even that silver cloud has a dark lining: "Outcome was unrelated to the degree of cholesterol lowering, either among trials or among participants," says Ravnskov. In other words, you got heart disease or you didn't, whether or not you lowered, raised or did nothing to your cholesterol level.

Medical researchers cite studies that support the cholesterol-lowering-heart-disease theory six times more often than studies that don't support that theory, Ravnskov says. The numbers of pro and con studies are about equal, he says, or about what you would expect statistical randomness to produce. Anti-cholesterol researchers simply stopped referring to nonsupportive trials conducted after 1970.

"Supportive results are not only cited more often, they are also published more often," Ravnskov says. In two cases, researchers testing cholesterol-lowering as a heart disease preventor stopped trials and didn't publish full results because of "side effects." The main side effects were — you guessed it — coronary heart disease.

He found 16 reports published after 1970 that cited 40 supportive or inconclusive studies. But, those 16 pro-cholesterol-lowering studies failed to mention even one of the conflicting studies, even though the nonsupportive findings were nearly as common as the supportive ones. Articles questioning cholesterol reduction and coronary heart disease simply have been avoided by reviewers, the report says.

Length of trial follow-ups made no difference. Long trials over several years fared even worse than short trials, he says. The longer trials (over five years) showed more people dying or developing heart disease soon after cholesterol-lowering treatment was started than the shorter trials showed. The reason for that is unknown, but researchers do know that most of the drugs used to lower cholesterol have serious side effects affecting the heart and other body systems.

Overall, lowering "high" cholesterol made no difference in the rates of total deaths and deaths from heart disease, the reviewer says.

"The impression of success presented to doctors is false because the numbers of controlled cholesterol-lowering trials in which total mortality and coronary mortality were reduced equal the numbers in which they were increased," Ravnskov concludes.

A review in the professional newsletter *Journal Watch* calls

Ravnskov's findings "damning" and asserts that "a careful assessment of the literature casts doubt" on current medical belief about the benefits of lowering cholesterol.

Before you go on any prescription-drug treatment to lower your cholesterol, ask your doctor about these new, disturbing findings.

MEDICAL SOURCES ————————————————————

> *British Medical Journal* (305,6844:15)
> *Journal Watch* (10,5:33)

Lowering cholesterol below 160 seems risky

Very low cholesterol levels could be as harmful to your health as high cholesterol is believed to be, according to a growing number of large studies.

People with total cholesterol levels below 160 milliliters per deciliter have higher rates of cancer, stroke and violent death such as suicide.

Some large studies have even found that, in people with cholesterol levels under 160, deaths from other causes outnumber lives saved by lowering heart disease rates.

"The medical implications ... raise some interesting issues and strongly suggest the need for additional research," says the American Heart Association.

MEDICAL SOURCES ————————————————————

> *Medical Tribune* (33,17:1)
> American Heart Association news release (Sept. 3, 1992)

What is the right cholesterol level for you?

The question remains, "Should you lower your cholesterol

level or not?"

The American Heart Association still thinks you should. The AHA position on lowering cholesterol remains the same since the recommendation was first made in 1961: To eat a diet low in saturated fats and cholesterol. The AHA believes this remains sensible and safe advice for all healthy Americans over age 2.

The National Cholesterol Education Program, along with the American Heart Association, urges people with cholesterol levels at 200 or above to go on a low-fat, low-cholesterol diet. Cholesterol levels between 200 and 240 are borderline high, and levels greater than 240 are high risk.

You may even need to be under a doctor's care if you have cholesterol levels in the borderline range, particularly if you smoke, have high blood pressure, low HDL (the "good" cholesterol), or a family history of heart disease.

Be aware, though, that tens of millions of dollars have been invested in the notion that low-cholesterol, low-fat diets are the basis for good nutrition. The lower-cholesterol-is-better belief has become an article of faith for most doctors, nutritionists and food producers. It's going to take a lot of hard evidence and, probably, a lot of time before the medical and nutrition establishments even grudgingly acknowledge the shaky foundation of their anti-cholesterol argument.

Also be aware that cholesterol-lowering drugs have serious short-term and long-term side effects. Drugs like these should be used only as a last resort for extremely serious cases of hypercholesterolemia (too much cholesterol in the blood), many respected medical researchers are beginning to warn.

According to Harvard Medical School researchers, people who normally eat high-fat diets might want to try to change to a traditional Mediterranean diet: In other words, a diet low in saturated fats and cholesterol. For those of you who eat a traditional Mediterranean diet, 30 to 40 percent of your calories come from monounsaturated and polyunsaturated fats, but studies show that your heart-disease risks are as low as people whose diet contains very low amounts of fat (less than 10 percent of total calories).

MEDICAL SOURCES ———————————————————

The Merck Manual, Sixteenth Edition, Merck Research Laboratories, Rahway, N.J., 1992
American Heart Association news release (Sept. 3, 1992)
The New England Journal of Medicine (325,24:1740)

Cast of characters in cholesterol drama

Cholesterol is a waxy, fat-like substance found in animal tissues, meats, dairy products, egg yolks and some oils.

There are two main proteins that carry cholesterol in the blood. They are LDL or low-density lipoprotein, also known as the "bad" cholesterol, and HDL or high-density lipoprotein — the "good" cholesterol. Added together, LDL and HDL make up total cholesterol levels.

Many doctors have begun to focus more on raising HDL levels compared to LDL than on lowering total cholesterol levels.

For years, doctors have believed that excess cholesterol in your blood contributes to buildup of plaque on your artery walls. Too much plaque creates a plug, strangling blood flow to muscles, especially the heart muscle.

MEDICAL SOURCE ———————————————————

1992 Heart and Stroke Facts, American Heart Association, Dallas, Texas, 1991

Vitamin Quiz: Test your vitamin, mineral knowledge

Questions:

1) Which vitamin is found in egg yolk, cod-liver oil and yellow or green, leafy vegetables?

2) Which vitamin is in vegetable oils, wheat germ, egg yolk, leafy veggies and legumes such as peas and beans?

3) Which vitamin occurs in citrus fruits, tomatoes, cabbage and green peppers?

4) Which vitamin, taken in excess, can cause peeling of the skin and loss of hair?

5) With what vitamin is your margarine probably fortified?

6) Name two essential nutrients that tend to be lowered in the blood of cigarette smokers.

Answers to vitamin quiz:

1) Vitamin A

2) Vitamin E

3) Vitamin C

4) Vitamin A

5) Vitamin A, beta carotene

6) Vitamin C, carotene

MEDICAL SOURCE ——————————————————

Vitamin and Mineral Encyclopedia, FC&A Publishing, Peachtree City, GA, 1987

OVEREATING

How to overcome your cravings

Everyone has experienced it at least once in their lives — a feeling of I've-got-to-have-that-food-and-I've-got-to-have-it-now!

It's known as a craving. We've all experienced it from time to time, and some people get cravings more than others.

What are the things that people crave most? The number-one choice is chocolate. After chocolate, cravings range from pizza to pretzels, cookies to chips, and doughnuts to peanuts.

So, why the cravings? you ask.

Most cravings are a mix of emotional and physical factors. Many people reach for food for comfort, celebration or company. It's not uncommon for people to binge on their "craved food" when they are tense, depressed, lonely or celebrating.

Other people begin to crave foods when they don't have anything else to do or when they're bored.

However, there are some true physical reasons why some people experience cravings. One big reason is hormones.

Researchers have found that women crave and eat more sweet, high-fat foods about 10 days before the onset of their menstrual period than they do during the rest of the month. Estrogen levels are very low at this point in the cycle, and scientists think that might influence the cravings.

The scientists think that high levels of estrogen take away the appetite. But when the level of estrogen drops 10 days before the period starts, that appetite suppression is gone and the cravings start.

Other causes behind cravings could be related to your

health. People with blood-sugar problems might crave sweet things. Those with low blood pressure might crave salty things. And those people with vitamin deficiencies could very well crave the foods that contain those needed vitamins.

Those cravings could be your body's way of getting the food it needs.

But, if you suspect that your cravings are not because of medical reasons (your body probably doesn't need that chocolate fudge pie), what can you do to overcome the cravings?

1) The first step is to figure out why the craving hits. Look for patterns: Do you reach for the ice cream after every stressful visit from your in-laws? Do you bake and eat cookies every time your husband leaves on a business trip? Does a stressful day at work cause you to want chocolate — anything chocolate? Try to nail down what your "triggers" are.

2) Once you think you've nailed down the trigger for your cravings, think of other pleasurable activities that you could do instead of eating. That could be as simple as catching a few minutes of your favorite TV show, buying a new book or magazine, or calling up an old friend. You should also consider going for a walk. Walking will not only get you away from the kitchen, it will also decrease your appetite and keep those extra pounds off your legs and waist.

3) Another key to overcoming your cravings is to give in to them. Yes, give in to them. Many people make the mistake of completely avoiding the food they crave. Then after a few days or weeks, they break down and binge. For example, you deny yourself any chocolate for two weeks, but then you go crazy, buy two dozen chocolate eclairs and eat them all. You then feel guilty, deny yourself chocolate for another two weeks and repeat the same process. If you will allow yourself occasional treats of the

food you crave, you won't have to break down and binge.

4) Try substituting the foods you crave with more healthy choices. For example, if chocolate-covered peanuts are your weakness, try carob-covered peanuts instead. The carob tastes like chocolate, but it's much better for you. Try frozen yogurt instead of ice cream. Try pretzels or butter-free popcorn instead of chips or nuts. You can get rid of the craving without eating unhealthy foods.

Learning to control your cravings will let you enjoy the pleasures of a treat now and then without the guilt of a binge.

MEDICAL SOURCES ───────────────────────

Lick the Sugar Habit, Avery Publishing Group Inc., Garden City Park, New York, 1988
Better Homes and Gardens, *Women's Health & Medical Guide*, Meredith Corp., Des Moines, Iowa, 1981

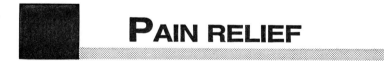

PAIN RELIEF

Natural remedies to ease your aches and pains

They have been around for hundreds of years, but researchers have only recently begun to rediscover their value. Herbs — they can provide relief for many common ailments, and you can grow many of them in your own backyard.

Here is a list of some of the more well-known herbs that many researchers think might become popular remedies.

Horseradish is usually thought of as a sauce or spice, but herb specialists claim that it is useful in helping your digestion. This member of the mustard family can also be used as a pain-relieving remedy for neck and back pain. Or you can use a gargle mixture of grated horseradish, honey and water as a way to ease hoarseness.

Rosemary is a member of the mint family, and the oil from this herb can be rubbed on the skin to help ease the pain of arthritis, bruises, cuts, sores and skin problems like eczema.

Catnip is Mother Nature's version of Alka-Seltzer. It helps soothe and relieve upset stomachs, headaches and baby colic. Catnip tea causes the body to sweat, so it can be used to help reduce fever.

This herb with the heart-shaped leaves also helps bring relief from the coughing and congestion of the common cold, and it even helps as a sleeping aid.

Peppermint is known far and wide for its minty smell, but few people know of its ability to relieve indigestion, upset stomach, colic, flatulence and even menstrual cramping. Rubbing oil from peppermint herbs on the skin can help soothe aching muscles and joints, and a cup of warm peppermint tea will help clear your sinuses.

Garlic is also a well-known herb that many chefs refuse to cook without. Keep up the good work, chefs — garlic seems to be helpful in lowering high blood pressure, lowering blood cholesterol levels, and helping to unclog arteries that are coated with atherosclerotic plaques. Garlic can also be applied directly onto the skin to get relief from insect stings.

Chamomile is one of the oldest known herbs with an age-old ability to relieve inflammation of the skin. Applying the ground-up leaves directly to the inflamed area helps reduce swelling and tenderness. Tea made from the oil of the chamomile plant is helpful in treating digestion problems, colic and menstrual cramps. You can even add the oil to your bath water if you want a natural relaxer, or you can use chamomile oil as a natural insect repellent.

Comfrey is another herb that can be used to reduce inflammation, especially around cuts and sores, insect bites, burns, bruises, sprains and skin problems. Grinding the leaves in a blender makes an ointment that you can rub directly on the skin to help reduce pain and swelling.

Sage is a member of the mint family that is unbeatable in its relief of sore throats, mouth and gum problems, cuts and sores, bruises and skin problems. Sage tea is even used to bring relief for nervousness or irritability — its relaxant effects can help you settle down after a long day at work.

Many amateur gardeners have been enjoying the benefits of herbs for years. Fortunately, doctors and researchers are beginning to rediscover the medicinal value of herbs, and we soon may see a return to more natural ways of dealing with common, everyday ailments.

MEDICAL SOURCES —————————————

Alive (106:6)
The Lawrence Review of Natural Products (February 1991, February 1992, July 1990, January 1991, January 1988, March 1991, October 1990, August 1992)

'Take two aspirin . . .' and only two aspirin — How to use pain relievers safely

Everyone is familiar with the coined phrase "Take two aspirin and call me in the morning." But not everyone understands the importance of the word "two."

Many people think that "If two aspirin are good, think of what four could do."

Unfortunately, that's where many people get into trouble with their over-the-counter drugs and their prescription drugs.

Whether you're taking pain relievers for a headache, a strained muscle or a stiff, arthritic joint, it is very important that you take your pain medicines safely.

Overdosing with aspirin or other similar drugs can lead to serious stomach problems and sometimes hearing problems. Other over-the-counter drugs can cause poisonous effects in your body if you take too many at one time. And prescription drugs can be even more dangerous and deadly if not taken according to the instructions.

If you are taking prescription pain relievers, be sure to talk with your doctor or pharmacist so you fully understand the correct way to take your medicine.

If you use over-the-counter pain relievers, follow these tips to get the best and safest results from the medicine:

❑ Always read the label carefully. Follow all instructions, cautions and warnings.

❑ Look for a drug information sheet inside the box. (Not all drugs contain a drug information sheet.) This often contains information that is not listed on the medicine box. Read this insert carefully and follow all instructions, cautions and warnings.

❑ Never take more than the maximum dosages listed on the package label. Overdoses can cause side effects, serious illness, hospitalization and even death.

❑ Always wait the full amount of time suggested on the label before taking your next dose. Taking the correct dosages too close together has the same effect as taking too many pills at one time.

❏ Adults should not take pain relievers for more than 10 days at a time (unless instructed to do so by their doctors). Taking drugs for too long can sometimes hide symptoms or problems that need to be checked by your doctor. Taking drugs for a long time can also cause other health problems. (Too much aspirin can cause bleeding in the stomach.)

❏ Adults should not take drugs for fever longer than three days at a time.

❏ Parents should limit the use of over-the-counter pain relievers in their children and teen-agers to five days for pain and three days for fever.

❏ Children and young adults (ages 2-20 years) should not take aspirin for chicken pox, flu or flu-like symptoms because of the danger of Reye's syndrome. (Reye's syndrome is a dangerous, and sometimes deadly, condition in children and young adults.)

❏ People who are allergic to aspirin should not take any other pain relievers that contain ingredients that are similar to aspirin, such as carbaspirin calcium, magnesium salicylate, sodium salicylate and choline salicylate.

❏ Pregnant women should avoid taking aspirin during the last three months of pregnancy unless advised by their doctors. Aspirin can cause dangerous bleeding in the mother and unborn child. If you begin to experience side effects (dizziness, hearing problems, stomach pain, vomiting, bloody stools or difficulty breathing), stop taking the drug immediately and call your doctor.

MEDICAL SOURCE ————————————————————

FDA Consumer (23,2:28 and 25,9:35)

Caffeine makes aspirin more effective

Taking aspirin for that headache? Then make sure it has caffeine in it, some researchers say.

Caffeine has been added to analgesics (pain relievers) for years. But experts have been slow to admit that the caffeine has any beneficial effect.

In a study, people with sore throats were separated into three groups. One group was given aspirin with caffeine, another group given aspirin without caffeine, and a third group took a placebo.

Researchers chose to test the aspirin on a sore throat because a sore throat is something that people routinely take aspirin for, and because it's easy to evaluate the effectiveness of the pain killer.

Not only did the aspirin with caffeine start to work faster, but the pain-killing effect lasted longer than aspirin alone.

The scientists concluded that caffeine acts as a kind of "catalyst."

It speeds up the action of the pain killer and makes it more effective.

Some cautions about caffeine — caffeine is a stimulant and can make your heart beat faster. Also, caffeine interacts with some medicines and can produce bad side effects.

If you have heart disease or you are taking medicines, check with your doctor about using medicines or foods containing caffeine.

MEDICAL SOURCE ───────────────────────────
Archives of Internal Medicine (151,4:733)

Play a tune to ease the pain

The timeless classic "Moon River" might be more than a

nostalgic tune from Audrey Hepburn's "Breakfast at Tiffany's."

It could be a good source of pain relief! And so could any other one of your favorite musical tunes.

Music might be an inexpensive, drug-free, safe addition to traditional methods of pain relief.

Researchers from the University of Pittsburgh School of Medicine conducted a study on about 40 people who were going to undergo mild surgery (laceration repair). About half of the people in the study were allowed to listen to their choice of music through a headset during the procedure.

Compared to the other half of the group who didn't listen to music, the group that listened to music appeared to suffer from the same level of anxiety.

However, the music group reported significantly lower pain scores than the group that had no music.

Afterwards, the music group filled out questionnaires about the music during their surgical procedure. Based on the answers on the questionnaires, 63 percent of the people in the music group felt the music was "very beneficial," and 32 percent of the group thought the music was "slightly beneficial."

When asked if they would want music again in a similar situation, the unanimous response from the music group was "Yes!"

If the idea of listening to music during medical (or dental) procedures appeals to you, consider asking your doctor to allow you to do so.

Your doctor will probably be eager to help you feel as relaxed and pain-free as possible.

MEDICAL SOURCE ─────────────────────────────

Modern Medicine (59,7:39)

Ice pack tips

Whether you've got a headache, a sprained ankle or a swollen joint, ice packs come in handy for bringing quick relief to your aches and pains and reducing swelling in minor injuries.

But often, the ice pack is no more than an old bread bag with some ice in it. And the usual scenario involves a hole in the bag and a big mess.

To avoid the mess and the rush of trying to make an ice pack, keep one or two in your freezer, ready to be used at a moment's notice.

For a "handy," reusable ice pack, fill a rubber glove (like the ones doctors use during surgery) with water, and tie the opening just as if you were tying a water balloon. Stick it in the freezer, and, presto—you've got a handy ice pack that can be used again and again.

For a more flexible ice pack that will bend and conform to the shape of your body, make a mixture of alcohol and water: one part rubbing alcohol to two parts water.

Put this mixture in a sealable plastic bag (or a glove) and put in the freezer.

The mixture won't harden completely to solid ice, so you can mold the bag to fit any part of your body. The bag (or glove) will also stay dry on the outside instead of "sweating" like other ice packs do. Use it again and again.

MEDICAL SOURCES ————————————————

Emergency Medicine (24,3:163)
Postgraduate Medicine (91,4:84)

Searing pain from a bowl of soup? How you can avoid this 'spicy' hazard

Watch that spoonful of soup for hidden dangers! Most people

remove bay leaves from their soups and stews before serving them
— and with good reason.

One lady forgot to do that and accidentally swallowed the bay
leaf.

She thought she had swallowed a chicken bone and went to the
local emergency room. She was in great pain; even normal breathing was excruciating.

The doctors found the bay leaf wedged into the esophagus
walls about halfway down the tube connecting the stomach and the
mouth. The edge of the leaf had cut and damaged the muscles in
the esophagus. Doctors easily removed the sharp leaf and sent her
home the same day.

Bay leaves are very rigid and have sharp edges. In some cases,
swallowing a bay leaf can be like swallowing a razor blade.

The moral of the story: Make sure you remove the bay leaf from
the entrée before you serve it!

MEDICAL SOURCE ————————————————————————

Annals of Internal Medicine (113,6:483)

PHYSICAL EXAMINATIONS

Do I need a physical?

It's the day after your fortieth birthday bash, and you're feeling the aftermath of too much food and drink. Ten years ago, you wouldn't have thought twice about it. But now, you're starting to wonder if that headache is hanging on a little too long.

Or, you think that your upset stomach is a bit more troublesome than it used to be. And, by the way, how come you're starting to feel a little winded after climbing the stairs?

So you ask yourself, Should I go in for a checkup? Now that I'm past age 40, should I have checkups more often?

Those are very natural questions to ask yourself. In fact, many people have questions about when or how often they should see their doctors for routine checkups.

The answer is simple: It depends. It depends on your age, sex, family history and general health.

There are certain tests and "warning flags" that doctors look out for in different age and sex groups. For example, a newly married 25-year-old woman probably will need to have a Pap smear at her annual checkup, but she's probably too young to be worried about a mammogram.

A 40-year-old man should certainly have his blood pressure checked at his routine checkup, but he doesn't really need a prostate exam until he reaches his fifties.

Or, a healthy person with no family history of high blood pressure probably only needs to check his blood pressure every couple of years, whereas persons with a family history of high blood pressure or who are overweight might want to have their blood pressure checked every year.

Well, if I get a complete physical, what should I tell the doctor? you ask next.

The answer: Everything. You need to tell your doctor about your eating habits, how often you exercise, whether or not you smoke, any family history of diseases like heart disease or diabetes, any changes in your health, any unusual symptoms or complaints, and so on.

All of that information helps the doctor form a complete picture of your health and provide you with the best care.

What if I feel fine? Do I still need regular checkups? The answer is yes, but probably not every year. There are certain tests that your doctor should run based on your age, health and sex.

The following chart will give you a ballpark estimate of when you should see your doctor for routine tests.

Blood Pressure

Age:		
	20-29	every 2 years*
	30-39	every 2 years*
	40-49	every 2 years*
	50+	every 2 years*

Cholesterol

Age:		
	20-29	—
	30-39	once
	40-49	every 4-5 years*
	50+	every 4-5 years to age 65*

Breast Exam

Age:		
	20-29	every 2-3 years**
	30-39	every 2-3 years**
	40-49	every 2 years**
	50+	annually

Mammogram

Age		
	20-29	—
	30-39	—
	40-49	every 1-2 years
	50+	annually

Pap Smear

Age:		
	20-29	every 1-3 years***
	30-39	every 1-3 years***
	40-49	every 1-3 years***
	50+	every 1-3 years to age 70***

Prostate

Age:		
	20-29	—
	30-39	—
	40-49	—
	50+	annually

Fecal Occult Blood (checks for colon cancer)

Age:		
	20-29	—
	30-39	—
	40-49	—
	50+	every 1-2 years

Blood Tests

Age:		
	20-50+	as needed

Urine Tests

Age:		
	20-50+	as needed

*Check more often if the person is overweight, a smoker or has a family history of heart disease.

**Check more often if the woman has a family history of breast cancer.

***Check more often if the woman takes the Pill, has been exposed to the drug DES, has multiple sexual partners, or has a family history of cervical cancer.

There are other "routine tests" that doctors run that are more dependent on your health status than on your age or sex. For example, smokers should have chest X-rays taken to help detect lung cancer. And middle-age people who never exercise should have a stress test done before starting an exercise program just to see if the heart is strong enough for the new exercise.

People who suffer from diabetes will need to have their blood sugar checked regularly, and chronic alcoholics might want to have their liver functions checked every now and then.

Although the chart above gives you a rough estimate of how often you need certain tests, the bottom line is this: Your body does a good job of telling you when something is wrong. If you are not feeling up to par, don't wait for your checkup in two years. Go on in and have your checkup early.

On the other hand, if you feel fine, you probably are. So, follow the chart for the basic tests, and trust your body to tell you if you need any additional attention.

MEDICAL SOURCES —————————————————————————

In Health (4,2:78)
FDA Consumer (26,6:26)

Poisoning

How to identify heavy metal poisoning

If you think that heavy metal poisoning is what your teen-age son gets from listening to his rock music too loud, you'd better think again. It is a kind of poisoning that can happen to you or members of your family and cause very serious problems.

Heavy metal poisoning is just what it sounds like — getting too much heavy metal in your body is poisonous.

If you're envisioning long steel beams, change your thinking to things like lead, arsenic or zinc. These and other types of heavy metals can be found everywhere, including inside your own home or workplace.

Exposure to heavy metals can occur in industries such as smelting, mining, metal refining and alloy production. In those kinds of industries, workers can inhale metal fragments, dust and vapors. In smelting companies or refining industries, the process of purifying one metal could release and expose workers to other kinds of metals, including dangerous ones.

Farmers and other agricultural workers are routinely exposed to pesticides and fertilizers that might contain metals such as arsenic or zinc. And people who build, repair or recycle car batteries are sometimes exposed to poisonous levels of lead and zinc.

At home, acidic liquids like juices or wines can release copper, zinc or lead from lead crystal, pewter pots or utensils, improperly glazed pottery or improperly galvanized iron cookware.

Family members can get zinc or arsenic poisoning by accidentally inhaling fumes or smoke caused by burning dry-cell batteries or specially treated wood.

The first thing to do in avoiding heavy metal poisoning is to recognize where the possible dangers are. The chart below will help you understand some of the possible dangers.

Sources of Heavy Metal Poisoning			
Metal	**Workplace**	**Neighborhood**	**Home**
Arsenic	Smelting, production of arsine gas, fertilizers, pesticides, producing treated lumber	Pewter plates and utensils, seafood, fertilizers or pesticides	Burning treated wood
Gold	—	—	Treatment of rheumatoid arthritis
Lead	Making batteries, producing pottery, smelting or soldering	Use of poorly glazed pottery, using pewter plates or utensils, emissions from cars	Eating or inhaling chips or dust of old paint
Zinc	Making batteries, fertilizers, pesticides, alloy metal production	Fertilizers and pesticides, use of poorly galvanized iron pots or utensils	Eating weird foods, known as food faddism
Copper	Pesticides, algaecides, fungicides, producing alloy metal products	Drinking acidic drinks from copper pipes or containers	Intrauterine device (IUD)

Now that you know where and how you can be exposed to these potentially dangerous metals, you need to recognize the symptoms that might suggest poisoning.

Some of the symptoms that can be caused by heavy metal poisoning include vomiting, diarrhea, abdominal pain, weight loss, fatigue, memory loss, difficulty walking (unsteadiness), loss of consciousness and coma.

Although there are certainly other things that can cause these symptoms, exposure to metals should cause you to question these symptoms.

The following chart will give you an idea of which kinds of metal poisoning causes which symptoms.

Symptoms Caused by Heavy Metal Poisoning			
Metal	**Stomach or intestines**	**Skin problems**	**Mental problems**
Arsenic	nausea, vomiting, diarrhea and abdominal pain	eczema, dermatitis, discolored lesions, warts and unusual growths	—
Gold	diarrhea, stomach pain	contact dermatitis	—
Lead	vomiting, constipation, severe weight loss (anorexia)	—	Convulsions, coma
Zinc	vomiting and bloody diarrhea	—	Unsteadiness, loss of reflexes, tremors, paralysis
Copper	vomiting, nausea, diarrhea, abdominal pain	contact dermatitis, eczema	—

If you suspect that you or any of your family members is suffering from mild heavy metal poisoning, see your doctor immediately. Catching metal poisoning early is often the key to the most effective treatment.

To avoid heavy metal poisoning, follow a few commonsense steps that will help you reduce your exposure to these harmful metals.

❑ To avoid poisoning from pesticides, fungicides and algaecides, wear long sleeves, long pants and gloves when using the chemicals or when working in fields or other areas where these chemicals are sprayed. Also use a face mask (like doctors use in surgery) to cut down on any fumes or vapors you could inhale.

❑ Always shower thoroughly after working with or around pesticides and other similar chemicals. Bathing will help get rid of any chemicals that accidentally got on your skin.

❑ If you use gold salts for rheumatoid arthritis treatment, talk to your doctor or pharmacist about the correct way to use it and the proper dosages. Contact your doctor immediately if you notice any unusual changes or symptoms.

❑ If you work in factories or industries where you could be exposed to heavy metals, be sure to wear your protective clothing if the company provides it (suits, gloves, masks, safety glasses, etc.).

❑ If your company does not provide safety clothing for the employees, contact your local Occupational Safety and Health Administration. They can determine if your working conditions are unsafe. If the conditions are unsafe, OSHA will require the company to create the proper safety measures.

❑ Check with your local fire department or OSHA before burning things in your yard (trash, old lumber, etc.). They can help you determine if the things you are burning will produce harmful smoke or fumes.

❏ If you live in an old home that has lead-based paint on the walls, consider repainting with some lead-free paint. Don't allow your children to play on the floor in rooms painted with lead paint. Dust and chips from the paint settle to the floor where the children could eat the chips or inhale the dust.

❏ Make sure you and your family use plates, pots, pans and utensils for eating that are certified as safe. The pottery bowls your child made at school should probably be decorations instead of serving bowls to avoid the possibilities of metal poisoning.

❏ Watch your children carefully. Make sure they aren't eating or drinking from old plates or cups they might have found outside or in an old building or garage.

❏ Have your car inspected regularly to make sure it meets the proper emissions requirements.

MEDICAL SOURCES ─────────────────────

Emergency Medicine (21,8:81)
Southern Medical Journal (81,9:1132)

Lead crystal beverage containers 'leak' poisonous heavy metal

Lead crystal admirers, beware!

The lovely lead crystal decanters that you use to store and display your wines and brandies are beautiful to look at, but they might contain some serious dangers. Researchers fear that dangerously high levels of lead can "leak" from the crystal decanters into the beverages they contain.

Lead is a very toxic heavy metal and can cause neurological

damage. And lead crystal contains a high 24- to 32-percent lead oxide.

Researchers tested this "leak" effect with a lead crystal decanter and white wine. They found that within one hour after the wine was poured into the lead crystal decanter, the concentration of lead in the wine had doubled. The wine had "leached" the lead from the lead crystal container.

When the researchers tested some brandy that had been stored in lead crystal decanters for over five years, they found over 20,000 micrograms of lead per liter of brandy.

The EPA's (Environmental Protection Agency) lead standard for regular drinking water is only 15 micrograms of lead per liter of water. So the brandy contained more than 1,000 times the regulation amount!

And the danger extends beyond decanters for alcoholic beverages. Researchers caution against the use of lead crystal baby bottles. Apparently, baby formula and apple juice also seem to leach the lead from the lead crystal. And infants are much more sensitive to the effects of lead poisoning than adults.

At this point, there seems to be almost no risk involved with storing beverages in lead crystal decanters for short time periods, such as during one meal. However, researchers are suggesting that storing any liquid in a lead crystal container for an extended period of time would be unwise.

Lead poisoning, known as "plumbism," has a sequence of symptoms that may develop over several days or weeks. Lead poisoning is characterized by personality changes, headaches, anorexia, constipation, metallic taste, vomiting and vague abdominal pain.

If you suspect lead poisoning, contact your physician immediately.

MEDICAL SOURCES ───────────────

Science News (139,4:54)
Georgia Environmental Protection Agency, Atlanta, Ga., 1993

Wine contains high lead levels

"Would you like a glass of lead with your dinner?"

That hardly sounds like a question a good waiter would ask at a fine restaurant, but that might be exactly what you're getting if you have wine with your dinner.

The federal government reports that wine sold in the United States might contain dangerous levels of lead. The Bureau of Alcohol, Tobacco and Firearms has been conducting tests for the past two years on many domestic and imported wines.

The findings were the same for domestic and imported wines. Many contained levels of lead that surpass Environmental Protection Agency recommendations for safe amounts of lead in drinking water. The agency found lead levels from 50 parts per million to as high as 700 parts per million. Those levels are dangerously high compared with the Environmental Protection Agency's recommendation that lead content not exceed 15 parts per billion.

Although scientists found high levels of lead in both domestic and imported wines, the levels generally were higher in the imported wines.

If you drink wine and think you might be suffering from mild lead poisoning, see your doctor right away.

MEDICAL SOURCE ————————————————

Wall Street Journal (June 6, 1991,B1)

Recycling hazard in your kitchen

Recycling is good for the environment, but is it good for you?

Possibly not, if you recycle plastic bread bags. Many people save and reuse bread bags to store their homemade bread or sandwiches in.

The problem arises when they turn the bags inside out.

Researchers have found that the ink on the printed portions of most plastic bread bags contains a large amount of lead. The lead can soak into food that touches the ink and increase the amount of lead in your diet.

Generally, the amount of lead that is consumed is not extremely dangerous, but it certainly isn't healthy.

Too much lead in the diet can lead to lead poisoning and symptoms such as vomiting, diarrhea, headache and convulsions.

If you reuse plastic bread bags, be sure to use them with the printed side out.

MEDICAL SOURCE ─────────────────────────

Science News (139,23:367)

Are your carpets 'healthy'? Beware of these hidden hazards

Unless you take your shoes off at the front door every time you enter your house, your carpet may contain poisonous chemicals.

Many carpeted houses, especially those built before 1950, may have dangerous levels of lead and pesticides ground into the carpet.

Apparently, you can pick up lead, pesticides and other dangerous chemicals on the soles of your shoes on the outside and track them into your home. Once inside, the poisonous stuff becomes trapped in the carpet fibers. The thicker the rugs, the higher the amounts of dangerous chemicals that may be trapped.

Homes built before 1950 have higher levels of these poisons than more modern houses due to the use of lead-based paints in the older homes.

Gardeners, too, may build up hazardous levels of chemicals in their carpets. That's because they track in dirt from the garden after applying heavy concentrations of pesticides and weed killers.

Carpets and rugs hold up to 100 times as much dust and debris as bare, uncarpeted floors.

The good news is that vacuum cleaners with powered carpet beaters can remove up to five times as much dust as regular suction vacuum cleaners.

You may want to ask your guests to remove their shoes at the front door and offer them a pair of slippers when they enter the house. That's a nice gesture of comfort and hospitality, and it also will help keep your carpets cleaner and healthier!

MEDICAL SOURCE ─────────────────────────────

Science News (138,6:86)

Contact these agencies for consumer information

❑ Food and Drug Administration (FDA) has information on foods, drugs, cosmetics, biological products, medical devices, radiological devices and veterinary products sold in interstate commerce. For information, call 301-443-3170, or write FDA, Consumer Inquiries Staff, HFE-88, Room 16-63, 5600 Fishers Lane, Rockville, MD 20857.

❑ Treasury Department's Bureau of Alcohol, Tobacco and Firearms gives information on the labeling and quality of alcoholic beverages. For information, call 202-566-7135, or write ATF, Room 4402, Ariel Rios Federal Building, 1200 Pennsylvania Ave., N.W., Washington, D.C. 20226.

❑ Alcohol, Drug Abuse, and Mental Health Administration gives information on drug and alcohol abuse, including counseling information. For information, call 301-468-2600, or write Alcohol, Drug Abuse, and Mental Health Administration, P.O. Box 2345, Rockville, MD 20852.

❏ Consumer Product Safety Commission gives information on household appliances, baby furniture and toys. For information, call 1-800-638-2772, or write CPSC, Washington, D.C. 20207.

❏ U.S. Department of Agriculture's Food Safety and Inspection Service answers questions about meat and poultry, such as how to safely handle, prepare and store chicken, pork and beef. For information, call 1-800-535-4555, or write the Food Safety and Inspection Service's Meat and Poultry Hotline, Room 1163S, Washington, D.C. 20250.

❏ Environmental Protection Agency (EPA) gives information on pesticides and safe levels on foods. For information, call 202-382-4361, or write EPA, Room W311, Mail Code A-107, 401 M St., S.W., Washington, D.C. 20460.

❏ Nuclear Regulatory Commission answers questions about hazards arising from nuclear materials in power reactors, hospitals, research laboratories or other commercial facilities. For information, call 202-492-7715, or write NRC Office of Public Affairs, Washington, D.C. 20555.

❏ Centers for Disease Control answers questions on most illnesses and associated subjects. For information, call 301-443-5287, or write Centers for Disease Control, 5600 Fishers Lane, Rockville, MD 20857.

MEDICAL SOURCE ―――――――――――――――――――

FDA Consumer (24,10:28)

POSTURE

Perk up your posture

Posture refers to the upright position of a person who's standing. The person who stands with his shoulders held back and his head upright, looking forward, is practicing good posture.

Poor posture can be the result of disease, spinal deformities, bad habits or a combination of all three. Bad posture, standing or walking with the stomach and pelvis thrust out, for example, can affect internal organs.

Parents should encourage good posture habits in their children, both for appearance's sake and to prevent permanent deformities.

The most common reason for seeking the help of an orthopedist (specialist in bones and joints) is the lower backache and pain that often accompany poor posture habits. A postural backache, which is worse when you stoop, can be treated with a combination of physical therapy, manipulation of the lower spine, and wearing a support garment, such as a girdle.

MEDICAL SOURCE ————————————————

The Good Housekeeping Family Health and Medical Guide, Hearst Books, New York, 1989

PREGNANCY

'B' happy — morning sickness might be a thing of the past

Expectant mothers, you can now say goodbye to morning sickness during your pregnancy. Taking a simple vitamin can help reduce the ill feelings that sometimes come with the joys of pregnancy.

Vitamin B6 (known as pyridoxine) seems to help relieve the nausea and vomiting of morning sickness during the first few months of pregnancy, researchers are saying

In a recent study, 31 pregnant volunteers took 25-milligram doses of vitamin B6 every eight hours for three days. Fifteen of these women had experienced morning sickness before the study began.

Twenty-eight other pregnant volunteers took sugar tablets instead of vitamin B6. Of the 28 women, 10 had complained of morning sickness before the study.

After the three days of treatment, only eight of the 31 women who had taken the vitamin-B6 supplements had any vomiting. Fifteen of the 28 women who had taken sugar pills still suffered from vomiting.

Overall, the vitamin-B6 supplements seemed to ease the nausea and reduce the vomiting during the first few months of pregnancy.

The recommended daily allowance of vitamin B6 for pregnant women is 2.2 milligrams a day. Nonpregnant women who are not nursing should get 1.6 milligrams of vitamin B6 each day.

The amount of vitamin B6 that the volunteers in the study took each day is 34 times greater than the Recommended Dietary Allowance for B6 for pregnant women. Talk to your doctor before taking large doses of vitamin B6.

Other tips to relieve morning sickness symptoms:

❏ Avoid large meals. Instead, eat small meals throughout the day.

❏ Avoid meals that are heavy in fats. Eat meals and snacks that are high in carbohydrates (pasta, bread, cereals).

❏ Take iron tablets cautiously. Iron tablets seem to cause nausea in some women. Talk to your doctor about your need for iron supplements — you might be getting plenty of iron in your diet and could avoid taking iron supplement tablets.

Good natural sources of vitamin B6 include chicken, fish, kidney, liver, pork and eggs. These foods provide almost a half milligram of vitamin B6 per four-ounce serving. Good plant sources include unmilled rice, soy beans, oats, whole-wheat products, peanuts and walnuts.

Most studies have shown that, for most people, short-term megadoses up to 50 times the RDA cause no toxicity or bad side effects.

However, in one report, women who dosed themselves with about 55 times the RDA every day for more than six months came down with some severe mental and nervous system problems. Check with your doctor before taking extra vitamin B6.

MEDICAL SOURCES ───────────────────────────────

Medical Tribune (32,15:4)
Recommended Dietary Allowances, 10th Edition, National Academy Press, Washington, D.C., 1989

Protect your unborn baby from birth defects

Several studies suggest that taking folic-acid supplements

before and during pregnancy can help prevent neural tube defects (a defect of the tube from which the brain and spinal cord develop), such as spina bifida and anencephaly.

Researchers believe that in some cases, the B-vitamin, folic acid, offers protection from neural tube defects when women take folic-acid supplements before conception and during pregnancy. This is especially important if you have already had a child with a neural tube defect.

Although folic acid does seem to help prevent defects in high-risk pregnancies, folic acid does not prevent all spinal cord defects.

Researchers conducted a study to determine whether folic acid or a mixture of seven other vitamins taken near the time of conception can prevent neural tube defects. The study involved 1,817 women who were at high risk for neural tube defect pregnancies. Researchers divided them into four categories: those who took folic acid, those who took folic acid plus vitamins, those who took other vitamins, and those who took neither.

Out of 1,195 who completed their pregnancies, only six people from the folic acid groups delivered babies with neural tube defects, compared to 21 in the other two groups.

If you've had past pregnancies with neural tube defects and are planning to get pregnant, researchers suggest you include folic acid in your daily diet. If you are planning a pregnancy and don't have children with neural tube defects, researchers believe your diet should also contain adequate amounts of folic acid.

The RDA for folic acid (other forms of this nutrient are known as folate and folacin) is 180 micrograms for women. If you are pregnant, the RDA jumps to 400 micrograms daily. Since the average daily intake of folate through regular eating habits for most people in the United States is under 300 micrograms, you might need to consider supplements during pregnancy. Be sure to talk to your doctor about how much folic acid is right for you.

Some natural sources of folic acid include raw spinach, cabbage, broccoli, lettuce, frozen peas, rice, bread, fruits and nuts.

MEDICAL SOURCES ————————————————————————

Medical Tribune (33,16:20)
The Lancet (338,8760:131)
British Medical Journal (303,6796:209)
Recommended Dietary Allowances, 10th Edition, National Academy
Press, Washington, D.C., 1989

Vitamin A linked to birth defects?

Vitamin A is an important part of a healthy diet — for adults, children, babies and unborn babies. However, too much vitamin A could cause serious birth defects in those unborn children.

Vitamin A is one of the active ingredients in many new medications that are used to treat skin problems (acne, psoriasis, etc.). Although the vitamin-containing treatment works wonders on the skin problems, scientists have noticed an increase in the number of problem pregnancies among the women using these pills, ointments and creams.

According to a recent report, the use of one particular brand of a vitamin A-containing acne treatment drug among 154 pregnant women resulted in 21 cases of malformed babies, 26 cases of serious defects in the babies, and 12 cases of miscarriage.

Researchers estimate that pregnant women who use this acne treatment have a 25-percent chance of having a baby with serious birth defects.

To help reduce the risk of birth defects from excess vitamin A, the Food and Drug Administration has recommended that a woman of childbearing age not use skin treatments that contain vitamin A unless her doctor determines that she meets all of the following requirements:

- She has a serious or disfiguring case of acne.
- She can understand and carry out her doctor's instructions.
- She is able to effectively use contraceptive measures to prevent becoming pregnant.
- She has received both written and verbal warnings of possible birth defects if she gets pregnant while using the drug.
- A pregnancy test is performed within two weeks of starting the vitamin-A drug therapy, and the test is negative.
- She will not begin the drug therapy until the start of her next normal menstrual period.

The FDA hopes that these guidelines will help women avoid the tragedy of serious birth defects that might come with the use of vitamin A-containing medications.

MEDICAL SOURCE ————————————————————

The Western Journal of Medicine (152,1:68 and 78)

PREMENSTRUAL SYNDROME

Does a vitamin a day keep your PMS away?

Oh, no, it's "that time of the month again." Do your family and friends avoid you at "that time of the month," speculating that your mood swings, anxiety and depression have hit once again?

Twenty to 50 percent of all women who have not yet reached menopause suffer from premenstrual syndrome (PMS).

Researchers conducted a study to find out if taking multivitamin and mineral supplements would help ease PMS symptoms. The researchers studied 44 women with PMS. Some women were given six to 12 vitamin supplements each day for three menstrual cycles, and the rest received a placebo, a fake, ineffective pill.

Scientists evaluated menstrual symptoms before the study and for three menstrual cycles during treatment.

The 12 supplement tablets reduced practically all the PMS symptoms including anxiety, mood swings, weight gain, swelling, headaches, fatigue, increased appetite and depression.

Those taking only six vitamins reported relief for most symptoms except swelling and weight gain.

But, according to Dr. Jeannette South-Paul of Uniformed Services University of Health Sciences, women should increase the length of time they exercise and remove caffeine, sugars and alcohol from their diet before beginning daily dietary supplements to relieve PMS symptoms.

Twelve supplements a day is too many, the U.S. Food and Drug Administration said. So, the supplement manufacturers have subsequently revised the recommended PMS dosage to six per day, according to Dr. Guy E. Abraham, medical director for Optimox

Corp., the California-based manufacturer of Optivite vitamin and mineral supplements. Optivite is the brand used in the clinical trials, he said.

The vitamins contained in the recommended six pills and how they compare to the daily Recommended Dietary Allowances are as follows: vitamin A, three times the RDA; vitamin E, eight times the RDA; vitamin D3, half the RDA; folic acid, one RDA; vitamin B1 (thiamin), 23 times the RDA; vitamin B2 (riboflavin), 19 times the RDA; niacin (as niacinamide), one-and-one-half times the RDA; vitamin B6 (pyridoxine), 187 times the RDA; vitamin B12 (cyanocobalamin), 31 times the RDA; pantothenic acid (one of the B-complex vitamins), three-and-one-half times the Estimated Safe and Adequate Daily Dietary Intake (ESADDI); and vitamin C, 25 times the RDA.

For minerals, the six-pills-a-day group got one RDA for magnesium; one-half RDA for iodine; one RDA for iron; under one ESADDI for copper; twice the RDA for zinc; two times ESADDI for manganese; two RDA for selenium; and one-half ESADDI for chromium. The group also got small amounts of potassium, calcium and choline bitartrate.

Although taking multiple supplement tablets every day was successful for the women in this study, researchers say you should talk to your doctor before doing the same.

MEDICAL SOURCE —————————————————————————

Journal of the American College of Nutrition (10,5:494)

Raynaud's syndrome

Tips for sufferers of Raynaud's syndrome

Here are the symptoms: In chilly weather, if you hold a cold can of soda, your fingers become pale, then turn blue and feel numb.

After you get warm, your fingers gradually regain normal color and feeling. Sound familiar?

You're not alone.

About one out of every 10 women may have these symptoms at times. Men have these symptoms also, but at a much lower percentage.

Raynaud's syndrome is an illness that causes blood vessels in different parts of the body to close up and slow down the flow of blood to those areas of the body. The areas most commonly affected are the hands and feet.

In most people, the body has a way to keep from losing too much heat when exposed to the cold. The blood vessels near the skin narrow just a bit to keep heat from being released from the blood through the skin. That is why your hands, feet, nose, ears and face feel so cold when you are out in the cold weather.

In people who have Raynaud's syndrome, the body tries to do the same thing — only the response is exaggerated. Instead of the blood vessels narrowing a little, they narrow a lot. In some cases, all blood flow is blocked.

The areas of the body that are affected by these almost-closed vessels (usually the hands and feet) turn white because of the reduced blood flow.

After the white color, those areas start turning blue because the blood that is present in the veins is moving too slowly or sluggishly

Finally, after a while, the skin turns red. The red color is caused by blood rushing back into those areas when the narrowed blood vessels finally relax and loosen up.

Many people experience pain or a pins-and-needles sensation in the affected areas of the body as this is going on.

At first, these symptoms last only a few seconds, and the symptoms disappear as soon as the body is warmed. But over time, the "Raynaud's reaction" happens more often, lasts longer, and affects a larger part of the body (the whole hand instead of just the fingertips). In serious cases, people have lost the sense of touch in their fingertips. And if the flow of blood in those vessels is cut off for too long, the tissues can begin to die — resulting in gangrene.

It doesn't always take extremely cold or freezing temperatures to trigger the symptoms of Raynaud's syndrome. Even exposure to milder temperatures, like a walk on a cool autumn evening or reaching into the refrigerator, can trigger the symptoms.

People with certain kinds of jobs might be more likely to develop Raynaud's syndrome than others. For example, people who use vibrating tools (like jackhammers) are more likely to develop Raynaud's. Pianists, typists and other people who constantly use their fingers might also have an increased risk of developing Raynaud's syndrome.

For most people, Raynaud's syndrome is more of an inconvenience and nuisance than a serious health problem. And a few simple changes in lifestyle can help you to avoid an attack of Raynaud's symptoms:

❑ Dress warmly on cool or cold days, taking special care to cover your hands, feet, ears and face from the cold.

❑ Dress warmly when you are in an air-conditioned building. Sometimes the cool air from the air conditioner can trigger the symptoms.

❑ Keep a pair of gloves or mittens next to the refrigerator. Put these on when taking things out or putting things in the refrigerator or freezer.

❑ Avoid directly handling frozen items (frozen foods in the freezer). Try to handle them with your gloves on.

❑ Use holders for glasses or cans containing cold drinks.

❑ Keep a pair of gloves or mittens in your car for cool mornings and for pumping gas on cold days.

❑ If you work in an air-conditioned building, consider using a small space heater to take the chill off the air around your desk. (Make sure it does not violate fire safety or building standards.)

❑ Do not smoke. Smoking keeps your lungs from working as well as they should. This affects your heart and the amount of blood that circulates through your body.

❑ Do not stand or sit in the same position for long periods of time. Occasionally this cuts off circulation in some part of the body (usually the legs). Moving around or changing position will help your blood to circulate better.

❑ Get regular exercise. Keeping your heart, lungs and blood vessels healthy by exercising will improve your body's response to the cold.

❑ Wear battery-heated gloves and socks on particularly cold days.

❑ Learn coping techniques to reduce the impact of stress and emotional upset.

❑ Try to reduce the stress in your life. Sometimes stress can make your body tense and more likely to trigger the Raynaud's symptoms.

While Raynaud's syndrome is usually this manageable form, certain diseases may cause similar symptoms and should be considered to rule out serious problems.

Raynaud's syndrome can sometimes be more serious if associated with scleroderma, systemic lupus erythematosus, or mixed connective tissue disease.

Check with your doctor to make sure you don't have these serious disorders.

Mᴇᴅɪᴄᴀʟ Sᴏᴜʀᴄᴇs ─────────────────────────

Healthline (7,11)
Postgraduate Medicine (89,4:171)

Sɪɴᴜs ᴘʀᴏʙʟᴇᴍs

How to recognize sinusitis and some simple home remedies to treat it

Your head is pounding, your nose is dripping, and your throat feels like sandpaper. You think you're suffering from sinusitis, but how can you be sure it's not the flu?

Many people get confused when trying to decide whether they've got the flu, sinusitis or just the common cold. Some of the symptoms for the different illnesses are similar.

Sinusitis is defined as "the inflammation of the sinuses." It can be acute and last anywhere from one day to three weeks; subacute, and last from three weeks to three months; or chronic, and last longer than three months.

And any one of your four sinuses (or all four) can be infected: the ethmoid sinus, the maxillary sinus, the frontal sinus and the sphenoid sinus. Each of the sinuses has a drainage tunnel, and it is when that tunnel gets blocked that you begin suffering from a sinus infection.

The drainage tunnel can be blocked by any number of things, but one of the most common causes is swelling resulting from inflammation caused by an upper respiratory tract infection.

So, sinusitis often follows another illness. The tunnel can also be blocked due to swelling from a reaction to allergies or even trauma (getting hit in the nose or face).

Once the tunnel that drains the sinus gets blocked, the natural flow and drainage of mucus and other liquids gets blocked, and the mucus begins accumulating in the sinus space.

The mucus begins to harden, and that damages the cells that line the sinus cavity. The damaged cells get inflamed, and they begin swelling and causing pain. Then bacteria begin growing in the trapped mucus, and soon you have a full-blown bacterial infection.

The signs and symptoms of the resulting sinus infection usually occur pretty rapidly after the infection starts. One key factor is that most cases of sinusitis come soon after a different respiratory infection or some other kind of viral infection. You can tell the difference between the old infection and your new case of sinusitis because the sinusitis should have two or more of the following symptoms not found in other common respiratory infections:

- Fever
- Nasal congestion
- Pain in your upper jaw and teeth
- The feeling of facial pain or pressure, especially over your sinuses (across your nose, under your eyes, and across your forehead)
- Yellow or green nasal discharge
- Swelling of the eyelids or area just under the eyes
- Tenderness when you press on the areas just over the sinuses

If you have two or more of these symptoms, you've probably got a case of sinusitis.

Most cases of sinusitis require antibiotics from the doctor for complete healing.

However, there are a few things you can do in the meantime to make yourself more comfortable:

❑ Take a hot shower. The moist steam from the shower will help clear your sinuses and make you feel better.

❑ Wash out your nostrils. Take a syringe and fill it with warm water, then gently inject the water into one nostril. The water (and mucus) will drain out through your mouth into the sink. Repeat a few times on each nostril until the drainage is clean. It sounds kind of unpleasant, but it really will help clear your sinuses. If the plain water irritates your skin, try mixing two cups of warm water with a spoonful of salt and a pinch of baking soda.

❑ Drink lots of liquids. This will help loosen and "unharden" the mucus in your sinuses and help it drain out. This will relieve the pressure and infection in your sinuses.

❑ Try cold compresses on your face to ease the pain.

❑ Other people like to use warm compresses or heating pads on the face to relieve some of the pain and discomfort of sinusitis. Try both hot and cold compresses and pick the one that brings you the most relief.

❑ Use some over-the-counter sinus relief medicines. These medications seem to work better at relieving the pain and pressure than aspirin or acetaminophen. However, aspirin can help relieve some of the inflammation and fever.

❑ Avoid using nasal sprays to relieve your symptoms. Although these will relieve your symptoms at first, after three days the spray will begin making your congestion worse instead of relieving it. Use decongestant tablets that you take by mouth instead.

❑ During the day, avoid lying down. Sitting or standing upright is usually more comfortable than lying down in most cases of sinusitis. If you want to rest, or even nap, try sitting in a recliner instead of lying down. This doesn't put as much pressure on the sinuses.

MEDICAL SOURCE ─────────────────────

Postgraduate Medicine (91,5:281)

Skin problems

Dry skin got you down? Here's simple relief

Does your skin remind you more of an alligator's hide than it does of smooth, supple baby's skin? Are you tired of dry, chapped or itching skin? Well, you don't have to suffer forever.

You and millions of other people are plagued with dry skin from time to time.

In fact, about eight out of 10 people over age 60 suffer from dry skin, and half of all women over age 40 suffer from dry facial skin. Even children experience dry skin from time to time.

Fortunately, there are some simple remedies that should help soothe and smooth out your skin:

❏ Try to avoid rubbing or scratching your skin — this only makes it worse. Instead, try using an over-the-counter anti-itch medication such as Benadryl.

❏ Avoid wearing clothes that aggravate your skin, such as wool and other rough fabrics. When you wear clothing made from rough or coarse fabrics, wear a cotton shirt, blouse or garment under it.

❏ Cover your skin with a scarf and gloves when you go outside in the winter to protect yourself from the chapping effects of the cold wind and chilly air.

❏ Drink about six to eight glasses of water each day to keep enough moisture in your body. Try to avoid caffeine and alcoholic drinks — they pull moisture out of your system.

❏ Keep the air in your home moist. You can do this by putting a bowl of water on your heater during the winter months or using a humidifying machine that you can buy at your local pharmacy.

❏ Wear rubber gloves when washing your car, washing dishes or other chores that involve putting your hands in soapy water.

❏ Avoid using strong detergent soaps when bathing. These soaps strip away natural oils and moisture in your skin. Try mild, unperfumed soaps instead.

❏ Try to avoid bathing or showering too often (more than once a day). This also robs your body of natural moisturizing oils. Don't sit in whirlpools or hot tubs, and avoid saunas and steam baths.

❏ Try some oatmeal. Put some colloidal (powdered) oatmeal in your bath water, much like you would put bath oils in the water and soak for a while. You can find colloidal oatmeal at most pharmacies or supermarkets. Just follow the instructions on the label and let the oatmeal do its thing.

❏ If possible, avoid putting makeup or other perfumed products on your dry skin.

❏ After bathing, do not rub your skin with a towel. Instead, gently blot your skin dry.

❏ Try the "soak-grease" method of soothing dry skin:

1) Soak your dry skin in water for about five to 10 minutes. You can do this in the bathtub or the sink, depending on how much of your body has dry skin. Soaking in water allows your skin to pull in water, much like a sponge.

2) Dry the skin gently with a soft towel—remember not to rub the skin with the towel.

3) Apply a thin layer of lotion, oil or petroleum jelly on your skin to keep the moisture from escaping. These things form a kind of shield against the environment and keep water

from being pulled back out of your skin. Some lotions and creams work better than others. The thicker and more oily, the better — but these kinds of creams can stain your clothes. So, if you do this in the morning before work, you might want to use a thin, nonoily lotion. However, before you go to bed, try the soak-grease steps again and use a thicker cream or some petroleum jelly.

If your dry skin doesn't get better after trying these remedies, call your doctor. Sometimes dry skin is a warning sign of a more serious illness, like diabetes or thyroid problems.

MEDICAL SOURCES ─────────────────────────

> *U.S. Pharmacist* (17,6:30 Supplement)
> *Medical Tribune* (32,20:14)

Have you found splotches of itchy, crusty scabs on your skin?

It could be a common skin condition called contact dermatitis.

You'll know when you have contact dermatitis because you'll probably develop an area of eczema somewhere on your skin. That means you'll have an itchy patch of blistered skin that eventually begins to scale and crust.

Contact dermatitis usually occurs on the hands, eyelids or genitals. Usually, you can look for one of two causes.

The most common cause of contact dermatitis is coming in contact with something that irritates your skin. This is called irritant contact dermatitis, and the good news about it is that you won't necessarily have a reaction the next time you come in contact with the substance.

It just means that this time your exposure was long and strong enough to cause a reaction. It is possible to develop irritant contact dermatitis the first time your skin comes in contact with a substance.

Less common is allergic contact dermatitis. If you have this form of contact dermatitis, you have developed an allergy to something.

And, be forewarned: You might have the same reaction whenever you come in contact with this substance again.

The hard part is identifying the cause of your contact dermatitis. It could be anything that your skin has come in contact with.

Sometimes you can determine that a chemical, or something at home or work, has irritated your skin. Your doctor might test a patch of your skin to see what kinds of things cause an allergic reaction. But it can be hard to pin down the source and to decide whether it is an irritant or an allergen.

Your doctor can treat your contact dermatitis with a corticosteroid cream or tablets, but the best way to avoid a repeat performance is to stay away from the substance that bothers you.

And if you know what causes your contact dermatitis, wear gloves or wash your hands immediately after exposure.

MEDICAL SOURCE ───────────────────────────

Modern Medicine (59,11:38)

Herbal tea for serious skin problems?

Herbal tea is nice for a rainy day and a good book, but is it any good for treating serious skin disorders? It could be, if it's the right concoction.

Scientists are excited about the possibilities of treating difficult cases of skin disorders with a Chinese mixture of herbs and spices. The troublesome skin disorder is known as "atopic dermatitis."

This is a disorder that is usually inherited from your parents (50 to 75 percent of the time), and it is characterized by serious skin reactions to common environmental products (detergents, fabrics, etc.).

Atopic dermatitis usually begins in early childhood, and it causes reddened, itchy splotches on the skin that can become thickened and leathery. The sores often become infected or inflamed, resulting in blisters and pus buildup.

People who suffer from atopic dermatitis usually try to treat it by avoiding the things that cause the reaction, regular use of soothing creams and lotions, and the careful use of corticosteroid creams and medications. Unfortunately, most of the treatments don't work very well, and many people with this disorder suffer from the social embarrassment as well as the physical discomfort of the disease without any relief.

It turns out that some Chinese doctors were treating this disorder with herbal tea remedies and seeing good results. So the U.S. scientists "borrowed" the recipe from the Chinese physicians and ran a study to test the effects of the herbal formula.

The herbs that the Chinese doctors recommended included the Chinese herbs Ledebouriella seseloides, Potentilla chinensis, Clematis armandii, Rehmannia glutinosa, Paeonia lactiflora, Lophatherum gracile, Dictamnus dasycarpus, Tribulus terrestris, Glycyrrhiza glabra and Schizonepeta tenuifolia. These herbs, grown in mainland China, were ground up into a fine powder and mixed in a certain mixture that could be freshly brewed each day.

The American researchers conducted a study that included 40 volunteers (between the ages of 19 and 57) who suffered from atopic dermatitis and had not received much relief from standard treatments.

Half of the group of volunteers were given the herbal mixture to prepare and drink daily for eight weeks. After the first eight weeks, they had a four-week rest period with no treatment. Then they had an additional eight weeks in which they drank an herbal drink every day that tasted like the Chinese mixture but actually contained an ineffective placebo of no medicinal value.

The other half of the group of volunteers reversed that schedule: For the first eight weeks, they drank a "placebo tea" each day. Then they had a four-week rest period, followed by another eight weeks in which they drank the Chinese mixture every day.

Neither group knew which drinks contained the real herbs from China. However, each volunteer kept a diary in which they recorded any improvements or problems with the therapy. And the scientists tested each volunteer every four weeks throughout the entire 12-week study.

At the end of the study, the volunteers reported that they experienced improvement in their skin conditions while taking the Chinese herbal formula. Many reported that they itched less, some reported less redness and irritation, and several even reported sleeping better while taking the Chinese herbal tea.

Although many studies are still needed before doctors will begin prescribing herbal tea for serious cases of dermatitis, researchers are excited about the possibilities. This could offer a new and natural remedy for an age-old, difficult-to-treat problem.

MEDICAL SOURCE ————————————————————

The Lancet (340,8810:13)

The bug from the hot tub — how to avoid whirlpool folliculitis

Whirlpools, hot tubs and saunas have become more and more popular in the 1990s. Health clubs, tanning parlors and even private homeowners are installing more of them than ever before.

Unfortunately, the increase in the number of whirlpools has increased the number of people suffering from an infection known as whirlpool folliculitis.

Whirlpool folliculitis is a skin infection caused by the bacteria Pseudomonas aeruginosa. This bacteria is extremely hearty and can grow in a variety of settings, including the water in hot tubs and whirlpools.

Although the high water temperature in whirlpools and hot tubs kills many types of molds and bacteria, the Pseudomonas aeruginosa bacteria can survive the high temperature and the high chlorine content in the water.

The bacteria will cause a skin infection only if it enters the skin — through tiny breaks in the skin, open sores or even through the tiny pores in the skin around each hair follicle.

If the bacteria enters the skin, you will usually notice a rash within one to four days after your exposure to the bacteria in the whirlpool.

The rash usually is hives-like in nature, and it involves all areas of the body that were exposed to the bacteria except the head and neck. The hive-like bumps sometimes look very much like insect bites.

Often people who are infected also suffer from a low-grade fever, headaches, general fatigue and achiness, breast tenderness (in men and women), and upper respiratory complaints (coughing, wheezing, etc.).

If you get the aggravating skin infection, don't bother with any antibiotic creams or pills — the bacteria is not affected by the antibiotics.

Fortunately, the infection clears up on its own in about two to 10 days. It does not leave scars, and it rarely occurs in the same person twice.

So should I avoid whirlpools from now on to avoid getting this infection? you ask.

No, not exactly.

Scientists believe that there are three situations that seem to promote infection with Pseudomonas aeruginosa:

• Too much time in contaminated water in whirlpools
• Too many people in the water
• Inadequate pool care

These three situations can be avoided by following these simple tips:

❏ Limit the amount of time you spend in the whirlpool.

❏ Avoid bathing or sitting in hot tubs or whirlpools that have had a lot of people in them. Don't use them late in the day after people have been in the water all day.

❏ Stay out of any whirlpool or tub that has cloudy water.

❏ Maintain the proper amount of chlorine in the water to help discourage the growth of the bacteria. The Centers for Disease Control's Suggested Health and Safety Guidelines for Public Spas and Hot Tubs suggests a free chlorine concentration of 1 to 3 milligrams per liter and a pH of 7.2 to 7.8. Sometimes the bacteria will grow in water that contains the proper amount of chlorine, but the recommended amount of chlorine certainly helps to discourage it.

❏ If you have used a pool late in the day or a pool that did not have clear water, don't scrub yourself in the shower trying to get rid of the bacteria. Vigorous scrubbing and bathing with anti-bacterial soap can actually break the skin and alter the normal protective skin barrier. Remember that the bacteria have to get into the skin to cause infection, so try to avoid breaking the skin while bathing.

MEDICAL SOURCE ─────────────────────

   Cutis (45,2:97)

Good sense and bad cents — how to avoid nickel dermatitis

We used to find it in our five-cent pieces, but now it seems to pop up everywhere else. And for many people it leaves pain and irritation in its path.

"It" is the metal nickel. And although it is no longer used to make a five-cent money piece, nickel is present in many household articles, such as jewelry, cooking utensils, glass dyes, ceramics, batteries and magnets.

Nickel is even found in some food products because of the nickel found in fungicides and in the equipment used in food processing and packaging.

The problem with nickel is that it can cause an allergic skin reaction known as "nickel dermatitis." Now, just like not everyone is allergic to bees, not everyone is allergic to nickel.

But for those who are, simple skin contact with nickel can cause a skin lesion that is red, swollen and blistered. The skin lesion may go on to become discolored and leathery. The skin cells involved in the lesion become dry, itchy and bark-like.

In some people, the skin reaction then progresses to become a hives-like reaction, with red bumps that have crusty tops on them. The bumps are ugly, itchy and irritating.

Women suffer from nickel dermatitis more often than men. Women seem to get the aggravating skin problem because of their contact with household articles, whereas men seem to come in contact with nickel at work in industrial settings.

The best way to avoid getting nickel dermatitis is to avoid coming in contact with nickel.

How do I do that? you ask. A lot of my jewelry and cooking utensils contain the metal nickel!

Follow these simple tips on how to avoid skin contact with nickel:

- Try coating any nickel-containing jewelry with clear nail polish.
- Replace buttons that contain nickel with brass, wooden or plastic buttons.
- Consider replacing your nickel-containing kitchen utensils with stainless steel utensils.
- If you are getting your ears pierced, avoid anything except stainless steel needles and posts.
- After your ears are first pierced, leave the stainless steel posts in your ears for about three weeks to make sure your ears have healed completely. Then try different earring posts to see which ones you might react to.
- Even gold earring posts occasionally contain nickel, so be sure to test all your jewelry around the house before wearing it out to a fancy occasion.
- If you work in an industrial setting where you might be exposed to nickel, wear protective clothing like long pants and sleeves and heavy-duty vinyl gloves.

Although you probably can't avoid nickel 100 percent of the time, following these simple tips will help decrease your exposure to nickel and cut down on your problems with nickel dermatitis.

MEDICAL SOURCE ———————————————

Cutis (45,2:87)

Apply simple vitamin cream to reduce extra pigment that causes 'darkened' age spots

If the darkened "age spots" that have begun to appear on your hands and face are not your idea of attractive, help could be as simple as the letter "A."

Research indicates that a cream containing the drug tretinoin — a powerful form of vitamin A — might help remove age spots.

Tretinoin — also known as Retin-A — is a form of vitamin A that is currently rubbed on the skin to help fight acne, but researchers suggest that it also helps reduce the production of the skin pigment melanin.

These "liver spots" that are often referred to as "age spots" are actually areas on the skin that have been damaged by years of exposure to the sun.

The skin responds to the damage by producing more melanin, the pigment that gives the skin its color and produces the sought-after summertime tan. The extra pigment in a small area produces the age spot.

Until now, any attempts to remove the spots have been less than successful. Some bleaching agents even left the skin under-pigmented.

What remained after the liver spot was removed was a "bleached" portion of skin that was much lighter than the surrounding skin. Most people would rather have the age spots.

Scientists conducted a test with 60 people between the ages of 36 and 86 who had age spots. Half of the people in the group used a "placebo cream" that did not contain any medication. The other half applied the vitamin-A cream to their age spots once a day for 10 months.

The scientists examined the age spots once a month for the whole 10 months. The color of the age spots was compared to the color before treatment, and the scientists graded the color as much darker, darker, slightly darker, unchanged, slightly lighter, lighter, much lighter or absent.

After 10 months of treatment, eight out of 10 people who had used the tretinoin cream experienced some lightening of their age spots.

Among that group, the spots were "much lighter" in 23 percent and "lighter" in 65 percent. Some of the people who responded well to the first 10 months of tretinoin therapy were assigned to treatment for another six months.

Four people who had experienced a complete clearing of an age spot during the first 10 months maintained these results for the next six months of treatment.

Although the results were positive, the scientists also reported some side effects associated with the use of the tretinoin cream.

Up to 82 percent of the people using the cream developed redness and scaling of the skin in the areas that came in contact with the cream.

Redness and scaling began between one and four weeks after the start of tretinoin treatment, but the symptoms usually started to decrease in severity over time. The skin reactions improved with the use of moisturizing creams and with a decreased amount of tretinoin cream.

The Food and Drug Administration has approved tretinoin cream only for use as an acne treatment. However, many doctors are already prescribing the cream to lighten age spots and freckles.

A big caution: Tretinoin, a prescription drug, has caused birth defects when used by pregnant women.

MEDICAL SOURCE ——————————————————

The New England Journal of Medicine (326,6:368)

Simple tips to help bring relief to your nails

If your fingernails used to be a point of pride, but lately they've become an embarrassment, you're not alone. And you don't have to suffer without relief.

Most people think that as we get older, our nails become dry, brittle and cracked.

Not so. Brittle nails, in people who are otherwise healthy, are almost always due to external causes.

These include excessive use of solvents, soap and detergents. These substances can also soften your nails and cause the ends to split and flake. Sometimes, the nail splits so badly it comes off completely.

Just staying away from detergents for a while should considerably help nails return to normal.

If not, apply lotion containing formalin daily for a few weeks. However, this lotion can irritate the skin, even causing an allergic skin reaction in some cases, so take care when applying.

Ridges in nails may develop across the width, or along the length of the nails, and they occur for different reasons.

Ridges across the nails are called "Beau's" lines. These are due to bodily upsets, such as severe infection.

Surgery can also cause ridging, because the nail growth may be temporarily interrupted due to the anesthesia. These lines will eventually grow out, although the nail can break off if the groove is deep enough.

Ridges along the length of the nail are due to a growth irregularity and are often more pronounced in the elderly.

There is really no treatment for this, and the severity will vary from time to time.

A single groove, running the length of one nail, may be produced by a tumor at the base of the nail.

Check with your doctor if you have any concerns about your nails.

MEDICAL SOURCE ———————————————

British Medical Journal (301,658:973)

Problems with nails and hands? It could be your hair spray

If you are having problems with your fingernails, you might need to check out your hair spray. Hair spray is a probable cause of nail disorders.

A 46-year-old woman had been using a new hair spray when she discovered some problems with her nails and hands.

Apparently, she was in the habit of spraying with one hand while running the other hand through or smoothing her hair.

She noticed that her fingernails began to "turn loose, peel and hurt." Also, the skin on the backs of her fingers began to peel.

She stopped using her hair spray and her fingers and nails both returned to normal. The distinctive ingredient in the hair spray that caused these problems is unknown.

Cosmetics are one of the most common causes of contact/irritant nail abnormalities. So, if you have "sensitive" nails and fingers and must continue to use your hair spray, try to keep the hair spray from actually touching your nails and fingers.

MEDICAL SOURCE ———————————————

Cutis (47,3:165)

Fitness ailments — what to do for exercise-related skin injuries

Are you a weekend warrior when it comes to sporting or

recreational activities? On the weekends you give it all you've got, then you retreat to the quiet safety of the house during the week to recover?

Well, weekend warrior or dedicated athlete — you still might experience skin problems that are directly related to your exercise and fitness activities.

Below are some common athletic ailments and what you can do to treat them and prevent them.

❑ Runner's rump. This embarrassing affliction is caused by jogging and long-distance running. You'll find redness and soreness (and possible swelling) in between the buttocks caused by the constant friction between the buttocks when running or jogging. You might also experience redness and raw skin on your upper thighs and groin area. This can be caused by your pants rubbing against the skin. Runner's rump will disappear by itself in a day or two if you'll cut back on the running for a few days. If your pants are the problem, consider buying some of the silky, nylon running shorts or some Lycra leggings to run in. These fabrics are not as rough or coarse as some other fabrics and might be easier on your skin.

❑ Jogger's nipples. This is another embarrassing ailment that plagues runners. This can happen to almost anyone who jogs, but it is more common in long-distance and marathon runners. Jogger's nipples result from the rubbing of the nipples against coarse fabric for long periods of time. The problem can be as simple as a mild irritation or as serious as actual hemorrhaging. If your case is serious, you need to see your doctor. Otherwise, most cases of jogger's nipples will go away if you'll take a few days off the running schedule. To avoid this problem, put some good lotion or tape on the affected areas before running. Men should try to avoid shirts made from rough fabrics. Wear soft cotton or silky nylon shirts to cut down on the friction and irritation. Women should buy proper sports bras made with soft fabric. Make sure the bra fits correctly to avoid the bra shifting and moving while you are running.

❑ Surfer's nodules. These are small tumor-like bumps that appear on your kneecaps, shin bones or ankles where your skin comes into contact with the surfboard. The nodules are your body's attempts to heal damaged tissues. Stay away from the surfboard for a while to let them heal.

❑ Black palm. Golfers, tennis players, basketball buffs and weightlifters all have this kind of problem from time to time. Black palm is just what it sounds like — a bluish-black discoloration of the palm of the hand. In other words, the palm of your hand looks like one huge bruise. This results from sudden, choppy movements that rip and tear the delicate blood vessels in your palm. Just like a bruise, these will go away over time on their own. To avoid this problem in the future, weightlifters should consider buying some padded gloves to help cushion their hands. Golfers and tennis players can use athletic gloves (like batting gloves used in baseball).

❑ Tennis and skier's toe. This painful ailment is the bruising and discoloration of the big toe due to repeated and sudden starts and stops that jam the big toe into the front of the shoe. Joggers and racquetball players also have this problem occasionally.

For relief, soak your feet in warm water after your activity, then get off your feet. Take a pain reliever (aspirin or acetaminophen) if the pain is too bad.

To avoid this problem, keep your toenails trimmed and wear properly fitting shoes.

Sporting shoe salespeople can help you pick out a shoe for your activity that fits you properly.

MEDICAL SOURCE ————————————————————

U.S. Pharmacist (17,6:31 Supplement)

'Leaf' these three-leafed plants alone

It's as common as baseball and hot dogs during the summer months, but not nearly as much fun.

It's poison ivy, and it (along with poison oak and poison sumac) affects from 10 to 50 million Americans every year. Many researchers estimate that about 50 to 85 percent of the nation's population is allergic to these pesky plants.

And unfortunately, it's hard to get away from them. They grow as vines on trees, bushes, fences and telephone poles, or they can grow as ground shrubs of different sizes. They each contain an oil called urushiol. It is the urushiol oil that reacts with your skin to produce an itchy, blistering red rash several hours, or even several days, after you have come in contact with the plants.

Most people come into contact with poison ivy, oak or sumac during the summer months when the sap in the stems and leaves of the plants is most abundant. But you can get the telltale rash from these plants any time throughout the year.

The best treatment for the dermatitis that these poisonous plants cause is to avoid coming into contact with them. To avoid them, you need to know what they look like.

For poison ivy and oak, the rule of thumb is "Leaflets three, let it be." These plants are easy to recognize because of their distinct three-leaflet design. Each stem of poison ivy contains three, perfectly identical, shiny, pointed leaves. And remember that it can grow as a plant, bush or vine.

Poison oak looks very much like poison ivy with the three leaflets on each stem. But poison oak has "hairy" leaves that look like oak leaves instead of the shiny leaves in poison ivy.

Poison sumac is not nearly as common. Its leaves consist of seven to 13 smaller, paired leaflets along a straight stem. Poison sumac grows best in the swamps of the Eastern United States.

It's not just the leaves on these three plants that you need to avoid. All parts of the plants, including leaves, stems, roots and berries, contain the urushiol oil that causes the skin reaction.

If you have poison ivy, oak or sumac growing in your yard, you can get rid of it, but you need to do it carefully.

To get rid of the irritating plants, wear clothes that cover nearly all of your skin and wear plastic gloves. Uproot the plants and put them in plastic bags in the trash. Or you can spray herbicides on the plants about every three weeks.

But never burn the plants. The oil from the plants that causes the rash can rise with the smoke. If you inhale it or it comes in contact with your skin, you could be looking at a serious problem. After uprooting the plants and throwing them away, take a bath, wash your clothes, and clean off your tools with soap and water.

If you are planning to spend some time outdoors and you think you might come in contact with poison ivy, oak or sumac, follow these precautions:

❑ Wear clothes that will cover your skin. Always wear boots or shoes and long pants when walking through the woods. Wear gloves and long sleeves if you are weeding or pulling vines.

❑ As soon as you get back inside, wash your skin with soap and water, including under your fingernails. Sponging your skin off with rubbing alcohol will also help remove any remaining urushiol oil. Also remember to wash your clothes, shoes and any garden tools and even any pets that came in contact with the plants. Never sponge off your skin while you are still in the woods. This can strip your skin of its protective oils. Wait to sponge off until you get out of the woods.

❑ You might not develop a rash after your first exposure to poison ivy, oak or sumac. Some people are exposed many times before they have a reaction. But if you do react, the degree of your reaction will depend on how much urushiol oil got on your skin. The reaction first appears as an itchy area of redness and mild swelling. Soon, blisters develop, and the blisters often become crusty. The reactions are always located on thin skin — arms, face, neck, trunk, groin or legs. You'll never get a rash from poison ivy on the palms of your hands or the soles of your feet — the skin is too thick.

❑ Extremely sensitive people might develop a rash within a few hours of touching the plants. Less sensitive people might not develop the rash for several days to a week. In fact, many people think that their poison ivy rash is spreading to other parts of their body because new areas of rash pop up every day. But the rash is not spreading or even contagious — it's just that some areas of your skin took longer to react. The old myth—that scratching will spread the rash — is just that: a myth.

❑ The rash will clear up on its own, so the only thing you can do is stop the rash from itching so badly. Applying a soothing lotion or cream will sometimes relieve the itch, and you can buy over-the-counter cortisone creams that will help severe itching.

❑ Calamine lotion is a tried and true remedy for a bad case of poison ivy, oak or sumac. The calamine lotion cools your skin and makes the itching feel better. It also leaves a powdery film on the rash that helps absorb any oozing from the rash and helps keep your clothes or dirt from sticking to the oozing blisters. But only use the calamine lotion until the blisters stop oozing and dry up. Using the calamine lotion beyond that point will only dry out your skin and make the area itch more.

❑ If the rash covers a large part of your body, a cool bath will help soothe the itching and discomfort.

❑ Cool compresses will also help relieve the itching. Put a cotton cloth soaked in cool water or Burow's solution (aluminum acetate) over the rash and let a fan blow over it to cool the skin. Your compress should not be more than a layer or two thick. If the compress is too thick, the water will not evaporate from it, and you won't get the benefit of the cooling process on your skin.

❑ Forget the myth that the liquid from the blisters can cause the rash to spread — it doesn't. In fact, when blisters form, it might be a good idea to drain them. If they are drained, the anti-itch creams you are using can get to the underlying skin easier.

❑ To drain a blister, insert a sterile needle into the edge of the blister. Then gently press the top of the blister to remove the fluid. Hold a piece of tissue or gauze onto the skin to absorb the liquid. Then wash the skin well and put on your anti-itch cream. But do not remove the skin covering the blister — this skin protects the delicate layer of skin underneath. And do not open any blisters on your face or genitals. Let your doctor take care of that.

❑ Try using antihistamines to cut down on the itching. You can get over-the-counter antihistamine lotions (Benadryl) or antihistamine pills (Benadryl or Chlor-Trimeton).

❑ Try some oatmeal. Colloidal oatmeal mixtures will help absorb and dry up the oozing blisters. You can get over-the-counter brands of colloidal oatmeal mixes — just follow the instructions on the label.

❏ Try not to scratch. Scratching doesn't spread the rash, but it increases your chances of getting infected.

❏ If you have a serious case, your doctor can prescribe some cortisone pills or give you a cortisone injection. See your doctor if you have a rash on or around your genitals, on your face, in your eyes, or in your mouth or nose.

MEDICAL SOURCES

Emergency Medicine (24,7:171)
The Physician and Sportsmedicine (20,5:163)
Healthprint (7,4:1)

Tartar-control toothpaste — friend or foe?

That rash around your lips and mouth might not have been caused by something you ate. It could be from your toothpaste.

Tartar-control toothpaste seems to cause a skin reaction in some people, scientists reveal. The skin reaction is a red, scaly rash around the mouth that causes itching and burning.

Researchers recently studied 20 women who had the rash around their mouths. Apparently, all of the women had been using tartar-control toothpaste several times each day.

The researchers instructed the women to use different kinds of toothpaste without tartar control. The rash cleared up in over half the women after they stopped using the tartar-control toothpaste.

Later studies showed that the women who used tartar-control toothpaste just once a day had no more problems with the rash. But if they used the toothpaste up to three times a day, the rash reoccurred.

The researchers suggest that if you use tartar-control tooth-paste and you develop a rash around your mouth, try switching brands of toothpaste. If the rash doesn't clear up after a few days, try using regular toothpaste that doesn't contain the tartar-control ingredients.

MEDICAL SOURCE —————————————————————————————

Consumer Reports Health Letter (September 1990,72)

How to cope with skin reactions that are drug side effects

Your doctor prescribed some medicine for your respiratory infection, and it has started to clear up. But now your skin is breaking out in a strange rash. What are you to do?

That's a question many people ask when they experience skin reactions from drugs. Listed below are some common skin reactions and what to do for them.

❑ Urticaria. This is a skin reaction that causes inflammation of the skin and raised areas of redness and swelling. The skin lesions vary in size, and they usually last no longer than 24 to 48 hours. (A lesion is a sore, an inflamed area, a reddened bump, or other abnormal patch on the skin.) Some of the drugs that can cause this reaction include penicillins (methicillin, nafcillin, ticarcillin, ampicillin, amoxicillin, etc.), sulfonamides (sulfacytine, sulfadiazine, sulfisoxazole, sulfapyridine, etc.), barbiturates (phenobarbital, secobarbital, pentobarbital, etc.), anticonvulsants (phenytoin, mephenytoin, etc.), salicylates (aspirin, etc.) and opiate analgesics (morphine, fentanyl, levorphanol, methadone, etc.).

The best treatment for drug-induced urticaria is to stop taking the offending drug. Then take antihistamines (or use antihistamine skin cream) to clear up the skin reaction. Cool, wet compresses will bring relief to the irritated skin while the antihistamine starts working. You could also try an oatmeal bath. Pour two cups of colloidal (powdered) oatmeal into a tub of warm water and take a soothing bath. You can get colloidal oatmeal at your local pharmacy or supermarket.

❏ Contact dermatitis. This skin reaction results in a papular eruption, raised, solid skin lesions less than a half-inch in diameter. The lesions are red and itchy and can form small blisters. Chronic contact dermatitis results in the thickening of the skin, until it becomes leathery. The local dermatitis might spread to the whole body, which is referred to as "exfoliative dermatitis." If this happens, you could experience fever and chills. Serious cases of whole-body dermatitis should be treated by a doctor.

Some drugs that might cause contact dermatitis include topical anesthetics (lidocaine and benzocaine), neomycin and penicillin. The immediate therapy for this skin reaction is to stop using the drug causing the problem. Then use a corticosteroid lotion or spray on the irritated skin. You can get these over-the-counter products at your drug store. Also take some antihistamines to relieve the itching, and use some cool, wet compresses to bring immediate relief to your skin.

❏ Photosensitivity. This is just what it sounds like — your skin becomes extra-sensitive to light (especially sunlight). The irritated skin looks as if it has been sunburned, and this condition can develop within minutes to hours after being exposed to strong light. Some drugs that can cause this reaction include thiazides and other diuretics (chlorothiazide, cyclothiazide, benzthiazide, etc.), antifungal drugs (amphotericin, flucytosine, nystatin, etc.), tetracyclines (doxycycline, methacycline, etc.) and sulfonamides (see previous page for examples).

If photosensitivity results, call your doctor. Then take extra care to protect and shield the skin from strong light (especially sunlight).

Use sunscreens, light clothing, etc., to keep the light off the skin. If sunburn has already occurred, use some sunburn-relief tips: cool, wet compresses; aloe vera; hydrocortisone cream; or an oatmeal bath, using colloidal oatmeal in the bath water.

If you notice any other unusual reactions after taking any medications, such as dizziness, shortness of breath or difficulty breathing, a fluttering heart or racing pulse, call your doctor immediately. You could be suffering from a severe allergic reaction, and you might need medical care right away.

Always ask your doctor or pharmacist for a complete list of the side effects of the drugs you are using.

All doctors and pharmacists have this information available at their fingertips, so don't take "no" for an answer. Get the information you need.

If you're taking over-the-counter drugs, carefully read the package and the package insert.

These usually contain information on special cautions and side effects. If you are not satisfied with that information, ask the pharmacist in your local drug store to give you a list of the side effects.

The pharmacist usually has a big book that contains all drugs and can tell you what you need to know.

MEDICAL SOURCE —————————————————

U.S. Pharmacist (17,7:33)

Hot tip for relief of shingles pain

If you're suffering from distressing skin pain from shingles or diabetes, get ready for some red-hot pain relief! It's natural, it's safe, and its active ingredient comes from the same red peppers you use to spice up your chili.

Remember the sudden, explosive sensation you get when you bite into a red pepper? The ingredient that causes that hot taste is the same ingredient that helps relieve skin pain.

This hot new medicine is capsaicin, and when used properly, it may relieve the skin pain caused by shingles and diabetes.

When applied to the skin, capsaicin causes a sensation of warmth. Generally, you can expect to experience pain relief after about two weeks of therapy. But, occasionally it might take up to four weeks of therapy before you begin feeling pain relief.

Many doctors prefer to use capsaicin for skin pain relief instead of other drugs.

Capsaicin has fewer drug interaction problems than many other drugs. Some capsaicin products are available in over-the-counter, nonprescription (lotion) forms.

MEDICAL SOURCE ─────────────────────

U.S. Pharmacist (15,12:27)

The bedtime blues — how to get rid of insomnia

It happens night after night. You and millions of Americans get into bed, hoping for a good night of sleep — only to toss, turn, wiggle and squirm until the wee hours of the morning.

You get up in the morning, cranky, irritable and sleepy.

You suffer from insomnia — the inability to fall asleep or to stay asleep at night. You and about 20 percent of Americans have recurrent insomnia. About twice that number of Americans have difficulty falling asleep or returning back to sleep after waking in the night.

For some, insomnia is an occasional nuisance. For others, it is a nightly curse — a problem that won't go away. In many cases, insomnia is only short-term, and it is frequently referred to as "transient insomnia."

Usually transient insomnia is directly related to some event going on in your life. Stress from a new job, loss of an old job, marriage trouble, a rebellious teen-ager, an impending retirement, financial problems, death of a loved one or anxiety over an upcoming relocation — these are examples of sources of stress in people's lives that frequently cause temporary sleeping problems.

Those sleeping problems are usually taken care of when the problem itself is resolved.

Insomnia is also caused by medications. Many prescription drugs and some nonprescription drugs have side effects that include insomnia.

And occasionally, a combination of drugs will produce insomnia as a side effect, even though no single drug in the combination causes insomnia.

Insomnia is frequently related to physical illnesses. People who suffer from illnesses or diseases that cause pain or discomfort are often unable to sleep due to their pain.

Many people with terminal illnesses such as cancer might be afraid to sleep because of the fear of nightmares or the fear of not reawakening in the morning. Although their bodies crave sleep, the fear of sleep keeps them edgy and awake.

Depression, like anxiety and stress, is a frequent cause of insomnia. As with stress, the insomnia caused by depression usually disappears when the depression is resolved.

Another segment of the American population has trouble sleeping due to shift work. Most of the people who suffer from work-related insomnia or sleepiness have rotating work schedules — a day shift one day, and a midnight shift the next. Their "body clock" can't get adjusted to the changing schedule, and they can't sleep when they need to.

Other people who work straight evening or midnight shifts might have difficulty sleeping during the day even though their shifts are regular. The light from the windows or the noise of outside activity during the day is enough to keep them awake even though they are sleepy.

Many types of insomnia can be improved without the aid of sleeping medication. The following tips will help you deal with your sleeping problems:

❑ Avoid tobacco, caffeine, nicotine and alcohol in the evening. These "drugs" can interfere with your sleep.

❑ Avoid heavy meals late in the evening.

❑ Avoid hunger at bedtime. If you are hungry, get a light snack, remembering to avoid large or heavy snacks and meals.

❑ If possible, avoid taking naps during the day. If you must take naps, take one early in the day (soon after lunch) instead of late in the afternoon or early in the evening. The closer the nap is to your bedtime, the harder it will be for you to fall asleep at night.

❑ If possible, keep a regular sleeping schedule. Try to go to bed and get up at the same time each day. Do not oversleep on weekends or holidays. If you take naps, take them at the same time each day.

❑ Schedule time to "wind down" before going to bed. Take a warm bath, read quietly in a comfortable room, listen to some soothing music, meditate or pray before bedtime.

❑ Make certain the bed is comfortable. If the mattress is lumpy or soft, consider getting a newer one.

❑ Make sure the bedroom is comfortable — quiet, dark enough for you to sleep, a comfortable temperature, and safe.

❑ Get regular exercise during the day. Regular exercise helps you to sleep well as long as the exercising is not close to bedtime.

❑ Don't take your problems to bed with you. Schedule a time earlier in the day or evening to mull over any problems or stressful situations in your life, then do your best to put them out of your mind until the next day.

❑ Don't just toss and turn. Get out of bed if you don't fall asleep within 20 to 30 minutes. Get up, go to another room of the house where you can read quietly, watch TV, listen to music or find something else to do until you get sleepy. Then go back to the bed and try to fall asleep again.

❑ If you think your insomnia could be caused in part by a stressful family or work situation, follow the tips above and don't worry — that insomnia will probably go away as soon as the stressful event passes.

❑ If your insomnia is caused by a painful or uncomfortable illness, talk to your doctor about a pain medicine that includes a sleeping aid.

❑ Insomnia resulting from depression or anxiety can often be helped by the same things that might help the depression — family support, a friend to confide in, professional counseling or antidepression medicine. Talk to your doctor about how to best deal with your depression.

❑ If your insomnia is caused by crazy shift work, consider requesting a work schedule that moves gradually clockwise rather than shifts that change irregularly or rapidly. Also consider buying black-out shades for your windows to make the room dark. Many people also use "noise-making machines" to sleep with — radio-type devices that mimic the sound of falling rain, a waterfall, ocean waves, wind blowing through trees, etc. These sounds will help lull you to sleep as well as block out the regular outside noise that goes on during the day while you are trying to sleep.

❑ If you suspect that your insomnia is a side effect of a drug you are taking or the result of a combination of drugs, talk to your doctor right away. He probably can prescribe different medications that will perform the same therapy but won't have the same side effects. However, don't change your medication routine without checking with your doctor first.

If you can't fall asleep without medication, use the medication wisely:

- Take the lowest dose of the sleeping medication possible.
- Follow the instructions on the label as closely as you can. If you have difficulty understanding the instructions, ask your pharmacist for advice.
- If you are using an over-the-counter sleep aid, read the box or package insert about side effects and cautions.
- If you are using medicine that your doctor prescribed, make sure you ask him or your pharmacist about dosage, side effects, cautions, etc.
- Try taking the medicine for a week to two weeks, then stop taking it (unless instructed otherwise by your doctor). Your body might not need the medicine any longer.
- Don't drive or operate any type of heavy or dangerous equipment while you are using sleeping pills.

MEDICAL SOURCES ———————————————————

> *American Family Physician* (45,3:1262)
> *The University of Texas Lifetime Health Letter* (2,2:1)
> *U.S. Pharmacist* (17,1:26)

Amnesia from your sleeping aid?

Those of us who have insomnia sometimes feel we would do anything for a good night's sleep.

But sometimes the cure can be even worse than the problem!

This might be the case with a prescription sleeping aid called Triazolam.

Researchers believe that although Triazolam does help people who have problems sleeping, it often causes memory impairment and even amnesia.

So, although you might feel more rested after using Triazolam, it might cause you real difficulties in your daily life or work.

If you take Triazolam or other prescription drugs, check with your doctor or pharmacist about possible side effects.

MEDICAL SOURCE ───────────────────────

The Lancet (337,8745:827)

Prescription drugs: nightmares for some people

For most adults, nightmares are a thing of yesteryear: an unpleasant memory left behind with childhood. But for some adults, nightmares continue to be very real and scary experiences.

For one 33-year-old man, the nightmares started when he began taking 500 milligrams of the anti-inflammatory drug naproxen for some shoulder and arm pain. He took the drug for three days.

During those three days, he reported waking up with recollections of vivid nightmares of accidents and plane crashes and other terrifying events. The nightmares occurred every night that he took the naproxen.

When he stopped taking the drug, the nightmares went away. A few weeks later, he began taking the naproxen again, and again he suffered the same bizarre nightmares.

Many prescription medications have some related side effects that can be as simple as increased drowsiness and upset stomach or as frightening as nightmares and mental disorders.

In addition to naproxen, some other drugs that have been shown to cause nightmares (from use or withdrawal from the drug) include alcohol, doxepin, fluphenazine in combination with diphenhydramine, reserpine, thioridazine, thiothixene, buspirone, beta blockers and verapamil.

If you are currently taking any of these or any other drugs and are suffering from nightmares, talk to your doctor or pharmacist.

There might be another drug that you can take with similar therapeutic effects without the nightmares.

Don't change or stop taking your prescribed medicines without talking to your doctor first.

MEDICAL SOURCE ───────────────────

Southern Medical Journal (84,10:1271)

SMELLING PROBLEMS

'Wake up and smell the coffee' ... again

Can you still "wake up and smell the coffee" as well as you once did? Or have the taste and smell of your favorite things diminished in recent months?

Well, that might be because of a disorder known as "hyposmia" — a diminished sense of smell. And, although it isn't life-threatening, it is life-changing for some two million people in the United States who suffer from it or some form of smelling disorder.

A major complication involved is that problems with the sense of smell also affect the sense of taste. So, a loss of smell that results in taste disorders can cause mealtimes to become dreary, boring and even sickening.

Some people with taste or smell loss overeat to compensate for the lost sensation, which results in unwanted weight gain.

Others with diminished or distorted smell and taste will undereat or avoid food altogether, resulting in dangerous weight loss and vitamin deficiencies.

Loss of smell can even be dangerous. In fact, Dr. Robert Henkin of the Taste and Smell Clinic in Washington, D.C., recalls one man who died in a house fire because he couldn't smell the smoke.

What causes smell and taste disorders? Many things can.

Chronic infection in the nose or sinuses can contribute to problems in the senses of smell and taste.

Another common cause is zinc deficiency. Zinc deficiencies can result from a dietary deficiency, diarrhea, chronic infection or diuretic drugs.

Various drugs can cause problems with smell and taste. Drugs containing sulfur are known to suppress taste. Common, sulfur-containing drugs include the anti-inflammatory drug penicillamine, the blood-pressure drug captopril and transdermal (patch) nitro-glycerin to treat angina pain.

And, the antibiotics tetracycline and metronidazole can cause a metallic taste in the mouth.

Menopause can also cause changes in a woman's senses of smell and taste.

The good news is that many cases of smell and taste disorders can be solved.

Treating and clearing up nose and sinus infections usually help restore the senses of smell and taste. And problems caused by zinc deficiency can be solved by taking a zinc supplement.

Women suffering from smell and taste problems after menopause often find relief with hormone replacement therapy. And your doctor usually can prescribe different medications if a drug is contributing to such disorders.

If you have noticed changes in the way things smell or taste, talk to your doctor right away. You might be suffering from hyposmia or some other type of smell or taste disorder.

Medical Source —————————————————————

FDA Consumer (25,9:29)

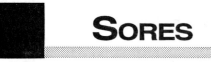

Sores

Apply regular table sugar to help heal minor sores and wounds

A spoonful of sugar might do more than make the medicine go down. Instead of helping it go down, the sugar might actually be the medicine!

Ordinary, granulated table sugar applied directly to sores or wounds helps heal sores.

Some hospital workers mix sugar with hydrogen peroxide to form a kind of paste and then put that paste directly on open sores, especially on bedsores. This "paste" seems to help the sores heal.

The sugar paste reduces the amount of water around the wound (the body naturally contains a large portion of water). The reduced amount of water helps prevent the wound from getting infected by bacteria, because the bacteria need water to live.

However, the sugar doesn't prevent the body from performing its normal healing process, such as new tissue growth — it just helps protect the area from dangerous bacterial infection.

The report cautions that the sugar paste is only effective in the early stages of the wound healing.

If doctors use the sugar paste in later stages of healing, the sugar grains can act like sandpaper. The abrasion caused by the sugar granules can cause unnecessary bleeding and actually prolong the healing process.

MEDICAL SOURCE ─────────────────────────────

The Lancet (338,8766:571)

Don't use aloe vera on cuts

Aloe vera might soothe and help heal burns, but it could double the healing time for cuts.

Surgeons found that applying aloe vera to surgical incisions instead of standard treatment significantly delayed the wound-healing process.

Incisions with standard treatment healed after 40 days. The same kinds of cuts treated with aloe vera took 84 days to heal.

MEDICAL SOURCE ─────────────────────────────

Science News (140,8:125)

STOMACH PROBLEMS

Cool your nausea with cola and soda crackers

It's worked for many pregnant mothers-to-be who suffer from morning sickness. The remedy is a noncaffeinated soft drink along with plain saltine crackers.

Some advise to let the cola lose its "fizz" first. Set out the opened container for an hour or so or overnight to let the carbonation escape, so that the cola will taste flat.

You also might try a pinch of powdered ginger root, a tested remedy for quashing that queasy feeling caused by motion sickness.

MEDICAL SOURCES —————————————————————

The Merck Manual, Sixteenth Edition, Merck Research Laboratories, Rahway, N.J., 1992
Popular Nutritional Practices, Sense and Nonsense, Dell Publishing, New York, 1988

Soothe upset stomachs with chamomile tea

It has been used since Roman times in teas and extracts to help soothe stomachaches and other digestive problems. The natural herb chamomile produces sweet-smelling flowers that can be dried and brewed for tea.

Take about a teaspoonful of the dried material, soak it in a cup of hot water, then strain to remove the solid particles.

MEDICAL SOURCE —————————————————————

The Lawrence Review of Natural Products (March 1991)

STROKE

Excessive use of salt can cause damaged arteries and stroke

You don't have high blood pressure, so you think you're safe. You really don't pay too much attention to how much salt you and your family consume.

Well, you might want to start paying close attention. High blood pressure isn't the only malady connected to excessive use of salt.

Too much salt in the diet can also damage the arteries — even if you don't have high blood pressure, warns an American Heart Association publication.

Over a period of time, salt causes the arteries to deteriorate.

This deterioration of the arteries that serve the brain can result in stroke.

In hopes of decreasing the dangerous effects of salt, the American Heart Association suggests that healthy people consume no more than 1.5 teaspoons of salt daily. That includes the amount of salt that is "hidden" in canned and frozen prepared foods.

For people who suffer from high blood pressure or other significant health problems, the recommended amount drops even lower — to one teaspoon each day.

MEDICAL SOURCE ————————————————

Heartstyle (1,1:8)

SUNBURN AND SKIN SAFETY

Simple tips to help protect yourself from the summer sun

Summertime means family vacations at the beach, outdoor volleyball and lounging by the pool. These and other summertime activities mean you and your family members will be out in the sun.

To get the most enjoyment from your outdoor activities with the least damage from the sun, be sure to follow a few simple summer safety tips:

❑ Begin your summer by spending small periods of time in the sun to avoid getting sunburned. In other words, don't spend three hours out in the sun on your first day of summer vacation. Start with short time periods (30 minutes or so) and increase that time daily.

❑ Use a sunscreen with a sun protection factor of at least 15 to avoid sunburn. Getting sunburned increases your risk of skin cancer, especially in children.

❑ Use a stronger sunscreen for sensitive areas: nose, lips and cheeks.

❑ Use a "broad spectrum" sunscreen that contains two or more UV (ultraviolet) ray blocking ingredients to block out both alpha and beta radiation from the sun.

❑ Always reapply sunscreen after swimming or showering.

❑ Try to avoid getting in the sun between 10 a.m. and 2 p.m. when the sun's rays are strongest.

❑ Wear a wide-brimmed hat to protect your face from the sun.

Check with your doctor immediately if you notice any unusual discolored splotches or lesions on your skin. Also see your doctor if you notice any changes in the shape or color of freckles or moles.

MEDICAL SOURCES ————————————————————

> *FDA Consumer* (25,4:16)
> *Medical Update* (15,2:4)

Armed with your favorite sunscreen for a day of fun in the sun?

You might be getting only half as much skin protection from your sunscreen lotion as you think.

The thickness of the sunscreen layer on your skin is the key to getting the sun protection promised on the bottle.

In a clinical study, 50 people applied a variety of brands of sunscreen the way they normally would. Scientists added fluorescent coloring to the sunscreens so the thickness could be measured. Most of the sunscreen-users rubbed on their lotion only half as thick as the recommended thicknesses.

Researchers say that when you apply sunscreen too thinly, you cut the skin protection in half.

To get the maximum protection, you need to apply your sunscreen in the thickness recommended on the bottle.

The best time to apply sunscreen is about 30 minutes before going out in the sun.

MEDICAL SOURCE ————————————————————

> *U.S. Pharmacist* (14,4:27)

Kiss sunburned lips good-bye

You've got your beach towel, your picnic basket, the beach ball and your suntan lotion, and you think you're all set for a day in the sun. But you're forgetting one important thing — your lip protection.

People are getting more and more careful about wearing sunscreen or protective clothing to avoid getting so many harmful rays from the sun, but most people neglect the one thing that is right under their noses, literally — their lips.

The lips burn easily from the harmful ultraviolet rays from the sun. And you don't even need to be in direct sun to get sunburned lips since reflective surfaces (water, sand, concrete) can flash you with up to 90 percent of the rays you thought you were avoiding by staying in the shade.

Too much sun on your lips can cause premature wrinkles because the ultraviolet sun rays damage the elastic properties of the skin. Sunburned lips can also lead to discoloration of the lips, lesions and cancerous growths.

You can get sunscreen for your lips in balms or creams. The best kind to get is a "sun block" formula. This kind of protectant deflects or scatters the UV rays that reach your lips instead of absorbing the rays. And it offers protection against many types of UV rays (some screens only filter out certain UV rays).

You can even use the sunscreen you use for the rest of your body on your lips. Most sunscreens don't contain any poisonous or harmful chemicals, so it's usually safe to wear sunscreen on your lips.

Some people with very sensitive skin might suffer from an allergic reaction, however. So, if your lips break out or begin itching with the use of regular sunscreen, stop using it and switch to a balm made especially for the lips.

You should always put on your lip sunscreen 30 minutes to an hour before you go outside. And remember to reapply to your lips every hour, and more often if you are eating, drinking, swimming or sweating.

MEDICAL SOURCE —————————————————————

U.S. Pharmacist (17,6:28 Supplement)

Vitamin-E oil might be the new kid on the beach

Sunbathers, get ready to smear on the oil. Not the coconut oil — the vitamin-E oil.

The natural oil from vitamin E might be a new type of sunscreen that can help protect you from the harmful ultraviolet sun rays that are known to cause skin cancer.

Investigators have been testing the cancer-protection benefits of vitamin-E oil on laboratory mice. In recent studies, researchers have found that smearing vitamin-E oil on the skin of mice kept under sun lamps reduced the expected number of skin cancer cases by half.

Scientists found that when exposed to ultraviolet light, 81 percent of the unprotected mice developed skin cancer. Only 42 percent of the mice protected with vitamin-E oil developed skin cancer.

More than 32,000 new cases of skin cancer develop each year — largely due to the harmful effects of ultraviolet radiation from the sun.

Scientists hope vitamin-E oil might help reduce the number of people suffering from skin cancer.

MEDICAL SOURCE —————————————————————

Atlanta Journal and Constitution (April 19, 1991,C3)

Shot in the arm for suntans — wave of the future?

Looking for a way to get a tan without suffering the savage effects of the sun?

If so, you're not alone. Millions of people who tan poorly or sunburn easily desperately wish for a way to get a tan without having to bake in the sun.

An answer might be closer than you think. And it doesn't include tanning salons.

"Suntan in a syringe" just might become the latest craze in tanning.

Recently, scientists began testing the effects of a drug known as melanocyte-stimulating hormone (MSH) in darkening human skin.

Melanocytes are the kinds of cells in human skin that make melanin. Melanin is the substance that gives your skin its color. People who have naturally darker skin produce more melanin that those with pale skin.

However, the melanocytes will produce more melanin if you expose your skin to the sun — thus, you get a suntan.

Scientists conducted a test to see if the melanocyte-stimulating hormone would cause — or stimulate — the melanocytes to make more melanin without exposure to the sun.

Twenty-eight male subjects between the ages of 19 and 41 volunteered to test the effects of the drug.

Twelve of the men had fair skin with histories of sunburning easily or tanning poorly (known as skin type I or II). And the other 16 men reported histories of easy tanning and little or no sunburning (skin type III or IV).

Half of the men received 10 injections of MSH over a 12-day period. The other half received injections of a placebo.

Both groups were advised to stay out of the sun while the scientists were conducting the test, and all of the men used a strong sunscreen to avoid any effects from the sun.

Scientists observed the effects of the injections for seven weeks. The men who received the placebo injections had no change in skin color.

However, all subjects who received the MSH injection developed darker skin, even those men with skin types I and II.

The men experienced the darkest tanning on the face and neck, with some lighter tanning on the arms and legs. However, the trunk and buttocks did not tan at all.

The scientists reported that the tanning appeared darkest during weeks three and five (one to three weeks after the last injection) and began to fade by week nine.

Scientists indicate that MSH would especially benefit those people who burn easily or tan poorly in the sun — people who have the greatest risk of getting skin cancer from the sun.

If MSH could produce more melanin in the skin, these people might have better protection from the dangers of ultraviolet rays from the sun.

As the ozone layer gets thinner, "suntan in a syringe" might help protect many people from the harmful effects of the sun.

MEDICAL SOURCE ————————————————————

Journal of the American Medical Association (266,19:2730)

'Tanning' pills may cause more than brown skin

The quest for the perfect pelt resulted in tragedy instead of a healthy tan for a woman who died several weeks after using the "tanning" pill, canthaxanthin.

Shortly after taking the tanning pills that she obtained from a tanning salon, she began suffering from headache, fatigue, easy bruising and weight loss.

She was hospitalized and diagnosed as suffering from aplastic anemia. This is a serious form of anemia that results from a disorder of the bone marrow.

She died 48 hours after leaving the hospital. Her death was associated with her use of canthaxanthin.

Although the Food and Drug Administration has issued a warning that canthaxanthin should not be used as a tanning agent, the drug is available through tanning salons and newspaper or magazine advertisements.

Scientists don't know how often this drug causes adverse side effects or what doses of the drug are dangerous.

However, even if there is only a small risk of this deadly side effect, the use of the drug as a cosmetic tanning agent does not justify the risk.

People who have used or are using oral tanning agents should see their doctor immediately if they develop questionable side effects.

MEDICAL SOURCE —————————————————————

Journal of the American Medical Association (264,9:1141)

TAMPER-PROOFING MEDICINES

Prevent product tampering — Examine your packages closely

Tamper-proof packaging is not a "sealed-tight" issue.

There is no such thing as a tamper-proof container. A better description would be tamper-evident packaging.

The tragedy of cyanide-laced Tylenol in 1982 spurred the Food and Drug Administration (FDA) to require that companies protect products from tampering by changing their packaging.

But that doesn't mean the remedies you buy over the counter are perfectly safe from mischief.

What is tamper-evident packaging? The key word in this description is "evident." That means companies now put at least one, and often two, protective barriers on a product, and you should be able to see whether or not these barriers have been broken.

Plastic wrap and other barriers on a product should alert you to look twice and read the label before you open a container. The FDA requires that package labels tell you exactly what the tamper-evident features are, so you can read the label to know what to look for.

One typical barrier is plastic wrap printed with a company logo or special picture. Another safeguard is distinctive packaging like individual foil pouches or blister packs. You've probably seen cold remedies or other pills packaged this way.

Shipping sometimes damages packaging. But when you buy a product, it should be in the same condition as when it left the company, with tamper-evident packaging intact.

Packaging for toothpaste, cough drops and skin products generally doesn't have to be tamper-evident because it's harder to tamper with these products.

Be sure to examine products closely before you open them.

MEDICAL SOURCE ─────────────────────────────
FDA Consumer (25,8:20)

Tips to foil tampering

To protect yourself against tampering, follow these simple guidelines for the products you buy without a prescription at your pharmacy or grocery store.

❏ Read the label to find out what the tamper-evident features of the product are.

❏ Look for torn, broken or damaged boxes, broken seals, puncture holes or torn wrapping.

❏ Never take medicine in the dark or when you're sleepy. Turn on the light and wait until you are awake enough to examine the product.

❏ If a product has a bad odor or is discolored, don't take it.

If you suspect that someone has tampered with a product, take it back to the pharmacist or manager of the store where you bought it.

If you look through your drugstore, you'll find tamper-evident packaging on products like these:

• All mouthwashes and rinses.
• Vaginal products.
• Contact lens solutions and tablets.
• All drug products that you can buy without a prescription.

MEDICAL SOURCE ─────────────────────────────
FDA Consumer (25,8:23)

TEETH TIPS

Look, Ma — no tooth erosion

Cavities are a big concern among children, teen-agers and young adults. But middle-aged and older adults should be more concerned with maintaining the health of their teeth and protecting them from things such as tooth erosion.

Tooth erosion sounds painful, but most people don't even realize that it's going on in their mouths. Tooth erosion is the thinning of the teeth due to a loss of the protective enamel that covers your teeth.

Tooth erosion can be caused by several things. Acidic drinks (fruit juices and wines), foods or medications (aspirin) can cause your mouth to become more acidic than normal. The extra acid begins to eat into the enamel on your teeth.

For example, many vegetarians suffer from tooth erosion because their vegetable and fruit diets are more acidic than the average American diet.

People who work in factories or around acidic chemicals can suffer from tooth erosion because they inhale fumes from the chemicals.

Stomach problems can also lead to tooth erosion. Reflux of stomach juices into the mouth exposes the teeth to the strong acids found in the stomach that help break down food during digestion. Excess vomiting produces the same effects — the strong acids from the stomach fill the mouth and cover the teeth, leading to erosion of the enamel.

Usually the mouth creates enough saliva to wash the teeth and keep them free from erosion. However, people who suffer from dry mouth have an increased risk of tooth erosion because their teeth are no longer protected by the washing effects of the saliva.

Dry mouth can be caused by infected or poorly functioning saliva glands, some medications, X-rays to the head or neck region, or heavy open-mouth breathing, such as during athletic events or even while sleeping.

To reduce your risk of tooth erosion, be sure to brush your teeth after every meal, but especially after eating or drinking acidic foods and beverages. If you cannot brush your teeth right away, at least rinse your mouth out with water a few times to get rid of as much acid as possible.

If you suffer from dry mouth, check with your pharmacist or doctor to see if your medication is causing it. If so, ask your doctor if she could prescribe another medication that does the same thing without producing the dry-mouth side effect.

You can relieve dry mouth with sugar-free chewing gum, non-acidic hard candies or by drinking lots of liquids (especially water).

Getting rid of dry mouth and reducing the amount of extra acid in your mouth will help you keep your pearly whites strong and healthy.

MEDICAL SOURCE ———————————————————
Dr. Alexander Grant's Health Gazette (14,5:4)

Natural plaque remover found in the roots of this plant

You can find it growing in the forests between Florida and Oklahoma. You can also find it in some commercial toothpastes and mouthwashes.

It's known as bloodroot, and it's a natural way to control plaque.

This short, flower-producing herb grows close to the ground in the Southeastern forests of the United States. If you damage the root, a red juice oozes out of the wound, hence the plant's name, bloodroot. The juice contains the substance sanguinarine, and it's this substance that you can find in your toothpaste.

Scientific studies show that sanguinarine begins removing plaque buildup on teeth in as little as eight days. The natural substance also helps reduce some common forms of bacteria that promote the buildup of plaque on the teeth.

So, if you want a natural plaque-fighter, look at the list of ingredients on your toothpaste box, and choose the one with the natural ingredients.

MEDICAL SOURCE ───────────────────────────

The Lawrence Review of Natural Products (November 1990)

Can green tea help combat green teeth?

Look, Ma ... no cavities! If you haven't been able to say this in a while, you may want to add green tea to your diet.

Scientists can now "give you the green light" to drink Japanese green tea.

An organic chemist, Isao Kubo, has demonstrated that extracts from Japanese green tea can kill the bacteria Streptococcus mutans that cause dental cavities.

Green tea also contains tannin, which helps stop the bacteria's production of glucans. Glucans are sticky materials that help acid-generating bacteria stick to your teeth.

In addition to tannin, nine out of 10 of the extracts in green tea also slow the production of glucan, according to Kubo and his team of researchers from the University of California, Berkeley.

Even better, these extracts kill the bacteria when they are combined, as they are in the tea.

Kubo also found the extracts in green tea to be effective against other molds, yeasts and bacteria including some responsible for gastrointestinal diseases and acne.

But for those of you who don't like green tea, these active compounds are available in spices such as coriander, sage, thyme and are also used in some candy and chewing gums.

MEDICAL SOURCE ─────────────────────────
Science News (141,16:253)

Go nuts over this new toothpaste

You've had peppermint- and bubble gum-flavored toothpaste before. But there's a new flavor in town.

Cashew nut-flavored toothpaste might be the next novelty you find on your grocer's shelves. Sounds nutty, but it's true.

There has been an increase in the demand for all-natural products, so the food industry has found a way to use something that's ordinarily thrown away: cashew nut shells.

Two research chemists discovered that oil from the cashew nut shell helps fight bacteria that cause tooth decay. "It has anti-plaque activity, too," said Isao Kubo, one of the researchers.

Does it sound too good to be true? These scientists don't think so. Researchers expect cashew products to become the next safe element in toothpaste and mouthwash products on the market.

MEDICAL SOURCE ─────────────────────────
Science News (139,12:191)

TMJ PROBLEMS

Home remedies for temporomandibular joint dysfunction

It's a painful disorder that affects up to a quarter of all healthy people in the nation.

But the disorder is poorly understood, so many doctors and dentists won't treat it, and even if they do, many insurance companies won't cover the medical costs.

Temporomandibular joint dysfunction (TMJ) is a disorder that involves the structures you use when eating: the mandible (lower jawbone) and the temporal bone of the skull (bone above the jaw that covers your temples).

These two bones form a joint that is held together with ligaments.

In between the bones, there is a disc of cartilage that serves as a shock absorber during the motion of chewing. When any of the structures (bones, ligaments or cartilage) involved in this joint have problems, TMJ can result.

Most people describe the symptoms of TMJ as pain or muscle spasms in the temple and cheek, just in front of the ear. Many complain of limited jaw motion (they can't open their mouths as wide as they used to) and clicking or popping of the joint. Sometimes the pain radiates to the neck and back, and headaches are common.

Unfortunately, doctors and dentists don't really know what causes TMJ.

Some of the possible causes or triggers of TMJ are listed on the following page:

- External trauma to the joint or surrounding muscles — car accidents, contact sports (football or hockey accidents), dental treatments or procedures, neck or back injuries that require traction.
- Dental problems — poor bite, missing or malformed teeth, misaligned jaw.
- Personal habits — gum chewing, clenching the teeth, grinding the teeth during sleep.
- Psychological problems — stress, anxiety, tension.

Although these causes could be the culprits, there are other people who suffer from TMJ who don't seem to have any of these triggers. The bottom line is that the cause of TMJ is still largely unknown.

And so is the treatment. Doctors and dentists are not sure what to do for this mysterious disorder. Although some doctors will prescribe pain medication or muscle relaxants, most will suggest many of the following home remedies:

❑ Let your jaws rest. Avoid chewing gum. Try a soft diet that avoids foods requiring strenuous chewing (meats, chewy candies, crunchy vegetables like carrots) for a while.

❑ Try to limit the amount of action your jaws see. Avoid lengthy telephone conversations and long, uninterrupted talks or presentations. If possible, avoid wide yawning. And stay away from activities that will strain your vocal cords (voice lessons, singing in the choir, yelling at football games).

❑ Also avoid activities that strain your jaw and neck muscles: cradling the phone between your ear and shoulder, lying on your side with your head propped up to read or watch TV, carrying a heavy shoulder bag for long periods of time.

❑ Use a heating pad for chronic pain (pain that lasts and lasts) and try ice packs for acute pain (pain that comes and goes pretty quickly). Gently massaging your temples might relieve some pain. And a hot shower, sauna or steam bath might soothe your aching jaw.

❏ Try to relax. Tension and stress cause most people to tighten their jaw muscles. Take a deep breath and consciously relax those muscles. Try other stress-management techniques to help relieve your TMJ discomfort (exercising, listening to quiet music, taking a long walk, reading a good book, meditation and prayer).

❏ Check your posture. Many people sit at their desks or at the dinner table in a hunched-over position. Poor posture can put extra strain on your back, shoulder and jaw muscles and can trigger symptoms of TMJ.

❏ If you participate in contact sports (football, hockey, basketball, soccer, etc.), buy a mouthpiece that protects your teeth and prevents your jaw from taking too much pressure on impact.

❏ Take some over-the-counter pain relievers. Acetaminophen will help relieve the pain, but aspirin products will also help clear up any inflammation around the tender joint. Some people even recommend crushing an aspirin, mixing it into some lotion in your hand, and rubbing it into the aching joint.

❏ Ask your doctor if he can recommend a local doctor or dentist that specializes in TMJ therapy. Sometimes physical therapy of the jaw muscles will help relieve the symptoms of TMJ.

MEDICAL SOURCES ――――――――――――――――――――――

Journal of the American Dental Association (123,6:43)
Nutrition Today (26,1:37)

TODDLERS AND MEDICINES

How to get your toddler to swallow, not spit, medicine

Your pediatrician says your toddler needs two spoonfuls of medicine every four hours, and you cringe. Getting the medicine into your toddler's mouth and keeping him from spitting it out are not easy tasks.

Until now. Researchers recommend an easy trick.

Place your toddler on his back with his head tilted up. Physically hold his lips apart and pour the medicine into the corner of his mouth.

With his lips held apart, he can't spit out the medicine and will probably swallow it when he realizes this.

You can do the same thing using a syringe to dispense the liquid medication. Again, keeping the child's lips apart keeps him from spitting out the medicine.

MEDICAL SOURCE —————————————————————

Emergency Medicine (24,4:191)

TOXIC FUMES

Well-ventilated area prevents breathing scare

"Use only with adequate ventilation." You've seen this label on different products before, but do you always heed the warning?

Not paying attention to the warning label was almost a deadly mistake for this 42-year-old woman.

She had safely used products containing mineral spirits many times before with no problems. But this time she worked in a closed room with no outside air coming in, and didn't wear a protective mask.

She had been painting bathroom walls with water sealant and applying polyurethane finish to some furniture.

She suffered difficulty in breathing and chest pains that eventually led to fluid buildup in the lungs and pneumonia. She was in the hospital for 14 days before being released.

To protect yourself from these potentially toxic products, be sure to apply them outside or in a well-ventilated area. Open all doors and windows if you are inside. Turn off all open flames, including pilot lights.

Some petroleum-based products that require good ventilation during use are paints, paint thinner, stains, lacquers, resins, rubber cement, sealant, gasoline and kerosene.

Be sure to store products with the lid closed tightly and out of the reach of children.

MEDICAL SOURCE ————————————————

Archives of Internal Medicine (151,7:1437)

URINARY TRACT INFECTIONS

How to avoid urinary tract infections

You usually sleep through the whole night without having to get up. But last night you had to get up three times to go to the bathroom.

And this morning you notice a feeling of bladder fullness that won't go away, and it burns when you go to the bathroom.

You've probably got a urinary tract infection (UTI).

UTIs are not uncommon, especially in women. About 20 percent of all women suffer from at least one UTI in their life. About one-third of those women will have another episode in less than three months. And about three out of four of those women will suffer from another UTI within two years.

Women are more prone to suffer from UTIs because the female urethra (the tube connecting your urinary bladder to the outside of your body) is only about an inch long. That's a short distance for bacteria to have to travel, so any bacteria that might be present near the urethral opening can easily infect the bladder.

Men, on the other hand, have a long urethra, and they have significantly fewer urinary tract infections because the bacteria never make it up the urethra to the bladder.

Most people who suffer from urinary tract infections complain of urinary frequency (feeling as if you have to go to the bathroom a lot), urgency (the feeling of having to go immediately), stinging while urinating, and the feeling of bladder fullness or cramping.

Some people even experience blood in their urine. Others complain of low-grade fever, abdominal pain and a general feeling of "unwellness."

Most urinary tract infections require the use of antibiotics from the doctor for treatment. So, there really are not any effective home remedies to make your UTI go away once you've got it.

However, there are many ways that you can lower your risk of getting a urinary tract infection.

Following a few simple tips will help you avoid the pain and discomfort of a UTI. Many of the tips apply more to women than to men due to women's greater risk of UTIs.

❑ Don't "hold it" — never wait to go to the bathroom. Every time you urinate, your bladder gets rid of most of the bacteria that was present there. Urinating often helps keep any harmful bacteria from infecting the bladder. But if you delay urinating too long after you've noticed the urge, you are allowing the bacteria more time to multiply. The more bacteria that are present in the bladder, the harder it is to wash them all away. That sets the stage for infection. Studies show that women who work or who are on long car trips and can't get to the bathroom often enough have greater numbers of UTIs than women who urinate often.

❑ Delaying urination also tends to swell the bladder and thus to shorten the urethra. This gives the bacteria in the area easier access to the bladder. It also increases the chances that some residual, or leftover, urine will remain in the bladder. This allows the bacteria to multiply and cause infection.

❑ Drink lots of liquids every day. This will make you urinate more often, and that will decrease your risk of urinary tract infections.

❑ When you have a bowel movement, wipe from front to back. Wiping from back to front pulls bacteria from the rectum and feces up toward the urethral opening and increases the risk of infection.

❏ If possible, take a shower and bathe the rectal area after each bowel movement instead of wiping. This helps remove offensive bacteria from the area more effectively. But don't take a tub bath. Taking a tub bath exposes all the skin in the genital area to water that is contaminated with bacteria from the rectum and feces.

❏ Wear cotton underwear instead of nylon underwear. The cotton breathes better and keeps the groin area cooler. Hot, moist areas are perfect for bacterial growth, and the nylon underwear promotes the retention of heat and moisture. The cotton keeps the area cool and dry.

❏ Wear thigh-high panty hose instead of full panty hose to keep the crotch area cooler and dryer.

❏ Wear loose clothing, and avoid extremely tight pants. The tight clothes trap heat and moisture, promoting the growth of bacteria.

❏ Women should always urinate soon after sexual intercourse. The act of intercourse doesn't cause the bacteria to multiply, but it encourages the movement of the existing bacteria up through the urethra. Urinating soon after intercourse will wash away the bacteria that may have entered the urethra. Urinating before intercourse is also helpful — it helps flush away any bacteria that might get pushed up into the urethra during intercourse.

❏ Change tampons often. Waiting too long encourages the growth of harmful bacteria. This can cause vaginal as well as bladder infections.

❏ Avoid long tampons, or tampons that expand in length (instead of in width) when they absorb moisture. Long tampons can push against the urinary bladder and create the right conditions for an infection. Use shorter tampons that expand in width to absorb moisture.

❑ Avoid using genital deodorants. The chemicals can trigger UTIs in many women.

❑ Avoid douching so often. Douching disturbs the natural protective barriers that help prevent infection. If you do douche, use the most natural, chemical-free formula you can find.

❑ Make sure the genital areas of both sexual partners are clean to reduce the risk of a bacterial infection.

❑ If you use a diaphragm for contraception, try another method. Diaphragms press against the bladder and prevent the bladder from emptying all the urine it contains. This increases your likelihood of infection. Also, most women leave the diaphragm in for eight to 10 hours. This time span allows bacteria to multiply and cause infection.

❑ Drink some cranberry juice every day. Cranberry juice is very acidic, and it makes the urine more acidic. Many bacteria cannot survive in an acidic environment, so the cranberry juice cuts your chances of a urinary tract infection.

❑ Keep the area around the urethral opening as clean as possible. Showering daily and washing with a mild anti-bacterial soap will eliminate excess bacteria that might grow and multiply in the rectal and urethral area.

❑ To relieve the pain that sometimes comes with urinary tract infection, take an over-the-counter relief medicine specifically for urinary problems. Remember, however, that this kind of medicine only treats the symptoms and makes you feel better. It does not kill the bacteria. You need an antibiotic from your doctor for that. So don't trick yourself into thinking you are well after taking some medicine for your symptoms. And don't delay seeing your doctor. The longer you wait, the farther up your system the bacteria travels.

Eventually the bacteria could reach the kidneys and cause serious, and sometimes permanent, kidney damage.

❏ Aspirin or acetaminophen might also provide pain relief until the antibiotics start working. A heating pad on your lower abdomen can also soothe the discomfort.

MEDICAL SOURCES —————————————————————————

Emergency Medicine (24,4:30 and 24,2:33)
Complete Guide to Symptoms, Illness & Surgery, 2nd Edition, The Body Press/Perigee Books, New York, 1989

This juice can be 'berry' good for the kidneys

You have heard for years that cranberry juice fights urinary tract infections.

Sure enough, new studies show that its ability to fight infections is real.

Researchers believe that if you can keep bacteria from sticking to cell walls of the bladder by flushing them out, you can stop the development of urinary tract infections.

Cranberry juice contains two compounds that slow the growth of bacteria that cause urinary tract infections, according to researchers. One of the compounds is fructose, a natural sugar contained in many fruit juices, but the other compound is unknown.

These compounds seem to inhibit the sticking ability of the bacteria, Escherichia coli. Usually called E. coli, these germs normally live in the intestines, but can cause annoying infections if they take hold in the urinary tract.

Recent studies indicate that certain juices contain anti-sticking agents. In other words, they stop bacteria from "gluing" themselves to bladder walls by making the walls slippery.

Researchers tested seven juices: blueberry, cranberry, grape-fruit, guava, mango, orange and pineapple.

Only the blueberry and cranberry juices contained the anti-sticky substances.

MEDICAL SOURCE ─────────────────────────

The New England Journal of Medicine (324,22:1599)

Arthritis drug side effects can mimic cystitis

Most of the time, bacteria are the cause of the bladder infection known as cystitis.

And when you have cystitis, your doctor can prescribe an antibiotic that will clear up the trouble.

But antibiotics won't cure the form of cystitis that results from taking a drug called tiaprofenic acid.

When a number of older people took tiaprofenic acid for the pain and swelling of arthritis, they developed cystitis symptoms: the urge to urinate frequently, a burning sensation when they urinated, fever and low-back pain. Researchers don't understand exactly how tiaprofenic acid causes cystitis. But when these arthritis sufferers stopped using the drug, the cystitis went away completely.

If you are taking tiaprofenic acid, you might want to discuss this possible side effect with your doctor.

MEDICAL SOURCE ─────────────────────────

British Medical Journal (303,6814:1376)

Vaginal Infections

Help prevent stubborn yeast infections with this healthy food

There are over-the-counter drugs to treat this condition. But, have you tried the all-natural way to heal painful yeast infections?

Two recent reports show that eating eight ounces of yogurt every day might halt repeat attacks of vaginal yeast infections. However, not all yogurts are effective at preventing yeast infections. Only brands that contain active cultures of Lactobacillus acidophilus appear to control the candida fungus.

The fungus that causes candidal vaginitis (yeast) infections is present at all times in the vagina in many women. Most of the time, harmless bacteria that live in the vagina keep down the growth of this fungus.

Candidal vaginitis infections occur when the fungus grows out of control for one reason or another.

When a woman eats yogurt daily, bacteria from the yogurt stay in the gastrointestinal system and vagina and actually slow or stop the growth of the candida responsible for yeast infections.

To test this theory, researchers located women who averaged five to eight yeast infections per year and divided them into two groups. One group ate eight ounces of yogurt daily for six months, then crossed over to a yogurt-free diet for six months. The other group ate no yogurt for six months, then added yogurt to their diet for the next six months.

The group that started out eating eight ounces of yogurt each day experienced such relief from yeast infections, that some of the women actually refused to stop eating yogurt for the next phase of the research. Overall, while women were eating yogurt daily, they had three times fewer yeast infections.

Doctors don't know all the reasons why some women have recurrent vaginal yeast infections. But they do know that pregnancy, diabetes and the use of antibiotics and corticosteroids increase infection rates for some women.

Eating yogurt that contains active cultures of Lactobacillus acidophilus might be one natural way to prevent this problem.

Other diseases can mimic the symptoms of candidal vaginal infections, so check with your doctor to rule out other problems.

MEDICAL SOURCES ──────────────────────────

> *Science News* (141,10:158)
> *Annals of Internal Medicine* (116,5:353)

Acidophilus remedies

Yogurt is more than a healthy, midday snack, if you are female, that is. If your yogurt contains the bacteria Lactobacillus acidophilus, you're eating your own natural protection against vaginal infections and urinary tract infections.

You see, your body has its own natural supply of "good" bacteria. L. acidophilus is one of those "good" bacteria found in various places in the body. Eating yogurt (or milk, etc.) that contains the acidophilus bacteria helps guarantee your body has enough of the bacteria to fight off "bad" bacteria. That helps your body fight off vaginal infections and urinary tract infections.

Acidophilus is available in some yogurt and milk, and in commercial tablets, granules and capsules.

MEDICAL SOURCE ──────────────────────────

> *The Lawrence Review of Natural Products* (November 1991)

Strong link between cancer and douching

How often should I douche?

It's a question many women want to ask their doctors, but most are too embarrassed to bring up the subject.

The answer is surprising: Seldom, if ever.

Women who douche more than once a week might increase the risk of cancer of the cervix as much as fourfold compared with women who douche less often.

Researchers think that douching might set the stage for cancer because it removes natural vaginal secretions along with helpful bacteria.

The type of douching preparation made little difference in the outcome of the study.

Whether you douche with vinegar and water, baking soda and water, commercial solutions or plain water, you still have an increased risk of cancer.

As surprising as it may seem, women once commonly used household cleaning solutions such as Lysol or Pine Sol for douching until scientists reported a strong link between such substances and cervical cancer.

Now the commercial types of feminine cleansing might hold the same dangers.

If you ask how often you should douche, your doctor might recommend regular baths or showers instead.

MEDICAL SOURCE ─────────────────────────

Science News (139,11:175)

WALKING PROBLEMS

New chair-walker gives confidence back to elderly

"Goodbye wheelchair, hello independence," might soon be the cry of many older people who have been confined to wheelchairs due to hip, joint or muscle problems.

Older people need to maintain their independence and pride despite reduced mobility, and one New York surgeon has provided a tool that just might enable the elderly to do that.

The new creation is known as a "chair-walker." The chair-walker is a combination of the traditional wheeled walker that elderly people commonly use and the wheeled seat-walkers that babies use.

Dr. Julius Jacobson took a traditional walker and added a seat that helps users stand up. The seat then swings out of the way to let them walk freely and catches them if they fall.

It enables the elderly person who has suffered decreased mobility to walk confidently without the fear and danger of falling.

The chair-walker also helps avoid the weakening and degeneration of the muscles and bones that come with immobility.

Nursing home workers have used the new chair-walker in trial runs with positive reviews, and the chair-walker has even won an award from *International Design* magazine. The chair-walker will enable those who are permanently disabled to regain some independence and might also be helpful as a rehabilitation tool to help people learn to walk again after hip or joint surgery.

MEDICAL SOURCE ————————————————
The Wall Street Journal (July 16, 1991, B1)

How big is too big? Guidelines for desirable weight

Your doctor frowns at the scale and says you need to lose some weight.You frown because you weigh the same amount as your mother, and the doctor doesn't fuss at her.

What's the deal?

The deal is this: Being overweight can increase your risk of heart disease, diabetes and other dangerous illnesses. But "overweight" means different things for a 25-year-old and a 45-year-old.

Apparently, researchers are suggesting that gaining a little weight as you age is not a health hazard. The key word is little.

Although most people are concerned with how much they weigh, many researchers suggest that the big concern should be where you carry your weight.

People who carry extra weight around their waists (known as an "apple" shape) have greater risks of heart disease, high blood pressure and diabetes than the people who carry extra weight around their hips and thighs (known as a "pear" shape).

To find out if you are an apple or a pear, measure your waist right above your navel and your hips over the largest part of your buttocks. If your waist measurement is as big or bigger than your hip measurement, you are an apple.

To determine your "waist-to-hip" ratio, divide your waist measurement by your hip measurement. If the number is above 0.95 for men or above 0.80 for women, you are an "apple."

Remember that "apples" have greater risk for developing dangerous diseases. Talk to your doctor about a diet and exercise plan that will help you lose those extra pounds around your waist and get your overall weight back within the proper guidelines.

The following chart will give you an idea of your weight guidelines based on your height, sex and age.

Height and Weight (without shoes)			
Height	**Women over 25**	**Men over 25**	**All over 35**
5'0"	103-115	—	108-138
5'1"	106-118	111-122	111-143
5'2"	109-122	114-126	115-148
5'3"	112-126	117-129	119-152
5'4"	116-131	120-132	122-157
5'5"	120-135	123-136	126-162
5'6"	124-139	127-140	130-167
5'7"	128-143	131-145	134-172
5'8"	132-147	135-149	138-178
5'9"	136-151	139-153	142-183
5'10"	140-155	143-158	146-188
5'11"	—	147-163	151-194
6'0"	—	151-168	155-199
6'1"	—	155-173	159-205

MEDICAL SOURCES

Nutrition Action (18,4:1)
Heart Disease and Stroke (1,3:148)
Archives of Internal Medicine (150,5:1065)

Want to lose weight? Don't skip breakfast

You've always heard breakfast is the most important meal of the day.

Well, studies now show that eating breakfast might do more than just give you extra energy. Eating breakfast can also help you lose weight.

Researchers studied 52 overweight women ages 18 to 55 and assigned them to a weight-loss program for 12 weeks. They were divided into two groups. One was the no-breakfast group who ate only two meals a day, and the other was the breakfast group who ate three meals a day.

The results of the study showed that those who ate breakfast had a lower fat intake and a higher carbohydrate intake than those who did not eat breakfast.

Another advantage was that breakfast eaters ate fewer impulsive snacks and reduced the fats and calories that are associated with them, according to the report. Apparently, eating breakfast helps reduce impulsive snacking throughout the day and, therefore, can play a major role in weight loss.

Nutrition experts recommend breakfast as a vital part of a healthy diet. But despite this good advice, 24 percent of women ages 25 to 34 routinely skip breakfast.

Some people believe that not eating breakfast will help them lose weight because their calorie intake is less.

On the contrary, scientists say, eating breakfast helps to keep you from overeating throughout the day. Eating breakfast is also linked to improved strength and endurance, better attitudes in work and school, constant blood-sugar levels and hunger prevention.

Apparently, people who eat breakfast (especially ready-to-eat cereals) benefit from a more adequate supply of nutrients, lower amounts of calories from fat and higher intakes of fiber.

Skipping breakfast appears to be associated with overeating at other meals or increased between-meal snacking which, in turn, tend to increase your overall intake of calories and can cause you to gain weight.

If you are trying to lose weight, breakfast might be your best friend. Researchers recommend that you include a low-fat, high-carbohydrate breakfast as part of your weight-loss program.

This might include whole-grain cereals with skim milk, bagels or English muffins.

MEDICAL SOURCE ——————————————————————

The American Journal of Clinical Nutrition (55,3:645)

After you reach age 75, being fat might not be such a bad deal

Overweight? Worried about your health? If you're over 75, you might not need to be concerned. After you hit age 75, being fat doesn't seem to hurt your health. High body weight does not seem to be a factor in deaths among elderly men.

In a recent study of males aged 75 or older, researchers kept track of 162 men for over two years and recorded their survival rates.

During the follow-up period, 53 men died. Researchers in the study looked at height, weight, age, race, cigarette-smoking status, and presence of glucose intolerance and hypertension. Glucose intolerance and a low body weight were significantly associated with the death rates.

The researchers concluded that men with low body weight died earlier because they had pre-existing diseases or conditions that made them thin.

Talk to your doctor to determine if your weight is healthy for your age and height.

MEDICAL SOURCE ——————————————————————

Southern Medical Journal (83,11:1256)

Afraid to quit smoking because you'll gain weight?

Truth is, when you quit smoking, you might weigh no more than if you'd never smoked.

Many people think that the one positive side effect of smoking is weight control. However, a study about weight gain after you quit smoking shows that smoking is not necessary for weight control.

Researchers followed a wide variety of people over a 13-year period, including black and white, male and female, smokers, nonsmokers and former smokers.

The researchers found that, on the average, weight gain after a person quit smoking was about 4 to 9 pounds.

Half of the people studied didn't even gain that much. The weight of the people who had smoked and quit was now equal to the nonsmokers' weight. That means if you quit smoking, you might weigh no more than you would if you had never started smoking.

Truth is, whatever benefit smoking might have, it's not worth all the health problems that smoking causes.

Kick that smoking habit and find yourself a good low-fat diet.

Being a little thinner for a few years of life now is not worth giving up several years of life in the end.

MEDICAL SOURCE ————————————————

The New England Journal of Medicine (324,11:739)

USS Scott sailors fight the battle against body fat and weight

A crew of U.S. sailors aboard the guided missile destroyer USS Scott have been doing more than protecting their country.

They've also been protecting their hearts from heart disease and their bodies from cancer.

During a six-month tour of duty in the Mediterranean, the crew aboard the ship ate a low-fat, high-fiber diet prepared according to guidelines from the American Cancer Society (ACS).

Researchers compared sailors from the USS Scott who ate the ACS diet with sailors from another ship who ate a standard U.S. Navy diet that contains high-fat, low-fiber foods.

The researchers found that the USS Scott sailors lost an average of 12 pounds, while the other ship members gained about seven pounds.

The sailors from the USS Scott saw an average decrease of two inches in their waist sizes. But the other ship's crew had a waist-size gain of about one-and-a-half inches per person.

Seventy-four percent of the sailors on the USS Scott who weighed more than 200 pounds at the start of the deployment lost weight on the ACS diet.

Only 26 percent of the sailors who weighed more than 200 pounds on the other ship lost weight. Researchers also report that 89 percent of the USS Scott sailors whose body fat was too high showed a decline in body fat.

Most of the sailors who ate the ACS diet said that they liked the food on the diet, and most said they would maintain similar eating habits after they came home. The American Cancer Society recommends a diet that is low in fat and high in fiber to help protect against heart disease and cancer.

Talk to your doctor about a low-fat, high-fiber diet that will suit your needs and help protect your body from heart disease and cancer.

MEDICAL SOURCE ————————————————

Medical Tribune (35,5:19)

WRINKLES

How to prevent facial wrinkles

Remember how your mother used to say that if you make ugly faces, your face will freeze like that?

Well, she wasn't too far from the truth — when it comes to wrinkles, that is.

Although the process of aging will always cause some wrinkles to form on your face, there are some wrinkles that you might avoid. And one kind comes from the faces you make.

Place a mirror in front of your telephone and watch yourself as you talk on the phone. If you frown, grimace, wrinkle your nose or raise your eyebrows, you'll notice how wrinkles form on your face. Over time, those wrinkles become more obvious, and they don't always disappear when you stop frowning.

Sleeping on the side of your face can also cause wrinkles over time. The weight of your head against the pillow on your cheeks can push the skin on your face into little folds and wrinkles that could start to become more permanent.

Wrinkles are also formed because of damage caused by the sun. The ultraviolet rays from the sun damage the cells in the skin, and the skin becomes less elastic.

And just like an elastic waistband sags when the elastic band is damaged, your skin begins to sag and wrinkle when the elasticity of the skin is damaged.

Another less common cause of wrinkles is weight loss. Obese people who lose weight and become thin occasionally have more obvious wrinkles (as well as stretch marks) than people who have always been thin.

Cigarette smoking is another culprit behind wrinkle formation. Many smokers who are in their 40s have skin that looks like they are in their 60s. The cigarette smoke seems to increase the normal aging process, and wrinkles develop much earlier than they should. Wrinkles around the lips and mouth are especially common among smokers.

Follow these simple tips to help avoid premature facial wrinkles:

❏ If you smoke, stop.

❏ Try to avoid frowning, grimacing and making ugly faces — but don't go overboard. Having no expression is not worth the effort. Just avoid exaggerated ugly faces.

❏ Try to avoid sleeping on your side. Placing a pillow under your knees will make sleeping on your back more comfortable. (Many photography models do this to avoid getting premature wrinkles.)

❏ If you're losing weight, do it slowly and safely. Crash diets that cause you to lose too much weight all at once are both dangerous for your health and sure to cause wrinkling of the skin on your face.

❏ Take the recommended daily allowance of vitamins E and D to help reduce skin damage from the sun.

❏ Limit the amount of time you spend in the sun. If you have outdoor activities, try to schedule them in the morning or late afternoon when the sun rays are not as strong and harmful.

❏ Apply sunscreen to all areas of your skin that will be exposed to the sun 20 minutes before you go outside. Remember to reapply the sunscreen after you've been in the water, or if you have been perspiring.

❏ Make sure any tanning salons you visit don't use lights that give off type-A ultraviolet radiation. This type of ultraviolet ray damages deep skin tissue, directly causing wrinkles.

❏ Wear sunglasses on bright days. This helps protect your eyes, and it helps to keep you from squinting, which can cause wrinkles around your eyes.

❏ Take care of your skin. Wash your face daily with a mild cleanser and blot your skin dry. Avoid rubbing your skin dry with a towel — this is damaging to the tender skin on your face. Apply a moisturizing cream to prevent your skin from becoming dry and scaly. When applying makeup, try to blot on your foundation instead of rubbing, especially under your eyes. Rubbing can stretch and damage the skin, causing wrinkles.

MEDICAL SOURCE —————————————————————
Postgraduate Medicine (88,1:207)

How to protect your face from wrinkles: Break this habit

Wrinkle up, smokers — men and women who smoke are more prone to facial wrinkling than their nonsmoking peers, say researchers.

Donald P. Kadunce and his colleagues at the University of Utah Health Sciences Center in Salt Lake City conducted a study of 109 smokers and 23 people who had never smoked.

Researchers took pictures of people's brows and temples to determine how many wrinkles they had and compared it to their smoking history.

Result — **the more you smoke** and the longer you smoke, the more wrinkles you get. Heavy smokers have five times the rate of excessive skin wrinkling as those who don't smoke.

Smoking appears to damage collagen, a fibrous protein found in the skin, which represents 30 percent of the total body protein. Damaged collagen seems to lead to faster skin wrinkling.

Researchers also believe that eye irritation from smoke, especially in bright sunlight, can cause you to squint your eyes. Squinting, in turn, makes crow's feet around your eyes.

For years, researchers have known that prolonged exposure to the sun can cause premature aging of the skin and can also produce early wrinkles. But, this study shows that smoking ages skin excessively.

Smoking coupled with sun exposure is doubly bad; together these factors can lead to even more severe wrinkling.

So, for the best protection of your skin and face, stop smoking and stay out of the sun.

MEDICAL SOURCE ————————————————————————
Science News (139,20:309)

New wrinkle remover might offer sweet promises of smoother skin

Looking for a wrinkle remover? Want younger-looking skin? There might be a sweet solution on the way.

Researchers report that a substance made from sugarcane plants may be successful in removing wrinkles, age spots, small scars or areas of discoloration on the skin.

This promising solution, known as glycolic acid, seems to help increase the amount of natural collagen and elastin in the skin.

So far, more than 150 people have been treated with the glycolic acid, and researchers report great improvement in skin condition.

Glycolic acid seems to have a more specific effect on the skin than other anti-wrinkling solutions, making glycolic acid more effective than other less specific solutions.

Researchers will continue testing the effects of this new wrinkle remover before releasing it for commercial use.

MEDICAL SOURCE ————————————————————

Pharmacy Times (56,10:95)

INDEX

A

abdomen 536
abdominal cramping 242
abdominal pain 89, 454
abscess 72
acacia gum 162
Ace bandage 373
ACE inhibitors 215, 217
acetaminophen 179, 180, 187, 274, 276,
   348, 388, 423, 476, 492, 529, 536
acetate 90
acid indigestion 234, 283
acid rebound 288
acidic drinks 237, 523
acidophilus 539
Acne 5-9, 126, 466, 526
   and foods 6
   and menstrual cycle 6
   anti-acne creams 8
   blackhead 5
   causes of 5
   inflammatory acne 6
   noninflammatory acne 6
   oil glands 5, 7
   pimples 5, 6
   Retin-A for 487
   sebaceous glands 5
   treatment of 7
   vitamin-A treatment
      danger of birth defects 466
   whitehead 5
Actifed 235
actinic keratosis 142
activated carbon filters 391
acute pain 529
acute subungual hematoma 259

adenomas 118
adrenal gland 338
age spots 487, 551
aging 380, 548
AIDS 35, 246
airway obstruction 217
Albuterol 235
alcohol 125, 128, 129, 130, 269, 275,
   278, 284, 307, 319, 325, 333, 337,
   338, 352, 371, 388, 468, 477, 503,
   507
Alcohol, Drug Abuse, and Mental
   Health Administration 460
alcoholic drinks 235, 236, 238
alcoholism 353
algaecides 453
alginic acid 288
Alka-Seltzer 234, 440
Allergies 9-20, 93, 176, 214, 474. *See
   also* **Hives; Skin problems;
   Asthma**
   allergens 9, 12, 18, 36, 38, 45
   allergic contact dermatitis 480
   allergic reaction 18, 19, 363
   allergic reaction to sperm 353
   allergic rhinitis 9, 11
   and ACE inhibitors
      diuretics 217
      drug reactions 217
   and arthritis
      food allergies as cause 25
   and cosmetics 346
   and hair dye 18
   and heart attack 20
   and sunscreens 516
   and toothpaste 497
   antihistamines 235

E